Intensive Care

Intensive Care

Edited by

ERIC SHERWOOD JONES

Whiston Hospital, Prescot, Merseyside

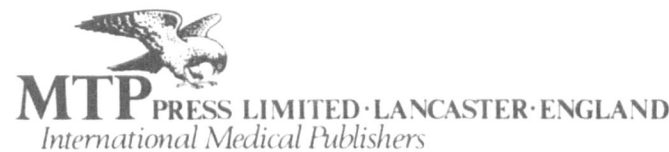

MTP PRESS LIMITED·LANCASTER·ENGLAND
International Medical Publishers

Published by
MTP Press Limited
Falcon House
Lancaster, England

Copyright © 1982 MTP Press Limited
Softcover reprint of the hardcover 1st edition 1982

British Library Cataloguing in Publication Data
Intensive care.
  1. Critical care medicine.
  I. Sherwood Jones, Eric
  616′.028   RC86.7
ISBN-13: 978-94-009-7315-2   e-ISBN-13: 978-94-009-7313-8
DOI: 10.1007/978-94-009-7313-8

Phototypesetting by Georgia Origination, Liverpool
Printed by Butler & Tanner Limited, Frome and London

Contents

Preface

A comprehensive text of intensive care would readily fill the equivalent of the *Shorter Oxford English Dictionary*. This is because the diseases treated are both numerous and varied; thus the patient can be medical, surgical, trauma or obstetric. It follows that the sum total of knowledge which needs to be available is truly encyclopaedic. This compact volume represents only a fragment of such information. The contributors were chosen because of their experience and because their methods were well-tried. The text therefore summarizes the best of current therapy and includes the controversial. The contributors come from four countries, adding an international flavour. One topic – The Recovery Room – outside the confines of intensive care has been included for two reasons. The recovery room is an important but neglected aspect of care, and it also seems important to define its relationships with the intensive care unit. It is hoped that the book will help the nurses and doctors involved in intensive care and, therefore, the patient.

ERIC SHERWOOD JONES

Contributors

P. M. ASHWORTH
Department of Nursing
University of Manchester
Stopford Building
Oxford Road
Manchester M13 9PT, UK

S. T. ATHERTON
Intensive Care Unit
Whiston Hospital
Prescot
Merseyside, UK

B. J. BAIN
Department of Haematology
St Mary's Hospital Medical School
Praed Street
London W2 1PG, UK

A. P. BALL
Infectious Diseases Unit
Cameron Hospital
Windygates
Fife, KY8 5RR, UK

F. W. BLAISDELL
Department of Surgery
University of California
Davis Medical Center
4301 X Street, Rm. 257
Sacramento
CA 95817, USA

K. CHATTERJEE
Medicine Cardiology Division
University of California San
    Francisco
Cardiovascular Research Institute
Moffitt Hospital Rm. 1186
San Francisco
California 94143, USA

E. M. COOKE
Department of Microbiology
University of Leeds
Leeds LS2 9JZ, UK

W. E. DAVIES
Spinal Injuries Unit
Princess Alexandra Hospital
Ipswich Road
Brisbane
Queensland
Australia 4102

R. S. EDMONDSON
Department of Anaesthesia
Leeds General Infirmary
Leeds LS1 3EX, UK

J. V. FARMAN
Department of Anaesthesia and
    Intensive Care Unit
Addenbrooke's Hospital
Cambridge CB2 2QQ, UK

M. W. FLOWERS
Accident and Emergency Department
Leeds General Infirmary
Leeds LS1 3EX, UK

D. S. HESS
Medicine Cardiology Division
University of California
 San Francisco
Cardiovascular Research Institute
Moffitt Hospital Rm. 1186
San Francisco
California 94143, USA

J. W. HOLCROFT
Department of Surgery
University of California
Davis Medical Center
4301 X Street, Rm. 257
Sacramento
CA 95817, USA

R. B. HOPKINSON
Intensive Therapy Unit
East Birmingham Hospital
Birmingham B9 5ST, UK

W. B. JENNETT
Southern General Hospital
Glasgow GS1 4TF, UK

H. S. KRISTENSEN
Departments of Infectious Diseases
 and Anaesthesia
Rigshospitalet – University Hospital
18 Tagensvej
DK 2200 Copenhagen
Denmark

P. G. P. LAWLER
Intensive Therapy Unit
South Cleveland Hospital
Marton Road
Middlesbrough
Cleveland TS3 4BW, UK

H. A. LEE
Department of Renal and Metabolic
 Medicine
University of Southampton
St Mary's Hospital
Portsmouth
Hants PO3 6AD, UK

J.-R. LE GALL
Service de Réanimation médicale
Hôpital Henri Mondor
94010 Creteil
France

A. R. LUKSZA
Intensive Care Unit
Whiston Hospital
Prescot
Merseyside L35 5DR, UK

R. P. F. PARKES
Intensive Care Unit
Princess Alexandra Hospital
Ipswich Road
Brisbane 4102
Queensland
Australia

T. A. PORTS
Medicine and Cardiology Division
University of California
 San Francisco
Cardiovascular Research Institute
Moffitt Hospital Rm. 1186
San Francisco
California 94143, USA

M. RAPIN
Service de Réanimation médicale
Hôpital Henri Mondor
94010 Creteil
France

W. SCHUMER
Department of Surgery
University Health Science
The Chicago Medical School at VA
  Medical Center
North Chicago
IL 60064, USA

D.J. WHITE
Bacteriology Department
Whiston Hospital
Prescot
Merseyside, UK

D.M. WRIGHT
Intensive Care Unit
Princess Alexandra Hospital
Ipswich Road
Brisbane 4102
Australia

N. WRIGHT
Regional Poisoning Treatment Centre
Dudley Road Hospital
Dudley Road
Birmingham B18 7QH, UK

Acknowledgements

Portions of Chapter 5, including Figure 5.1, are reproduced with permission from the following journals: *Comprehensive Therapy, Journal of the American Medical Association,* and *Surgery.* In Chapter 8 Figure 8.1 is reproduced with permission from *Surgical Forum.* In the recruiting of contributors the editor was helped by Dr Brian Davis, Dr Malcolm Wright and Professor Iain Ledingham. The edited version was typed by Miss Frances Twist, and help with the references was given by the Librarian of the Liverpool Medical Institution.

1
Intravenous feeding

HARRY LEE

The purpose of this chapter is to emphasize the practical aspects of intravenous feeding, rather than review the relevant pathophysiology. If such a therapy is to succeed, it must be capable of being practised both in specialized units and general wards which may be understaffed. In the last 20 years intravenous nutrition has advanced rapidly from being a somewhat erudite, complex form of treatment, to one that now should be considered commonplace, flexible and easy to manage. Indeed, unless it is accepted that any clinician can treat any patient on any ward at any time, the value of intravenous nutrition must be in doubt. The origins of intravenous feeding probably began following discussions and experiments by Sir Christopher Wren and Dr Robert Boyle. They experimented with ethanol and wine given intravenously to dogs, who actually survived! Fortunately, we have come a long way since then! Intravenous bolus feeding was probably first practised by Dr Latta in Scotland in the 1830s. Comprehensive parenteral feeding was first attempted by Frederich (1905) using a mixture of peptones, sugars, electrolytes and oils. Over the past century there has been a flurry of activity; first this dwelt upon the provision of electrolytes and water and then, at the turn of the century, the need to provide energy and nitrogen was recognized[1,2].

(I) AIMS AND OBJECTIVES

Intravenous nutrition must be seen as a therapy which provides complete nutritional support. It must be considered as the means of supporting nutrition for short or long periods when the gastrointestinal route cannot be used. As with any other form of therapy, an awareness of the specific need is essential and a team approach is vital if optimal patient care is to be achieved. A close analogy can be made with detection and treatment of infection. Here, the first line of observation and awareness often lies with the nurse, who notices the patient is unwell and records a raised temperature and tachycardia. The doctor is then informed, clinical examination and appropriate investigations are undertaken, and as a result antibiotics may be prescribed. Then a protocol is designed to assess the efficacy of the antibiotic. Why then should it be so different for the recognition of malnutrition? For it is true that in hospitals in 1981 'starvation in the midst of plenty' does occur and will continue to happen. This is because both medical and nursing staff fail to appreciate the importance of nutritional support for the critically ill and especially when there is partial or total gastrointestinal failure. One of the reasons for this lack of appreciation is the failure to adopt procedures by which malnutrition can be readily recognized. Furthermore, any treatment used to alleviate this malnutrition is not assessed by specific investigations and observations.

As a result of the metabolic response to trauma many critically ill patients will lose between 10 and 20 g of nitrogen per day. The greatest proportion of this nitrogen is lost in the urine as urea derived principally from the breakdown of muscle proteins. It is certain that any acutely ill patient who loses more than 30% of his initial body weight in an acute metabolic illness has only a small chance of survival[3]. Many of these patients will lose up to 20 or 30 g of nitrogen per day, which is equivalent to 0.6–0.9 kg of muscle. Is it surprising therefore that so many critically ill patients waste rapidly with resulting secondary complications? It is a shocking fact that, despite advances in medicine, improved surgical techniques and better anaesthesia, patients still die because of inadequate nutritional support.

Man, unlike the car engine, cannot switch off his metabolic processes because he is not provided with exogenous fuel. If fuel is not provided from without, then the body homeostatic mechanisms are so set that energy will be derived from the body tissues with harmful consequences[4,5]. That is why wasting is inevitable if substrates are not provided and why a negative nitrogen balance will occur. This latter is neither an ivory tower concept nor the repository of academic units. If only clinicians when doing ward rounds would recognize the condition of 'negative nitrogen balance', or perhaps, simply starvation, then appropriate treatment might follow.

What is the incidence of severe malnutrition requiring intravenous feeding? At this stage I must emphasize there is no competition between

2

Table 1.1 Tests for and evidence of malnutrition

Tests for malnutrition	Equipment required	Result in malnutrition
Body weight in kg and recent loss	various scales	$>$ 10%
Triceps skin fold thickness (TST) (fat energy reserves)	Holtain skin fold calipers	$<$ 10 mm in males $<$ 13 mm in females
Mid-arm circumference (MAMC) (muscle protein reserves) (MAMC = arm circumf. $- \pi$ (TST))	tape measure in cm	$<$ 23 cm in males $<$ 22 cm in females
Serum albumin (visceral protein)	routine lab. test	$<$ 35 g/l
Serum transferrin $\}$ short half-life proteins Complement C$_3$	routine lab. test	$<$ 2 g/l
Retinol binding protein	special tests	
Thyroxine binding prealbumin		
Urinary hydroxyproline	special test	$\uparrow$ collagen turnover
Lymphopenia	routine lab. test	$<$ 1.2×10^9/l
Plasma amino acid profile	specialized tests	changing valine/ glycine ratio
Urine 3-methylhistidine	specialized tests	increased muscle breakdown
Hair root morphology	tweezers and microscope	more telogens and dysplasic hairs
Visual assessment of patient	eyes! and clinical acumen	

3

enteral and parenteral nutritional methods. For parenteral nutrition there is only one absolute indication, namely gastrointestinal failure, which is also the only contraindication to enteral nutrition[6]. Of course, there will be times when partial parenteral nutrition combined with enteral nutrition can be given. Probably not more than 15% of all acute hospital admissions require active nutritional support by one way or another, of which probably only one third require intravenous nutrition.

(II) RECOGNITION OF MALNUTRITION

It is most important that malnutrition can be diagnosed as such[7]. In Table 1.1 some of the measurements are shown, and I wish to emphasize that these should be used in the assessment of all inpatients. It is an unfortunate part of modern hospital practice that the amount that a patient eats, or is offered, is not under the control of medical and nursing staff, but in the hands of ward orderlies or maids. This practice is to be condemned because the patient suffers as a result. It is considered routine for nursing staff to document temperature, pulse rate, respiration and, hopefully, weight on all hospital admissions, so I would advocate that the 'vital sign' charts should include additional measurements. These can be made equally well by nursing or medical staff, but not by non-professional staff. Furthermore, it might be argued that if dietitians were to pay more attention to the problems of hospital malnutrition and its diagnosis, they might improve the shining hour of many of our critically ill patients.

A careful history indicates how much weight has been lost recently, and weighing is mandatory. Whilst one knows that there are changes between the body cell mass and the fluid compartments in the critically ill patient, nevertheless, weight is a useful guide. In addition, simple measurements of mid-arm circumference and skinfold thickness provide useful indicators of muscle protein and adipose tissue (fat energy) respectively[7-9]. These measurements are capable of reproducibility in the ward and should not be regarded as research innovations. Then there are simple biochemical measurements of serum albumin, serum transferrin and C3 complement. The additional measurement of retinol binding protein and thyroxine binding pre albumin are probably of value[10]. Albumin has a relatively long half-life and is a crude indicator of severe malnutrition. The serum transferrin may take a week or 10 days before a fall will point to underlying malnutrition. The other two proteins referred to may be better indicators of rapid onset malnutrition, and, since their measurement is not too difficult, they should become part of routine hospital laboratory practice.

It is a fact that clinicians constantly underestimate the total nutritional requirements of their patients. Whilst it may be of some use to have so-called 'guestimate tables' (Table 1.2) [11,12], nevertheless the range within each

Table 1.2 Catabolic rates and estimated requirements

	Protein (nitrogen) (g/day)	Energy (kcal/day)	g N/kg body wt.	kcal/kg body wt.	kcal/g N
Apyrexial medical patient	45–75 (7.2–12)	1500–2000	0.16–0.20	30–37	= 170
Post-operative (uncomplicated)	75–100 (12–16)	2000–3500	0.20–0.22	37–45	= 190
Hypercatabolic, e.g. burns	>100 (> 16)	> 3500	0.22–0.30	46–52	= 210

1. Wide range of requirements for each group accentuates the risk of underestimating.
2. 1 g nitrogen ≡ 6.25 g protein ≈ 30 g muscle
3. Many patients breaking down 20 g nitrogen per day ≈ 0.6 kg muscle – hence potential for rapid wasting.

Table 1.3 Assessment of daily nitrogen losses and requirements

---

Urine urea nitrogen = 80% of total urine nitrogen across wide range
1 g (16.6 mmol) urea = 28/60 g nitrogen
(mol. wt. of urea = 60)
Total body water = 60% body wt. in kg
Urea equally distributed throughout body water
  (i) 24 h urine urea in $g \times 28/60 \times 6/5^* = X \times 0.56 = (A)g$
  (ii) Measure proteinuria, if any $= Y \times 4/25^{**}$
                                   $= Y \times 0.16 = (B)g$
  (iii) Correction for any rise of blood urea assuming no change in body
        weight in kg.
        Rise in blood urea $= Z$ g/l
        $Zg \times 60\%$ body wt. $\times 0.28 = (C)g$
        $(A) + (B) + (C) =$ nitrogen loss
                         $=$ minimal nitrogen requirement

---

* This factor is correct for untreated patients and those receiving synthetic crystalline amino acid solutions. Use 4/3 for patients receiving protein hydrolysate solutions, as only 60% of total urine nitrogen is present as urea nitrogen, some is excreted as peptide nitrogen
** 1 g nitrogen = 6.25 g protein
N.B. This formula takes no account of any extra renal losses e.g. intestinal fistula. 1 litre of such fluid loss can represent an extra 2–4 g of nitrogen requirement/day

Table 1.4 Consequences of a negative nitrogen balance

Loss of body weight
Less cold tolerance
Impaired humoral and cellular immunocompetence
Increased susceptibility to infections
Increased incidence of wound dehiscence
Loss of muscle mass – poor mobility – compromised ventilatory performance
Hypoproteinaemic oedema
Apathy, depression
Increased mortality

---

group is so wide that gross underestimates are inevitable. Central to the construction of any parenteral nutrition regimen is the daily nitrogen requirements. It is fortunate that there is a linear relationship over a wide range between total urinary nitrogen and urinary urea[13]. This applies both to the untreated patient and to those receiving crystalline amino acid solutions. The formula for estimating daily nitrogen requirements is given in Table 1.3. Clearly, such a formula assumes normal renal function and makes no allowances for extra renal losses. Studies have shown that for each litre of fluid lost daily from an intestinal fistula (the principal source of extra renal loss) an additional allowance of 3 g of nitrogen should be made[14].

A number of other tests have been examined, such as hair root morphology[15-17], skin testing with recall antigens, e.g. DNCB, candida[18,19], measurement of urinary 3-methyl histidine[20], and serum amino acid profiles. In the latter, the ratio of valine to glycine has been a useful indicator of impending malnutrition. Urinary hydroxyproline has also been used as an estimate of malnutrition[21] and, likewise, urinary zinc[22]. Whilst no one test is absolute in diagnosing malnutrition, those listed in Table 1.1, which are within the grasp of all clinicians, will suffice to measure the nutritional status and the response to intravenous nutrition.

It is important to emphasize again that intravenous nutrition is neither 'a drop of water with a dash of salt', nor 'nitrogen with a little sweetener'. It must be a comprehensive nutritional programme, which meets the requirements of water, electrolytes, nitrogen, energy, vitamins, essential fatty acids, essential biological elements and acid–base requirements. Let there be no misunderstanding; in the critically ill patient the first considerations are to maintain acid–base homeostasis and tissue perfusion. It is safe to let 48 hours pass before deciding on the need for intravenous nutrition. If, after 3 days of a critical illness, enteral feeding cannot be used, then failure to recognize the need for parenteral feeding and failure to start this therapy, are signs of clinical negligence. The metabolic response to trauma can be likened to the snowball going down the mountainside. If stopped early, little damage is done, but if it gathers momentum, not only may it be impossible to stop, but the damage becomes considerable. So too is the problem of an increasing negative nitrogen balance, as indicated in Table 1.4.

(III) DELIVERY SYSTEMS

Nowadays there should be little problem in gaining vascular access and in the last 5 years there has been a considerable improvement in the delivery systems. It is a matter of individual choice whether one uses a long peripheral catheter, e.g. Abbott's drum catheter[23] which ends centrally, or a central venous catheter[24,25]. My preference is to use the percutaneous infra-clavicular subclavian vein catheter with the tip ending just above the right atrium. This method has the advantages of allowing the patient unrestricted limb movements and furthermore, there is no limitation on the osmolar loading. I personally feel that there is little need nowadays for the short peripheral line delivery system[26]. Indeed, that method imposes certain limitations which are not permissible. For these patients vascular access is just as much a lifeline as the artificial kidney is for the patients on regular haemodialysis. Skilled insertion using an aseptic technique and meticulous after care are vital in the care of these lines[27,28]. I feel it is important for the clinician to familiarize himself with one method and then perfect it. It is sound medicolegal practice to take a chest X-ray immediately after inserting the catheter in order to check the location of the catheter tip. It should be mandatory that intravenous feeding is never begun without this investigation, otherwise avoidable complications will occur.

(IV) MATERIALS AND METHODS

The decision whether to deliver the nutrients from several bottles or to go for the 'big bag system' (2 or 3 litre) depends on personal preference, on the pharmacy support available at a given hospital, and the choice of ingredients[29]. It depends on whether additives can be made safely by the nursing staff. My personal preference is to use 1 litre bottles of nutrients, allowing more flexibility yet without too many bottles. The problem with a big bag system for the ICU patient is that, when based on the previous day's requirements and prepared early in the morning, the patient's condition may rapidly change, and a whole bag is wasted because the materials are inappropriate to the new situation. Of course, there is the question of the economics of such treatment. When properly prescribed for the right patients at the right time, this treatment can shorten the hospital stay by decreasing morbidity and mortality. At one time it was considered that the big bag system made an intravenous feeding regimen simpler. In a way this had its origins in the concept of 'one bottle for all patients at all times', which I believe is dangerous. I feel that in designing an intravenous feeding regimen, one must cater for the individual patient, based on measurements on that patient. If one does want to use a fat emulsion for providing part of the energy, then there are constraints on mixing a fat emulsion with other nutritional ingredients in a large bag. However, Solassol and Joyeux[30] have reported on the successful long term use of such mixtures. Thus, having gained vascular access in the duly identified patient, what are the ingredients one has to use to construct a comprehensive intravenous feeding regimen? Table 1.5 gives some indication of the solutions to be used. It is important to rationalize the materials and use only those with minimal complications and which give the best results[12,31].

(1) Energy

The ideal non-fat, non-protein energy substrate is glucose, which is normally used as a hypertonic solution through a central vein. Although sorbitol, xylitol or fructose alone or in combination with ethanol have been used in the past[32], it is now accepted that they do not have any advantages over glucose, and a glance at Table 1.6 shows why. At one stage it was

8

Table 1.5 Solutions and additives for complete intravenous feeding

Solution	Role	Principal contents
Normal saline (0.9%)	salt and water replacement	Na$^+$, Cl 155 mmol/l 310 mosmol/l
Sodium bicarbonate 8.4% (also 4.2% and 1.4%)	sodium and base replacement	Na$^+$, HCO$_3$ 1000 mmol/l
Glucose	water replacement	Glucose 205 kcal/l (0.86 MJ) 278 mosmol/l
Neutral phosphate solution (Boots)	phosphorus repletion and maintenance	Na$^+$ 162, K$^+$ 19, P 100 mmol/l
Hypertonic sodium chloride, e.g. 2.7% (3N)	salt repletion	Na$^+$, Cl 465 mmol/l 930 mosmol/l
Glucose 50%	high energy, low volume	Glucose 2000 kcal/l (8.4 MJ) 3800 mosmol/l
Soybean oil emulsion (Intralipid) 10%; 20%	high energy, low volume essential fatty acids	Fat (triglyceride, phospholipid) 1100 or 2000 kcal/l (4.6 or 8.4 MJ)
Vamin-N, Aminoplex 5 Aminofusin L1000, Synthamin 9	nitrogen source solutions – maintenance	Nitrogen content ranges from 5 to 9.26 g/l Variable electrolyte content Osmolality varies between 1000 and 1500
Intramin, Aminofusin L Forte Synthamin 17, Aminoplex 12	high nitrogen source solutions	Nitrogen content ranges from 12 to 17 g/l Variable electrolyte content Osmolality varies between 1000 and 1500
Multibionta Soluvit Parenterovite	water soluble vitamin preparations	B and C vitamins. Some need additional folic acid
Vitlipid	fat soluble vitamin preparation	A, D, K vitamins
Addamel	trace element solution	Ca, Mg, Zn, Cu, Mn, F, I, Fe
Plasma, HPPF, Buminate	for immediate restoration of serum oncotic pressure	Albumin, electrolytes

claimed that glucose could not be mixed with amino acid solutions, because of problems with sterilizing such solutions, but this is no longer true. Although 'stress diabetes' is common in critically ill patients, this is not a reason for avoiding glucose. Soluble insulin can be added to containers (plastic or glass) of hypertonic glucose and the dose adjusted to control the blood sugar. Hypertonic glucose can be delivered either through a metriset system, i.e. boluses every hour or through some form of constant infusion pump, e.g. Tekmar constant infusion pump. In some patients, quite large amounts of insulin are initially required to ensure adequate utilization although there is no evidence ever to exceed 240 units per day. One usually refers to these solutions as glucose–insulin–potassium mixtures. It is my practice to use half litre containers of hypertonic glucose and if the patient requires insulin, to add 60 units of soluble insulin to the first half litre of 40 or 50% glucose; 40 mmol of potassium are also added to each half litre. The nursing staff are instructed to measure the blood sugar every hour, using an Ames reflectance meter (or some similar method). If the blood sugar is above 10 mmol/1 a further intravenous bolus of insulin is given equal to 10% of the initial dose, i.e. 6 units. When after 10–12 hours the first 0.5 1 has been infused, the total dose of insulin would be 60 units plus a variable number of bolus doses. The second bottle of hypertonic glucose would contain 60 units plus the additions given during the first infusion. The frequency of blood sugar measurements can usually be reduced to 2 or 4 hourly over the next 48–72 hours. In many patients by about 72 hours the need for additional insulin may not be necessary and 1.25 1 of hypertonic glucose can be infused without added insulin. It is better to measure blood glucose rather than urinary glucose because this is far too crude. If urine testing is used, glycosuria simply indicates when the blood sugar must be measured; there is no other way of determining whether glycosuria '2%' is just 2% or 20%. Although some recommend the addition of albumin or polygeline to glucose solutions as a carrier for insulin, this is not my practice. When using the clinical titration, any insulin which adheres to the container surface will be compensated for by the monitoring. To use a separate pump for the constant infusion of insulin is, I believe, cumbersome, and makes nursing more difficult.* When giving intermittent glucose infusions, be wary of rebound hypoglycaemia. Nutritional support with glucose–insulin–potassium regimens not only provides nutrition, it maintains the functional integrity of cell membranes. In addition, most critically ill patients can utilize glucose–insulin regimens immediately, thus making glucose the energy substrate of choice.

Another excellent substrate which may be used, and which has an excellent clinical record, is the soya bean emulsion called Intralipid[33]. This

* Editor's note: Controversial! We prefer a separate infusion of insulin, using the method of McWilliam. (McWilliam, D. B. (1980). The practical management of glucose-insulin infusions in the intensive care patient. *Intensive Care Med.*, **6**, 2)

Table 1.6 Potential metabolic problems with energy substrates

Substrate	Lactate production with acidosis	α-Glycero-phosphate formation	Triglyceridaemia	Hyperuricaemia	Glyoxalate oxalate (-aemia: -uria)	Bilirubinaemia	Increased cell redox state
Glucose (a)	−	−	±	−	−	±	−
Fructose (b)	+	+	±	+	−	−	−
Sorbitol (c)	+	±	±	+	−	±	+
Xylitol (d)	+	++	+	+	+	+	+
Ethanol (e)	±	−	±	−	−	−	+

(i) Combinations b, c and d with e increase risk of metabolic complications.
(ii) Rapid infusion of glucose alone can produce hyperlacticacidaemia but extremly rarely lactic acidosis.

fat emulsion is basically a suspension of chylomicrons, the particles not exceeding 1 micron in diameter and comprising a triglyceride centre covered with phospholipid. This emulsion also contains approximately 8 mmol/1 of cholesterol. It is important to remember that, in comparison to glucose, a longer adaptation period is required for complete utilization whether the fat is given orally or intravenously. This is not a reason for excluding a fat emulsion as an energy source. The metabolic pathways of glucose or fat will differ but both are utilized to provide energy and to ensure the utilization of nitrogen given at the same time[34,35]. Table 1.7 shows some of the differences between these two energy substrates. Studies have clearly shown that these substrates are interchangeable in the moderately catabolic patient but during hypercatabolism the adaptation for the optimal metabolism of fat may be slightly longer, particularly when there is associated infection[36,37]. However, Table 1.8 shows there are certain advantages that accrue from using a combined energy regimen.

Table 1.7 Plasma profile related to energy substrate

Glucose	Fat
Pyruvate ↑	free fatty acids ↑
Lactate ↑	triglycerides ↑
Alanine ↑	ketones ↑
Immunoactive insulin ↑	pyruvate ↓
Free fatty acids ↓	lactate ↓
Ketones ↓	alanine ±
Triglycerides ±	immunoactive insulin ↓

A fat emulsion for most adults can be given in a dose of up to 3 g/kg body weight per day, and infants appear to have an even better tolerance. The evidence in man that fat emulsions are utilized is good and derived from (a) nitrogen balance studies (b) chylomicron kinetic studies (c) studies on the repiratory quotient (d) the elimination of ^{14}C labelled fat emulsions. It is generally accepted that during bacterial infection more caution is required before using a fat emulsion, or less fat should be used. In some patients with respiratory failure, in particular during IPPV, extra caution may be necessary but the use of fat emulsions is not precluded[38-40]. It is important to recall that Intralipid contains 50% weight/volume of the essential fatty acid, linoleic acid. It was formerly thought that essential fatty acid deficiency was a disease of experimental animals but this is now recognized in man and occurs far more readily than hitherto appreciated, particularly in the hypercatabolic patient. It has been suggested that essential fatty acids can be given percutaneously, i.e. rubbing sunflower seed oil on the skin[41], and it should really be a part of any comprehensive

Table 1.8 Sugg. IV energy regimen for 70 kg non-infected man requiring 3000 kcal/day derived equally from glucose and fat

Glucose	50% solution + potassium (usually 60 mmol/l) ± soluble insulin
	750 ml (32 ml bolus/h or continuous infusion via central catheter)
	365 g glucose (1500 kcal) per 24 h
	5.36 (g/kg body weight)/day
	0.223 (g/kg)/h (well within tolerance limits)
Fat	20% soybean oil emulsion (Intralipid)
	750 ml (allow 6–8 h fat free infusion period before morning blood sample)
	150 g fat-triglyceride 1500 kcal – (note extra energy from glycerol) per 24 h
	2.14 (g/kg body weight)/day
	0.089 (g/kg)/h
Total energy volume	1500 ml
Energy osmolar load	129 mosmol/h
% energy loss/day	less than 5%
Minimal monitoring required	

Rather than waste 0.5 l amounts of substrate use to nearest complete 0.5 l of either substrate or alternate between 1.0 l 50% glucose and 0.5 l Intralipid and vice versa.

intraveneous (i.v.) feeding regimen. For those who wish to use glucose only as the main energy source, a litre of 10% Intralipid should be given at least twice per week. When a fat emulsion is used as part of the intravenous feeding regimen it is important to make sure that there is a 6 hour fat-free period before the morning blood samples are taken. Then, by spinning down the blood samples one can determine whether or not the plasma is lipaemic. If the plasma is lipaemic this may alert the clinician to fat intolerance and may indicate the need for an alternative substrate. One of the advantages claimed for intravenous fat emulsions is that, because they are virtually isotonic with plasma, they can be given through peripheral lines[26]. However, it is my practice to give a fat emulsion with glucose through a central catheter although they are not mixed in the same container. A mixture has been used successfully on the Continent with a solution called Trivemil and some tentative research is already in progress in the UK. Since the metabolic response to trauma may inhibit the metabolism of ketones[42,43], the question is, could these patients receive a fat emulsion as part of their energy substrate? This remains *sub judice* and is an important area of research.

With respect to the total energy provision, a number of studies have shown that the optimum is 200 kcal/g of nitrogen, or 45 kcal/kg body weight. There is some evidence to suggest that in the hypercatabolic patient, the ratio may drop to 140:1 and in the less catabolic patient the ratio may be higher, approaching 250:1[44].

(2) Nitrogen

Another major constituent of intravenous feeding programmes is nitrogen; this clearly has to be provided as amino acids. It is useless to give plasma as a source of either essential biological elements, essential fatty acids, or amino acids. Over the years many different amino acid solutions have been manufactured but it is debatable whether the vast array from which one can choose offers an equal array of advantages. Provided a solution contains all eight essential amino acids and a fairly comprehensive profile of non-essential amino acids, then two solutions providing 10 g N/1 and 16–18 g/1 respectively are needed. For adult practice, these solutions should have 25% of their total nitrogen content derived from the essential amino acids. It is important that the non-essential amino acid profile is carefully balanced, and not filled with some cheap 'stuffing agent', e.g. glycine or glutamic acid. It was thought that the advent of the crystalline L synthetic amino acids would be a considerable advance upon the former casein hydrolysates. However, as far as nitrogen balance studies go, this has not been proved to be the case[45,46]. However, the newer solutions do contain much less ammonia, but are also deficient in trace elements and phosphorus which were present in the hydrolysate preparations. Whether the modern crystalline amino acid solutions should contain more branched-chain amino acids is debatable. Undoubtedly, leucine is the main determinant of amino acid metabolism in muscle[47] and possibly more should be added. In my opinion there is no need for a large number of amino acid solutions which are specifically made for individual diseases, though there is some evidence that a specific amino acid solution could be required for hepatic encephalopathy of cirrhotic origin[48,49].

When choosing an amino acid solution it is important to know its cost, and its electrolyte and energy content. A number of studies have shown that patients requiring intravenous nutrition need 0.2–0.24 g of nitrogen per kg body weight[50,23]. Alternatively, the amount of nitrogen required is derived from a formula (Table 1.3)[13]. It is important to emphasize again that there is no one ideal amino acid solution. There are a number of solutions which are adequate for intravenous nutrition, as evidenced by their capability of maintaining nitrogen balance, of correcting nutritional deficiences and an absence of toxic reactions[51]. It is not the brief of this chapter to go into the specific requirements for paediatric practice, when crystalline amino acid solutions must be used together with a comprehensive non-essential amino acid profile containing tyrosine and cystine/cysteine. This is because of the immaturity of the liver enzymes of sick infants. In adults, of course,

14

tyrosine can be obtained from phenylalanine and cystine/cysteine from methionine. It is necessary to have available solutions of high and low concentration of nitrogen. This is because fluid volume constraints will occasionally dictate the need for a concentrated solution. It is also probably preferable to use amino acid solutions without added sugars, thus allowing the clinician a choice of energy substrates.

(3) Electrolytes

Having decided on the energy and nitrogen requirements and the volume permitted, then attention is directed to basic electrolyte needs, ensuring that any regimen contains the optimal proportions of electrolytes to nitrogen. By careful monitoring of the patient and the plasma urea and electrolytes, a fair assessment of the requirements can be made. Unfortunately, serum potassium levels are but a poor indicator of body stores of potassium and the general rule should be that if the serum potassium concentration is below 3 mmol/l, there is a 10% deficiency of total body potassium[31]. A common mistake in intravenous feeding regimens is to under-estimate the needs for phosphorus. Although there is some phosphorus available in a fat emulsion, it is better to make an assessment of the patient's total phosphorus requirements and to add these as a neutral phosphate solution. The earlier casein hydrolysates contained appreciable phosphorus, but many of the modern solutions do not. Although the phospholipid phosphorus of a fat emulsion can be utilized in the body, it is unwise to rely solely on this for providing total phosphorus. The requirement has been estimated to be 0.5–0.75 mmol/kg body weight[14]. Magnesium deficiency should be avoided, especially in severe inflammatory bowel disease.

(4) Trace elements

Provision of essential biological or trace elements constitute another important feature. Although information is available about basic requirements in a healthy person, less is known about the critically ill patient[52]. No hard and fast rules can be made about the requirements, except that the basal requirements should be provided, and a commercial solution is available (Table 1.9). When a hypercatabolic patient becomes anabolic as a result of intravenous feeding, copper and zinc deficiencies may soon manifest themselves, unless additional amounts are given[53,54]. Zinc is an essential ingredient of tissue protein and protein synthesis is impaired during zinc deficiency. Zinc deficiency following intravenous nutrition is well-documented. It is my practice to use ampoules of zinc sulphate, each containing $40\,\mu$mol, and ampoules of copper sulphate providing $20\,\mu$mol.

Table 1.9 Composition of trace element solution 'Addamel'

Chloride	13.3 mmol
Calcium	5.0 mmol
Magnesium	1.5 mmol
Iron	50 μmol
Zinc	20 μmol
Manganese	40 μmol
Copper	5 μmol
Fluorine	50 μmol
Sorbitol	3.0 g
Sterile water	

Though there is some chelation between essential biological elements and amino acids, nevertheless, it is reasonable to add the trace elements to an amino acid solution, or alternatively, to saline or dextrose.

As previously implied, essential fatty acids (linoleic acid) should be provided. When a fat emulsion is used as part energy substrate of a regimen, the need will be covered[33,55]. Otherwise, it is estimated that 100 mg/kg body weight per day of linoleic acid have to be given intravenously to prevent a deficiency[41,52]. Since this deficiency is difficult to establish by laboratory tests, it is better to make provision for it in any regimen.

(5) Vitamins

Intravenous nutrition must include the supply of vitamins, both water and fat soluble. Fortunately, it is difficult to cause toxic manifestations by giving too much of vitamins C or B. Thus 75–100 mg daily of ascorbic acid should be given and adequate amounts of thiamine and riboflavin[52]. There are a number of preparations available which contain adequate amounts of vitamins B and C though some are deficient in folic acid, which may need to be added. From a practical aspect it should be remembered that the riboflavin in B vitamin compounds is light sensitive, and there is a choice of giving this as an intravenous bolus or adding the compound to bottles which are then protected from light. The timing of fat soluble vitamins is more difficult to establish. However, when an intravenous feeding regimen is to go on for more than 14 days, it would be logical to add fat soluble vitamins, using a preparation such as Vitlipid, which can be added to a fat emulsion[52]. Though problems of vitamin A excess are most unlikely, monitoring is necessary for hypercalcaemia due to vitamin D.

(V) DESIGN OF THE DIET

The ingredients of an intravenous diet have now been reviewed. How are these put together to meet the requirements of the individual patient? Table 1.10 provides the basis for constructing a regimen which is within the compass of any clinician. Having decided the fluid volume permitted, the solutions are chosen from a limited range (Table 1.5). The importance of limiting the choice is that the individual clinician becomes familiar with these solutions.

Table 1.10 Basis of an intravenous nutritional regimen

1. Nitrogen: 0.20–0.24 g/kg body weight
2. Energy: 40–45 kcal/kg body weight
3. Nitrogen: energy ratio 1:200
4. Energy derived from equal amounts of glucose and fat emulsion or from glucose–insulin–potassium regimen
5. Optimal potassium: nitrogen ration of 5 mmol: 1 g
6. Optimal magnesium: nitrogen ratio of 1 mmol: 1 g
7. Phosphorus intake 0.5–0.75 mmol/kg body weight
8. Water soluble vitamins, including folic acid
9. Adequate electrolyte provision
10. Essential biological elements, e.g. zinc, copper, magnesium, manganese
11. Energy and nitrogen given simultaneously
12. Essential fatty acids
13. Blood or plasma (or HPPF) for immediate restoration of haemoglobin or serum oncotic pressure
14. Even rate of infusion over 24 hour periods
15. Mobilize as soon as possible

Intravenous nutrition is no metabolic short cut to nutritional success; adequate monitoring of the patient is vital[12]. Many complications of intravenous nutrition have been reported (Table 1.11)[11] but the important fact is that they are all avoidable. Correct patient assessment, correct choice and appropriate monitoring can ensure this. Table 1.12 shows the monitoring required and its frequency. For some patients the monitoring of acid–base balance will need to be increased. For the difficult measurements, e.g. fat and water soluble vitamins, essential fatty acids and some trace elements, the plan is to include these in the regimen and thus prevent deficiencies. It is equally important to ensure that the diet will correct nutritional deficiencies as well as maintain nutrition. It is often queried whether i.v. feeding could be started in full on the first day, or whether there should be a gradual build up over 3 or 4 days. Although this method is proper when using enteral nutrition, there is no evidence to show that this is

17

necessary for i.v. feeding. It is preferable to have some form of flow chart for recording data on patients receiving i.v. nutrition. This is particularly so for those in the ICU. For other patients, once established on i.v. feeding, less monitoring is required since their requirements become stabilized.

Table 1.11 Complications of intravenous nutrition

Disturbance	Potential causal substrate
Metabolic acidosis: lactic acidosis	fructose, sorbitol, ethanol–carbohydrate combinations
Hyperosmolar dehydration syndrome	hypertonic glucose, sorbitol, xylitol
Hyperuricaemia	fructose, sorbitol, xylitol
Oxalaemia and oxaluria	? xylitol
Triglyceridaemia	fructose, sorbitol, xylitol, fat emulsion
Hyperlipidaemia	fat emulsion, particularly in bacterial infection or toxaemia
Essential fatty acid deficiency	fat free regimen
Hypophosphataemia	phosphorus free glucose regimens
Folate metabolism disturbances	ethanol
Hyperammonaemia	protein hydrolysate solution
Altered cerebration	poorly designed amino acid solutions
Vascular access complications: (i) thrombosis	hypertonic solutions given peripherally
(ii) infection	
(iii) damage to structures during central venous catheterization (e.g. haematoma, haemorrhage, pneumothorax)	
Fatty liver	glucose solutions

(VI) APPLICATIONS

The applications of intravenous feeding are boundless. It is important not to use intravenous feeding on the basis of some diagnostic index. It is better to be aware of those patients who, because all other routes of maintaining nutritional support cannot be used or prove inadequate, that parenteral nutrition must be used. For most adult patients requiring i.v. nutrition the materials and methods described are adequate. Debate surrounds the question of the amino acid solution to be used in hepatic failure[48,49]. But hepatic failure patients are heterogenous; Fischer and his colleagues[56] showed that branched-chain amino acids were particularly useful in reversing hepatic

Table 1.12 Optimal observations during intravenous nutrition

(A) Biochemical
    (i) Routine:
        Blood urea and electrolytes (daily)
        SMA 12/60 profile* (every 2nd or 3rd day)
        Serum lactate, pyruvate (in unexplained anion gap)
        Blood glucose (frequently with AMES meter according to i.v. regimen used)
        Liver function tests (at least weekly)
        Serum magnesium (weekly)
        Serum transferrin, complement C_3 (weekly)
        Serum and urine osmolality
        Observation of spun plasma each morning when using fat emulsion
        24 hour urine urea, sodium (daily)
        Acid–base balance
    (ii) Special:
        Serum amino acid profile
        Serum and urine, zinc and copper (especially in hypercatabolic patients)
        Any specific test determined by illness
(B) Haematological
        Hb, WBC, platelets, PCV (daily or less frequently depending on circumstances)
        BCR (prothrombin index)
        Serum folate (rarely)
(C) Physiological
        Vital signs - pulse, respiration, BP, temperature, colour
        CVP (line not mandatory)
        Weight (weigh bed invaluable)
        Fluid balance (urine volume, etc.)
(D) Mechanical
        Line inspection (filter changes, care with connections)
        Flow rates
        Catheter insertion point
        Pump checks
        Meniscus levels in bubble traps
        Back–flow up 'piggy-back' lines
          (particularly with solutions of low density, e.g. fat emulsion)
(E) Bacteriological
        Blood cultures (one a week at least)
        Viral agglut. titres (e.g. cytomegalovirus)
        Watch carefully for *Candida* or other fungus infections
(F) Radiological
        Chest X-ray
        (i) must have initial one immediately after catheter insertion
        (ii) subsequently one a week depending on clinical condition

* Includes albumin, calcium, phosphorus, bilirubin, urate, alkaline phosphatase, LDH, aspartate transaminase, creatinine.

coma, but this only occurred in cirrhotic patients. Thus it remains to be determined whether one should use solutions rich in branched-chain amino acids for all patients with hepatic failure. Although it is customary to provide glucose as most of the energy for such patients, it should be recalled that many such patients tolerate fat emulsions well, utilizing up to 1.5 g/kg body weight daily[57-59]. The debate over the use of branched-chain amino acids in hepatic coma raises the question whether these amino acid solutions should be regarded as nutrients or pharmacological agents.

Much has been written recently about the need for special solutions in renal failure, especially the acute type[60,61]. In my view such an approach is inappropriate and was based on false concepts[62,63]. Although these patients do have a high blood urea, there is little evidence to show that this has any nutritional significance. Indeed, my policy in acute renal failure with hyper-catabolism is to feed the patient as usual, either orally or parenterally[64], and then dialyse as necessary, both to maintain metabolic homeostasis and to provide 'space' for intravenous feeding. There is little doubt that the use of comprehensive intravenous feeding in acute renal failure during the past 5 years has improved the prognosis when dialysis techniques have remained stationary[65,66].

For patients with poor pulmonary function there is some evidence that parenteral nutrition impairs oxygen exchange and may reduce lung compliance[39]. The important point to stress is that a fat emulsion can be used in such patients, but with careful monitoring. There is no evidence that a fat emulsion is responsible for the adult respiratory distress syndrome (Chapter 8).

Parenteral feeding has been claimed to be of considerable value for patients with various types of neoplastic disease, particularly those affecting the gastrointestinal tract. It remains to be shown whether or not parenteral feeding has advantages over comprehensive enteral feeding. Certainly many cancer patients are anorexic, become malnourished and as a result have impairment of their immune mechanisms (Chapter 2). The work of Dudrick and his colleagues[67,68], suggests that intravenous feeding of such patients converts their skin anergic situation to a responsive state and makes them more amenable to chemotherapy. However, I believe that a note of caution is needed before one recommends parenteral nutrition for all cancer patients.

As indicated earlier, there is no conflict between enteral and parenteral nutritional support. Patients who have been on parenteral nutrition for some time should be gradually changed to the enteral route over the course of a week. In this way nutritional deficits are unlikely to occur and the risk of diarrhoea is lessened.

The aim of modern intravenous feeding should be to combine flexibility with simplicity, both in the design of the regimen, the monitoring required and the vascular access used. Unless this mode of therapy is used outside specialized units, the risk of patients dying from hospital malnutrition will continue. There can be no doubt about the efficacy of parenteral nutrition in appropriately selected patients. Probably the ultimate proof of this efficacy is in patients on the so-called 'artificial gut system'[30,35,69]. These patients have lost the major part of their small bowel and can be maintained for many months or years by means of intravenous feeding, at first in the hospital, and then in the home. Indeed, it has been from the study of these particular patients that much has been learned about the human requirements of essential biological elements, vitamins and essential fatty acids. These patients can be maintained in the home by simple apparatus, fed intravenously overnight, and lead a normal life during the day. If patients can be taught to look after themselves by this form of treatment, then it should not be beyond the comprehension of practising clinicians to do the same for hospital patients. The cost of intravenous feeding is undoubtedly high, but there is nothing more expensive than the cost of a hospital bed and the longer the hospital stay the greater the cost. Nevertheless one does need to select patients carefully for intravenous feeding and choose only those in whom enteral feeding is positively contraindicated. There is no doubt that in the past far too many patients were fed intravenously and could have been treated by cheaper alternative methods[70]. Also in earlier years there was a certain fear generated amongst clinicians by the ever increasing range of i.v. nutrients, particularly amino acid solutions, and by the potential complications of this treatment. I now believe that regimens have become far more standardized, monitoring is better understood and the value of nutritional support unquestionable. The practice of comprehensive feeding and the results obtained constitute one of the major advances in therapeutics.

In the appendix that follows details are given of nutritional support regimens for (1) a patient needing normal maintenance (2) a patient with a hypercatabolic state and (3) a patient with renal and hepatic complications.

APPENDIX

Example 1

Post-cholecystectomy 70 kg patient with ileus and ? intra-abdominal sepsis. Normal renal and hepatic function.

Vital details

Urine volume	=	2.1 l/24 h
24 hr urine urea excretion	=	218 mmol/l = 457.8 /day
	=	26.9 g urea = 15.1 g nitrogen
Temperature	=	38 °C (allow 1.0 l for insensible loss)
Gastric aspirate	=	0.5 l
Total fluid loss	=	3.6 l

Requirements

(a) Nitrogen   =   15.1 g

(b) Energy:-

    based on 200 kcal (0.84 MJ) per g N = 3016 kcal

    (or based on 45 kcal/kg body weight = 3150 kcal)

(c) Electrolytes:-

    Sodium 1.0 mmol/kg body weight and 0.5 l of normal

    Saline as replacement for gastric aspirate = 147 mmol

    Potassium 6.0 mmol/g nitrogen   = 91 mmol

    Magnesium 0.5 mmol/g nitrogen   = 75 mmol

    Phosphorus 0.5 mmol/kg body weight   = 35 mmol

Possible regimens

1 litre of Aminofusin L Forte providing 15.2 g N, 40 mmol sodium, 30 mmol potassium and 5 mmol magnesium or 1.5 litre of Vamin N (or Vamin-glucose with 600 kcal from carbohydrate content) providing 14.1 g nitrogen, 75 mmol sodium, 30 mmol potassium and 4.5 mmol magnesium.

1 litre of 50% dextrose (with 80 mmol potassium) = 2000 kcal (with or without added soluble insulin). 0.5 l of 20% Intralipid = 1000 kcal (this also provides essential fatty acid requirement, i.e. linoleic acid of 100 mg per kg body weight i.e. 7.0 g Intralipid contains 50% weight/volume linoleic acid; thus 14 g soybean oil are contained in as little as 70 ml 20% Intralipid or 140 ml 10% Intralipid. Also each 2 g fat in Intralipid 20% potentially yields 0.15 mmol phosphorus). 1 litre of normal saline = 155 mmol of sodium.

On alternate days substitute 0.5 l Boots Neutral Phosphate solution for 0.5 l normal saline. This provides 50 mmol of phosphorus, 81 mmol sodium and 9.5 mmol potassium. Thus a total volume of 3.5–4 litres over 24 hours will meet this patient's nutritional requirements. The extra 60 mmol of potassium can be added to the normal saline or neutral phosphate solution. Likewise, water soluble vitamins can be added either to the saline or 5% dextrose solution if substituted for normal saline because of fear of sodium overload. Ensure that 5–10 mg of folinic acid are added to the regimen each day. The trace element solution Addamel (see Table 1.9) can be added either to the amino acid solution, or glucose or normal saline. May need extra supplement of zinc sulphate or copper sulphate.

Example 2

A 68 kg man received multiple injuries in a road traffic accident. Injuries to chest with secondary infection. Fractured pelvis and compound fracture right femur. Abdominal injury resulting in intestinal fistula and ileus. Normal renal function.

Vital details

        Urine volume 2.4 litres/day
        24 hr urine urea excretion 643 mmol (268 mmol/l)
                        ≡ 37.8 g urea
                        ≡ 21.2 g nitrogen
        Fistula losses   = 0.7–0.9 l
        Gastric aspirate = 0.8 l
        Temperature 38.5 °C (allow 1.25 l insensible loss)
        Total fluid loss = 5.25 l

Requirements

Nitrogen (N) 21.2 g (urine) + 2.4 g (fistula loss allow 3 g nitrogen/l) = 23.6 g.
    Energy: based on 200 kcal/g N = 4720 (or based on 45 kcal/kg body weight = 3060 kcal).
    ∴ Compromise, since there is evidence that at higher catabolic rates the ratio of energy to nitrogen is less. Thus aim for ≈ 4000 kcal.
    Electrolytes: sodium 1 mmol/kg body weight + 1.5 l normal saline as replacement for gastrointestinal losses

                        = 68 + 233   = 301 mmol
        Potassium 6 mmol/g N   = 142 mmol
        Magnesium 0.5 mmol/g N   = 12 mmol
        Phosphorus 0.5 mmol/kg body weight   = 34 mmol

Possible regimens

(a) 1.5 l of Aminofusin L Forte providing 22.8 g N, 60 mmol sodium, 45 mmol potassium and 7.5 mmol magnesium; or (b) 2.5 l of Vamin-glucose providing 23.5 g N, 125 mmol sodium, 50 mmol potassium and 7.5 mmol magnesium and 1000 kcal, or (c) 1.5 l Intramin 11% providing 25.6 g N (electrolytes as for Vamin). Since, in this case, there is some evidence of infection, use energy based on 75% carbohydrate and 25% fat.

If using Aminofusin, then use 1.5 l 50% dextrose (with or without insulin but containing 80 mmol/l potassium) yielding 3000 kcal and 1.0 l of 10% Intralipid yielding 1100 kcal (total 4100) and also cover essential fatty acid requirements. Also use 1.0 l normal saline giving total of 215 mmol sodium (although a little under optimal amount, since renal function normal, sodium conservation will occur). Fat emulsion will provide approx. 15 mmol phosphorus daily, so on alternate days use 0.5 l of neutral phosphate (see Example 1). Total volume = 5 l. If using Vamin-glucose, then use 1.0 l 50% dextrose (± insulin and with 80 mmol potassium) and 0.5 l 20% Intralipid. Additionally 1.0 l normal saline, giving 280 mmol sodium; again alternate days substitute 0.5 l neutral phosphate for 0.5 l normal saline. Total volume = 5 l. If using 1.5 l Intramin, then use same regimen as for Aminofusin L Forte.

To all regimens additional potassium would be added to fulfil total requirements. Add water soluble vitamins (Multibionta, Soluvit, Parenterovite (1) and (2)) and the trace element solution Addamel'. The latter will bring magnesium up to 9.0 mmol for each regimen. Additions of zinc, copper and magnesium can be made with zinc sulphate, copper sulphate and magnesium chloride if indicated.

Example 3

Road traffic accident patient with multiple injuries; abdominal injuries including ruptured spleen and lacerated liver; associated chest infection; shock and acute oliguric renal failure. Also became jaundiced with serum bilirubin of 120 mmol/l, aspartic transaminase 147 units/l and alkaline phosphatase of 94 units/l. Associated ileus: Required daily haemodialysis for management of acute renal failure. Urine volume less than 50 ml/day.

Vital details

Patient's weight = 76 kg (total body water 60% of body weight = 46 l)

Daily rate of blood urea rise $= 15$ mmol/l
∴ Total daily urea increment $= 46 \times 15 = 690$
$= 40.6$ g urea
$\equiv 22.7$ g N
Gastric aspirate $= 1.2$ l daily
Potassium rising daily to 6.5 mmol/l
Temperature 38 °C (allow 1 litre for insensible losses)
Total fluid losses $= 1.2$ l $+ 0.05$ l (urine) $+ 1.0$ l
$= 2.25$ l

Requirements

Nitrogen $22.7 + 3.6 = 26.3$ g
Energy based on 200 kcal/1 g N $= 5260$ kcal (based on 45 kcal/kg body weight $= 3420$)
Compromise aim $= 4400$ kcal
Sodium 1 mmol/kg body weight $= 76$ mmol $+$ only 0.5 l normal saline for aspirate (in view of renal failure) $= 154$ mmol
Potassium – none extra added until indicated by serum concentrations, because of hyperkalaemia in renal failure. Potassium is added only to hypertonic glucose solution.
Magnesium is added only as ingredient of either amino acid solution or 'Addamel' solution. Trace elements will be lost during dialysis and these must be replaced.

Possible regimen

Since patient has some liver insufficiency, the fat energy should not exceed 1.5 g/kg body weight. Initially, potassium was omitted apart from half dosage added to glucose. Similarly, initially do not add any phosphorus to regimen. However, in regard both potassium and phosphorus, additions of both may have to be made once patient stabilized on haemodialysis protocol and intravenous feeding and then becomes anabolic. In view of the constraints on volume, it is advisable to use concentrated amino acid solution, although Vamin is probably the best from hepatic viewpoint. Currently, there is no ideal amino acid solution for acute hepatic insufficiency. The uraemic patient may need more insulin to control the blood sugar.

Thus, use either 1.5 l of Aminofusin L Forte or 2.5 l Vamin-glucose (see contents in example regimens 1 and 2). For energy use 1.5 l of 50% dextrose (with 40 mmol/l potassium ± insulin) and 0.5 l 20% Intralipid if using Aminofusin or 1 litre 50% dextrose (with 40 mmol potassium ± insulin) and 0.5 l 20% Intralipid.

Add usual additions of water soluble vitamins and trace elements to regimen, for these will be lost during peritoneal or haemodialysis.

Use appropriate ultrafiltration or haemfiltration to ensure that the fluid removed will accommodate the feeding regimen. Give amino acids between haemodialyses rather than during, to avoid unnecessary losses. Intralipid can be infused during dialysis. Since amino acids are inevitably lost during dialysis, infuse 0.5 l Vamin N over last 3 hours of haemodialysis to compensate for these losses.

References

1. Wilkinson, A. W. (1963). Historical background of intravenous feeding. *Nutr. Dieta*, **5**, 295
2. Lee, H. A. (1974). Historical review of parenteral nutrition. In Lee, H. A. (ed.). *Parenteral Nutrition in Acute Metabolic Illness*, pp. 3–10. (London: Academic Press)
3. Keys, A. (1948). Caloric undernutrition and starvation, with notes on protein deficiency. *J. Am. Med. Assoc.*, **138**, 500
4. Cuthbertson, D. P. (1932). Observations on the disturbance of metabolism produced by injury to the limbs. *Q. J. Med.*, **25**, 233
5. Moore, F. D. (1959). *Metabolic Care of the Surgical Patient*. (London: Saunders)
6. Lee, H. A. (1979). Why enteral nutrition? In Johnston, I. D. A. and Lee, H. A., (eds.). *Developments in Clinical Nutrition. Res. Clin. Forums*, **1**, 15
7. Blackburn, G. L., Bistrian, B. R., Maini, B. S., Schlamm, H. T. and Smith, M. F. (1977). Nutritional and metabolic assessment of the hospitalized patient. *J. Parenteral Nutr.*, **1**, 11
8. Bistrian, B. R., Blackburn, G. L., Hallowell, E. and Heddle, R. (1974). Protein status of surgical patients. *J. Am. Med. Assoc.*, **230**, 858
9. Bistrian, B. R., Blackburn, G. L., Vitale, J., Cochran, D. and Naylor, J. (1976). Prevalance of malnutrition in general medical patients. *J. Am. Med. Assoc.*, **235**, 1567
10. Shetty, P. S., Jung, R. T., Watrasiewicz, K. E. and James, W. P. T. (1979). Rapid turnover transport proteins: an index of subclinical protein-energy malnutrition. *Lancet*, **2**, 230
11. Lee, H. A. (1974). Planning intravenous nutrition – techniques and principles. In Lee, H. A., (ed.). *Parenteral Nutrition in Acute Metabolic Illness*, pp. 307–331. (London: Academic Press)
12. Lee, H. A. (1979). Principles of intravenous nutrition. *Int. J. Vitam. Nutr. Res.*, **18**, 45
13. Lee, H. A. and Hartley, T. F. (1975). A method of determining daily nitrogen requirements. *Postgrad. Med. J.*, **51**, 441
14. Tovey, S. J., Benton, K. G. F. and Lee, H. A. (1977). Hypophosphataemia and phosphorus requirements during intravenous nutrition. *Postgrad. Med. J.*, **53**, 289
15. Bradfield, R. B. (1972). A rapid tissue technique for the field assessment of

protein-calorie malnutrition. *Am. J. Clin. Nutr.*, **25**, 720

16. Jordan, V. E. (1976). Protein status of the elderly as measured by dietary intake, hair tissue and serum albumin. *Am. J. Clin. Nutr.*, **29**, 522

17. Tanphaichitr, V., Kulapongse, S. and Kominor, S. (1980). Assessment of nutritional status in adult hospitalized patients. *Nutr. Metabol*, **24**, 23

18. Bistrian, B. R., Blackburn, G. L., Scrimshaw, N. S. and Flatt, J. P. (1975). Cellular immunity in semi-starved states in hospitalized adults. *Am. J. Clin. Nutr.*, **28**, 1148

19. Meakins, J. L., Pietsch, J. B., Bubenick, O., Kelly, R., Rode, H., Gordon, J. and Maclean, L. D. (1977). Delayed hypersensitivity: indicator of acquired failure of host defences in sepsis and trauma. *Ann. Surg.*, **186**, 241

20. Long, C. L., Haverberg, L. N., Young, R. V., Kinney, J. M., Munro, H. N. and Geiger, J. W. (1975). Metabolism of 3-methyl histidine in man. *Metabolism*, **24**, 929

21. Picou, D., Halliday, D. and Garrow, J. S. (1966). Total body protein, collagen and non-collagen protein in infantile protein malnutrition. *Clin. Sci.*, **30**, 345

22. Kay, R. G. (1981). Intravenous nutrition – trace metals. In Hill, G. L. (ed.) *Nutrition and the Surgical Patient*. Ch. II, pp. 168–189. (Edinburgh: Churchill Livingstone)

23. Hartley, T. F. and Lee, H. A. (1975). Investigations into the optimum nitrogen and caloric requirements and comparative nutritive value of three intravenous amino acid solutions in the post-operative period. *Nutr. Metabol.*, **19**, 201

24. Parsa, M. H., Ferrer, J. M. and Habif, D. V. (1972). *Safe Central Venous Nutrition. Guidelines for Prevention and Management of Complications*. (Springfield: Charles C. Thomas)

25. Dinley, R. J. (1976). Venous reactions related to indwelling plastic cannulae: a prospective trial. *Curr. Med. Res. Opin.*, **3**, 607

26. Deitel, M. and Kaminsky, V. (1979). Total nutrition by peripheral vein – the lipid system. *Can. Med. Assoc. J.*, **3**, 1

27. Phillips, K. H. (1976). Nursing care in parenteral nutrition. In Fischer, J. E., (ed.). *Total Parenteral Nutrition*, pp. 101–110. (Boston: Little, Brown & Company)

28. Colley, R. (1977). Nursing in parenteral nutrition. In Greep, J. M., Soetors, P. B., Wesdorp, R. I. C., Phaf, C. W. R. and Fischer, J. E. (eds.). *Current Concepts in Parenteral Nutrition*. pp. 85–98. (The Hague: Martinus Nijhoff Medical Division)

29. Cosh, D. G., West, K. P., Thomas, M. P. and Sanson, L. N. (1979). The preparation of parenteral nutrition solutions. *Aust. J. Pharm. Sci.*, **6**, 97

30. Solassol C. and Joyeux, H. (1976). Ambulatory parenteral nutrition. In Fischer, J. E. (ed.). *Total Parenteral Nutrition*. pp. 285–304. (Boston: Little, Brown & Company)

31. Lee, H. A. (1979). Fluid balance and parenteral feeding. In Gray, T. C., Nunn, J. F. and Utting, J. E. (eds.). *General Anaesthesia*. 4th Ed., pp. 1591–1610. (London: Butterworth and Co. (Publ). Ltd.)

32. Lee, H. A. (1974). The alcohols – ethanol sorbitol xylitol. In Lee H. A. (ed.). *Parenteral Nutrition in Acute Metabolic Illness*. pp. 37–52. (London: Academic Press)

33. Lee, H. A. (1977). The rationale for using a fat emulsion (Intralipid) as part

energy substrate during intravenous nutrition. In Greep, J. M., Soetors, P. B., Wesdorp, R. I. C., Phaf, C. W. R. and Fischer, J. E. (eds.). *Current Concepts in Parenteral Nutrition*. (The Hague: Martinus Nijhoff Medical Division)

34. Greenburg, G. R., Marliss, E. B., Anderson, G. H., Langer, B., Spence, W., Tovee, E. B. and Jeejeebhoy, K. N. (1976). Protein sparing therapy in postoperative patients. Effects of added hypocaloric glucose or lipid. *N. Engl. J. Med.*, **294**, 1411

35. Jeejeebhoy, K. N., Anderson, G. H., Nakhooda, A. F., Greenburg, G. R., Sanderson, I. and Marliss, E. B., (1976). Metabolic studies in total parenteral nutrition with lipid in man. *J. Clin. Invest.*, **57**, 125

36. Bistrian, B. R. (1977). Interaction of nutrition and infection in hospital setting. *Am. J. Clin. Nutr.*, **30**, 1228

37. Blackhurn, G. L. (1977). Lipid metabolism in infection. *Am. J. Clin. Nutr.*, **30**, 1320

38. Wilmore, D. W., Moylan, J. A., Helmkamp, G. M. and Pruitt, B. A. (1973). Clinical evaluation of a 10% intravenous fat emulsion for parenteral nutrition in thermally injured patients. *Ann. Surg.*, **178**, 503

39. Sundstrom, G., Zaunner, C. W. and Arborelius, M. (1973). Decrease in pulmonary diffusing capacity during lipid infusion in healthy man. *J. Appl. Physiol.*, **34**, 816

40. Greene, H. L., Hazlett, D. and Demaree, R. (1976). Relationship between Intralipid induced hyperlipaemia and pulmonary function. *Am. J. Clin. Nutr.*, **29**, 127

41. Press, M., Hartop, P. J. and Prottey, C. (1974). Correction of essential fatty acid deficiency in man by the cutaneous application of sunflower seed oil. *Lancet*, **1**, 597

42. Smith, R., Fuller, D. J., Wedge, J. A., Williamson, D. H. and Alberti, K. G. M. M. (1975). Initial effect of injury on ketone bodies and other blood metabolites. *Lancet*, **1**, 1

43. Rich, A. J. and Whitehouse, M. E. (1979). The relevance of pre-operative nutritional assessment. In Johnston, I. D. A. and Lee, H. A. (eds.). *Developments in Clinical Nutrition. Res. Clin. Forums*, **1**, 83

44. Woolfson, A. M. J. (1979). Metabolic considerations in nutritional support. In Johnston, I. D. A. and Lee, H. A. (eds.). *Developments in Clinical Nutrition. Res. Clin. Forums*, **1**, 35

45. Tweedle, D. E. E., Spivey, J. and Johnston, I. D. A. (1972). The effect of four different amino acid solutions upon nitrogen balance of post-operative patients. In Wilkinson, A. W. (ed.). *Parenteral Nutrition*. pp. 247–254. (Edinburgh & London: Churchill Livingstone)

46. Tweedle, D. E. F., Spivey, J. and Johnston, I. D. A. (1973). Choice of intravenous amino acid solutions for use after surgical operation. *Metabolism*, **22**, 173

47. Buse, M. G. and Reid, S. S. (1975). Leucine: a possible regulator of protein turnover in muscle. *J. Clin. Invest.*, **56**, 1250

48. Aguirre, A., Funovics, J., Wesdorp, R. I. C. and Fischer, J. E. (1976). Parenteral nutrition in hepatic failure. In Fischer, J. E. (ed.). *Total Parenteral Nutrition*. pp. 219–230. (Boston: Little, Brown & Company)

49. Soetors, P. B. (1977). Parenteral nutrition in hepatic failure. In Greep, J. M.,

Soetors, P. B., Wesdorp, R. I. C., Phaf, C. W. R. and Fischer, J. E. (eds.). *Current Concepts in Parenteral Nutrition*. pp. 159-170. (The Hague: Martinus Nijhoff Medical Division)

50. Johnston, I. D. A., Tweedle, D. E. F. and Spivey, J. (1972). Intravenous feeding after surgical operation. In Wilkinson, A. W. (ed.). *Parenteral Nutrition*. pp. 189-197. (Edinburgh & London: Churchill Livingstone)

51. Jackson, M. A., Joshi, J., Talbot S. and Lee, H. A. (1979). Evaluation of a high nitrogen source amino acid solution (Aminofusin L'Forte). *Curr. Med. Res. Opin.*, **6**, 274

52. Shenkin, A. and Wretlind, A. (1978). Parenteral Nutrition. *World Rev. Nutr. Diet.*, **28**, 1

53. Kay, R. G., Tasman-Jones, C., Pybus, J., Whiting, R. and Black, H. (1976). A syndrome of acute zinc deficiency during total parenteral nutrition in man. *Ann. Surg.*, **183**, 331

54. Fleming, C. R., Hodges, R. E. and Hurley, L. S. (1976). A prospective study of serum, copper and zinc levels in patients receiving total parenteral nutrition. *Am. J. Clin. Nutr.*, **29**, 70

55. Meng. H. C. (1976). Fat emulsions in parenteral nutrition. In Fischer, J. E. (ed.). *Total Parenteral Nutrition*, pp. 305-334. (Boston: Little, Brown & Company)

56. Fischer, J. E., Funovics, J. M., Aguirre, A., James, J. H., Keane, J. M., Wesdorp, R. I. C., Yoshimura, N. and Westman, T. (1975). The role of plasma amino acids in hepatic encephalopathy. *Surgery*, **78**, 276

57. Lawson, L. J. (1965). Parenteral nutrition in surgery. *Br. J. Surg.*, **52**, 795

58. Zumtobel, V. and Zehle, A. (1972). Post-operative parentale Ernahrung mit Fettemulsiomen bei Patienten mit Leberschaden. *Arch. Klin. Chir. Suppl. Chir. Forum,* **1**, 179

59. Michel, H., Raynaud, A., Crastes de Paulet, P., Nalet, B., Orsetti, A. and Bertrand, L. (1976). Tolerance du cirrhotique aux lipids intraveineux. In Romieu, Solassol, Joyeux et Astric (eds.). *Comptes rendus du Congres. Int. de Nutrition Parenterale*. pp. 131-137. (Montpellier: Dehan)

60. Abel, R. M., Beck, C. H., Abbott, W. M., Ryan, J. A., Barnett, G. O. and Fischer, J. E. (1973). Improved survival from acute renal failure after treatment with intravenous essential L-amino acids and glucose: results of a prospective, double blind study. *N. Engl. J. Med.*, **288**, 695

61. Abel, R. M. (1976). Parenteral nutrition in the treatment of renal failure. In Fischer, J. E. (ed.). *Total Parenteral Nutrition*. pp. 143-70. (Boston: Little, Brown & Company)

62. Lee, H. A., (1977). The application of parenteral nutrition to renal failure patients. In Greep, J. M., Soetors, P. B., Wesdorp, R. I. C., Phaf, C. W. R. and Fischer, J. E. (eds.). *Current Concepts in Parenteral Nutrition*. pp. 217-226. (The Hague: Martinus Nijhoff Medical Division)

63. Lee, H. A. and Jackson, M. A. (1978). Parenteral nutrition in acute renal failure. *Infusionstherapie - Parenterale Ernahrung*, **1**, 153

64. Lee, H. A. (1976). The role of intravenous nutrition in the management of acute renal failure. *S. A. Med. J.*, **50**, 1703

65. Rainsford, D. J. (1977). Immediate care of acute renal failure. *Anaesthesia*, **32**, 277

66. Lee, H. A. (1980). The management of acute renal failure. In Chapman, A. (ed.) *Acute Renal Failure*. Ch. 6 (Edinburgh: Churchill Livingstone)
67. Copeland, E. M., MacFayden, B. V., and Dudrick, S. J. (1974). Intravenous hyperalimentation in cancer patients. *J. Surg. Res.*, **16**, 241
68. Copeland, E. M., MacFayden, B. V., Lanzotti, V. J. and Dudrick, S. J. (1975). Intravenous hyperalimentation as an adjunct to cancer chemotherapy. *Am. J. Surg.*, **129**, 167
69. Shils, M. E. (1975). A program for total parenteral nutrition at home. *Am. J. Clin. Nutr.*, **28**, 1429
70. Johnston, I. D. A. and Lee, H. A. (eds.). (1979). *Developments in Clinical Nutrition. Res. Clin. Forums,* **1**

2
Immunology

BOB PARKES

Recent years have seen a vast improvement in the care of critically ill patients. Aggressive initial resuscitation, early and appropriate surgical intervention and the availability of support systems have all contributed to an improvement in early survival. However, many patients ultimately succumb to overwhelming infection, despite the use of 'appropriate' antibiotics. This chapter will review aspects of clinical immunology relevant to a general ICU, particularly in regard to immunodeficiency syndromes and their impact on host defences.

(I) NON-SPECIFIC DEFENCE MECHANISMS

Before discussing cellular immunity, it is pertinent to review non-specific mechanical defence mechanisms and the way that these are breached in critically ill patients.

(a) Respiratory tract

IPPV is associated with a significant risk of pulmonary infection. The use of sedatives and relaxants causes depression or abolition of the cough reflex; furthermore, cilio-toxicity may result from tracheal intubation, repeated tracheal suction, or the use of high concentrations of inspired oxygen[1]. It is not surprising, therefore, that bacterial colonization of the respiratory tract, both with normal respiratory flora and enteric gram-negative organisms, occurs frequently. In addition, cellular clearance mechanisms are impaired. Alveolar macrophage activity is known to be compromised in a number of conditions, including persistent acidosis and shock, renal failure, pulmonary oedema, a high inspired oxygen concentration and excessive glucocorticoid activity[1].

(b) Gastrointestinal tract

The ability of the gastrointestinal tract to provide an adequate defence against infection depends not only on mucosal integrity but also on the presence of normal bacterial flora. Colitis has been shown to be associated with the overgrowth of *Clostridium difficile*, following the use of broad spectrum antibiotics, particularly lincomycin and clindamycin[2]. Permeability of the gastrointestinal mucosa may be altered in situations where the microcirculation is compromised, as in persistent shock or disseminated intravascular coagulation. Consequently, gram-negative bacteraemia or endotoxaemia is more likely to occur. This is compounded by depression of the reticuloendothelial system (RES) in a variety of clinical situations, and by shunting of blood away from the RES which may occur in portal hypertension from any cause.

(c) Genitourinary tract

Mechanical barriers to infection in the genitourinary tract are principally effected by the presence of a normal mucosa and the presence of an adequate urinary flow. Trauma to the urinary tract, as a result of infection or injury, may provide a portal of entry for bacteria. The association between the presence of an indwelling urinary catheter and infection is well established, but there is also evidence that oliguria may predispose to infection, particularly if an indwelling catheter is left *in situ* for a prolonged period of time[1].

(d) Integument

Breaching the integrity of the skin occurs not only in therapeutic situations, but also in trauma. The presence of a foreign body is particularly important in the pathogenesis of skin-related bacteraemia. Evidence to date suggests that skin flora are the major organisms cultured in cases of catheter-associated bacteraemia[3]. Bacteraemia may also result from illicit narcotic use. Finally, normal flora may be protective. Prolonged use of broad spectrum antibiotics has been associated with the emergence of mucocutaneous candidiasis.

(e) Reticuloendothelial system

The clearance of particulate matter of either host or foreign origin, is effected via the RES. Phagocytosis by reticuloendothelial cells does not occur in isolation; enhancement occurs with the aid of an α_2-globulin termed 'opsonic material'. Depression of the RES can occur acutely in a wide variety of clinical situations. These include shock, major trauma, operations, burns and the administration of large amounts of colloid[5]. RE depression appears, at least in part, to be related to depletion of opsonic material. A lowering of opsonic activity occurs soon after massive injury[5], and has been shown to correlate with an increased susceptibility to sepsis, both in human[5] and animal studies[6]. RES depression has significance when one considers the pathogenesis of gram-negative bacteraemia. Organisms isolated from patients with gram-negative bacteraemia are commonly enteric organisms. Traditionally, cross-infection has been invoked to explain this phenomenon, but it is likely that the portal of entry is via a compromised gastrointestinal mucosa, and this, coupled with depression of the RES, exposes the patient to a significant episode of bacteraemia or toxaemia. To date, opsonic material has not been available in sufficient quantity or purity to study the therapeutic benefits of artificial elevation of opsonic activity, and it remains to be seen whether reversal of this isolated defect could confer any significant benefit.

(II) DISORDERS OF CELLULAR AND HUMORAL IMMUNITY

A high incidence of anergic states has been found in infectious diseases, chronic inflammatory disorders and malignancy (Table 2.1). These are reviewed in major texts and will not be described in depth here. However, in recent years, a variety of immunodeficiency states have been described in patients suffering from major trauma, burns and in association with surgery. These may be classified into 'active' immunosuppression and 'passive' immunodepression. 'Active' suppression has been shown to occur within hours of an acute illness; its appearance correlates with the appearance of naturally occurring anti-inflammatory substances and disappears as the primary disease resolves. 'Passive' immunodeficiency occurs more as a result of therapy or nutritional deficiency. In many situations deficiency states correlate closely with morbidity and mortality of infection, and may, in some instances, be prevented or reversed by a rational approach to therapy.

Table 2.1 Acquired immunodeficiency

Conditions predominantly affecting cell mediated immunity
  Age
  Metabolic disorders
    Diabetes mellitus
    Dystrophica myotonica
    Hypothyroidism
    Renal failure
    Malnutrition
    Vitamin deficiencies (vitamin C)
                          (vitamin B_{12})
  Chronic inflammatory diseases
    Primary biliary cirrhosis
    Rheumatoid arthritis
    Sjögren's syndrome
  Granulomatous disorders
    Crohn's disease
    Whipple's disease
    Wegener's granulomatosis
    Sarcoid
  Malignant diseases
    Carcinomata
    Hodgkin's disease
    Lymphomata
  Infections
    E.-B. virus
    Measles
    Tuberculosis
    Leprosy
    Syphilis
    Viral hepatitis
  Pregnancy
  Trauma

Conditions predominantly affecting humoral immunity
  Metabolic disorders
    Malnutrition
    Nephrotic syndrome
  Malignant diseases
    Chronic lymphocytic leukaemia
    Multiple myeloma
    Hodgkin's disease
  Infections
    Malaria
    Trypanosomiasis

---

(1) Assessment of immune competence

A vast array of investigations of immune competence have been developed in recent years. However, most of these are unavailable outside specialized centres. In the study of acquired immunodeficiency in critically ill patients, cell mediated immunity (CMI) has been studied extensively due to ease of testing and the high degree of correlation between anergy and morbidity. CMI may be examined *in vivo* by skin testing. The afferent limb may be tested by exposing the patient to two doses, separated by 7–14 days, of dichloronitrobenzene (DCNB). Following the second exposure, localized erythema should occur within 24–48 hours. Efferent limb function may be studied by the intradermal injection of antigenic substances known to be processed via cell mediated immunity. Antigens commonly used are tuberculin (PPD), candida, streptokinase–streptodornase, mumps and trichophyton. Following intradermal injection of these antigens and a control solution, the sites are read at 24 and 48 hours. A positive result should show induration and erythema of greater than 10 mm diameter. It is important to note and exclude positive results at 6–18 hours, as responses occurring during this time are due to the Arthus phenomenon, a reaction mediated via humoral immunity. Delayed skin graft rejection is an unreliable test of CMI.

In vitro studies of CMI include quantitation of T-cell numbers, the ability of a purified preparation of T cells to proliferate in response to mitogens such as phytohaemagglutinin A (PHA) and pokeweed mitogen (PWM) and by allogenic lymphocytes (mixed lymphocyte culture, or MLC).

Humoral immunity, or B-cell function, may be assessed by quantifying the B cells, measurement of immunoglobulins, assessment of circulating antibodies to previously acquired antigens such as *Esch. coli*, and by assessing antibody response to a particular antigen. Flagella antigen from *Salmonella adelaide* (Flagellin) is most commonly used in this test. Secretory immunoglobulin activity, notably IgA, is relatively difficult to assay accurately, but techniques are available.

Neutrophil function is assessed on a qualitative rather than quantitative basis, as depression of absolute numbers of neutrophils is a relatively rare cause of neutrophil deficiency. Chemotactic activity in response to a given stimulus and phagocytic ability, and ability of neutrophils to kill ingested bacteria (neutrophil bactericidal index, or NBI) are the most commonly performed investigations.

(2) 'Active' immunosuppression

The presence of immunodeficiency in association with acute illness has been established for many years. Alexander[7] demonstrated an exaggeration in the normal cyclic variation in neutrophil function and showed an overall decrease in qualitative function compared with normal controls. Low levels of neutrophil activity were shown to correlate with the appearance of infection. As a significant depression occurred within 48 hours of injury, the presence of naturally occurring anti-inflammatory substances was sought. Later work by van Epps[8] demonstrated the presence of a β-globulin which appeared early in the course of an acute illness, and which was capable of inhibiting the function of normal neutrophils *in vitro*.

Active suppression of CMI is also known to occur. Early observers noted a prolonged survival of skin allografts in burned mice compared to controls, irrespective of histocompatibility antigen matching[9]. More recent and comprehensive evidence has been provided by Nineman[10]. He noted a significant depression of CMI in burned patients, the degree of which correlated with the severity of injury. Furthermore, an IgG appeared within 24–48 hours of injury, which was capable of suppressing PHA induced blastogenesis of normal T cells *in vitro*. On recovery, a second IgG appeared which was capable of reversing this depression. The authors postulated that active suppression of immunity occurred early in the course of injury; recovery was associated with the appearance of an IgG blocking antibody capable of restoring normal function.

Reference has been made to depression of non-specific opsonic activity in major trauma. Evidence also exists that active suppression of complement metabolism and activity occurs. Within 24 hours of a severe thermal injury, absolute depression of all components of complement is known to occur. This is thought to be consistent with protein loss through a wound. However, there is a parallel decrease in conversion of C_3 to C_{3a} which is not corrected by the addition of large amounts of normal serum[11], thus suggesting the presence of an inhibitor. To date, the nature of such an inhibitor has not been elucidated. More specific data exists regarding complement activity. The presence of an inhibitor of complement-augmented chemotaxis (chemotactic factor inhibitor or CFI) has been known for some time. The heterogenicity of CFI has recently been established. One fraction, a β-globulin, is directed predominantly against C_{3a}; the other, an α-globulin, has activity against C_{5a}. Both these substances appear within 24–48 hours of injury and are capable of blocking the opsonic and chemotactic activity of complement, with consequent indirect effects on neutrophil function.

The disorders described above do not occur in isolation. Numerous reports[8,10,11] have established the association between anergy, qualitative neutrophil dysfunction and disorders of complement activity and metabolism. However, it is difficult to establish their significance. Many reports demonstrating the presence of 'active' immunosuppression have noted an increased incidence of infection, but it is not known whether infection is the cause or result of immunodeficiency. It is tempting to speculate that 'active' immunosuppression is protective. At the time of injury, a vast quantity and variety of potentially antigenic material is released into the circulation. Should a failure of 'self-recognition' occur, it is possible for an autoimmune disease to develop at a later date. The presence of naturally occurring anti-inflammatory substances might prevent such a phenomenon; in addition, they might moderate the inflammatory response to shock, thereby maintaining intravascular volume at an optimum level. To date, little or no data exist on the effects of artificial stimulation of the immune response. Levamisole and transfer factor[13] have been shown to be capable of reversing anergy in a wide variety of clinical conditions. Experimental data are awaited to determine whether active immunosuppression can be reversed, and whether this will affect morbidity or mortality.

(3) 'Passive' immunodeficiency

In addition to 'active' immunosuppression, deficiency states are known to occur in circumstances which are unrelated to the host response to injury. With advancing age, a decline in activity of T-cell and T-suppressor cell function is known to exist[14,15] as well as an increase in autoantibody levels. Furthermore, anergic states in the elderly have been shown to be associated with significant increase in mortality, even in the absence of coexistent disease. However, immunodeficiency states may be induced in previously normal patients by therapy, or nutritional deficiency. These disorders have been closely linked with survival, and have significant therapeutic implications.

Protein calorie malnutrition (PCM)

Deficiencies in both affector and effector limbs of the immune response in PCM are well documented, both in the presence and absence of intercurrent illness. In malnourished children, studies have demonstrated abnormalities in T-cell function *in vivo* and *in vitro*[16-18]. Reduction in absolute levels of complement[19], and in immunoglobulin synthesis[20] have also been demonstrated both *in vivo* and *in vitro* defects in cell mediated immunity, and a reduced antibody response to 'Flagellin' in malnourished patients. Refeeding reversed these abnormalities.

The concept of PCM causing immunodeficiency is of more than theoretical interest. A significant association between anergy and morbidity and mortality due to infection has been demonstrated in trauma[22,23], malignant disease[24-26] and major surgery[24,27]. Furthermore, nutritional deficiency appears to correlate not only with defects in CMI, but with abnormalities of neutrophil function and immunoglobulin synthesis[28,23]. Skin testing appears

37

to provide a good guide to prognosis[27]. Patients who improve from an anergic state, or those who retain normal reactivity throughout the course of an illness, do better than anergic patients or patients whose immunological state declines[27]. Since the discovery of chronic granulomatous disease of childhood[29] techniques for evaluating neutrophil function have improved, and extensive work has been carried out on neutrophil function in critically ill patients. Two major facts emerge. Firstly, in PCM, there is a significant correlation between disorders of CMI and impairment of neutrophil chemotaxis; secondly, exaggeration of the normal cyclic variation in neutrophil function occurs in PCM, and depression of neutrophil function has been shown to correlate with the onset of bacteraemia[30].

Relatively little data are available concerning humoral immunity in PCM. Studies performed on children with kwashiorkor tend to be conflicting, but there is evidence that refeeding improves humoral immunity[20]. In a recent review of experimental data in animals, Law[31] suggested that PCM involves the primary rather than anamnestic immunoglobulin response, although both are affected. Depression of humoral immunity in PCM has a number of implications. If one considers the spectrum of bacteraemia seen in a general ICU, the pathogens commonly isolated are enteric gram-negative organisms, such as *Pseudomonas* and *Klebsiella* spp. Although these organisms exist in the normal gastrointestinal tract, bacteraemia is uncommon in the normal host, where defence is effected via gastrointestinal mucosal integrity, secretory IgA and the integrity of the reticuloendothelial system (RES). If one considers the compromised host, an immunological basis for gram-negative bacteraemia can be postulated. The combination of increased mucosal permeability and depression of the RES would be expected to predispose the patient to gram-negative bacteraemia. If the organism responsible has not previously appeared in the bloodstream, a primary IgG or IgM response would therefore be necessary for the formation of antibody–antigen-complement complexes to enable phagocytosis by neutrophils (IgA does not fix complement in appreciable quantities[32]). When one considers the spectrum of immunodeficiency described above, it is hardly surprising that gram-negative bacteraemia is so common. One might also postulate that elevation of IgG or IgM levels by active or passive immunization would cover the incidence of bacteraemia. In fact both *Pseudomonas* vaccine and hyperimmune globulin have been shown to reduce the incidence of *Pseudomonas* bacteraemia in burned patients[33].

Phosphate deficiency

Phosphate deficiency may occur in a variety of clinical situations. Deprivation of phosphate may occur in malnutrition, and malabsorption occurs during concurrent administration of aluminium based antacids. Excessive urinary excretion may occur after burns and major trauma, in diabetes mellitus, alcoholism and magnesium depletion. Phosphate depletion and hypophosphataemia develop within one or two days in the surgical or trauma patient admitted to the ICU unless inorganic phosphate is given.

Furthermore, inadequate phosphate repletion after malnutrition in malnourished patients has been linked to the 'refeeding' syndrome of sudden death seen in prisoners of war after the Second World War[34]. Impairment of neutrophil function is known to occur in phosphate deficiency. Phagocytic, chemotactic and bactericidal activity are impaired, and have been linked to both impairment of ATP synthesis [35] and to inadequate synthesis of organic phosphoinisotides[34].

Zinc deficiency

In patients undergoing parenteral nutrition, deficiency of trace elements may become clinically apparent. Zinc deficiency could develop in the intensive care patient on intravenous nutrition. The findings are dermatitis, diarrhoea, alopecia, a low serum zinc and a low alkaline phosphatase[36]. Zinc deficiency has also shown to be associated with defects in CMI, in both *in vivo* and *in vitro* studies, which are reversible with replenishment[37].

Vitamin deficiency

There is considerable difficulty in separating the effects of vitamin deficiency from other aspects of malnutrition. However, indirect evidence does exist implicating vitamin deficiencies in states of acquired immunodeficiency. Early reports drew attention to an increased incidence of infections in children suffering from scurvy and avitaminosis A. Selective deficiency of thiamine, biotin, nicotinic acid and pyridoxine have been shown to correlate with abnormalities of humoral immunity and neutrophil function.

Folic acid is incorporated into actively dividing cells, and deficiency is associated with megaloblastic marrow arrest and pancytopenia. Blackwell[38] reported three cases of acute megaloblastic arrest in patients receiving trimethoprim; all cases were associated with pancytopenia and gram-negative bacteraemia. Folic acid deficiency may be relative or absolute. Inadequate dietary intake is common, but relative deficiency may occur when intake is not increased to meet an increased metabolic demand, e.g. in pregnancy and hypercatabolic states. Acute folate deficiency develops in a few days in the surgical or trauma patient admitted to the ICU but is readily preventable.

39

Malabsorption of dietary folic acid is associated with alcoholism, the administration of anticonvulsants, metformin, colchicine and oral contraceptives. Antagonism occurs during administration of methotrexate, pentamidine, trimethoprim, pyrimethamine and triamterine. Folic acid losses are markedly increased by dialysis.

Therapeutic implications

If one examines data concerning malnutrition, immunity and morbidity, one does find a significant correlation between all three. However, it is necessary to examine certain aspects before accepting a cause and effect relationship. Because of the relative ease of skin testing, the anergic state has been most widely studied. Significant associations between anergy, malnutrition and infection do exist. It is important to remember, however, that the infections associated with anergy tend to be bacterial, particularly by gram-negative organisms. How then, does one invoke a defect in CMI to explain bacterial infection, particularly when the defence mechanism against these organisms is traditionally thought to be effected by humoral defence mechanisms? There are a number of possible answers. Firstly, there is evidence that T and B-cell populations do not operate in isolation. A subgroup of T cells are capable of stimulating or suppressing B-cell function. These are known as 'helper' and 'suppressor' cells respectively. It is possible that PCM affects the helper cell population, with subsequent suppression of humoral immunity. Secondly, as mentioned above, PCM affects not only T-cell function, but neutrophil activity, levels of complement and B-cell function. Therefore, it is reasonable to regard anergy as an easily estimated subgroup of a wider spectrum of disorders, just as liver function tests are used to follow the course of a patient with hepatitis, rather than relying on serial liver biopsies.

Does refeeding improve prognosis? This is a difficult question to answer. Because of the wide variation in the primary disease processes of patients studied, and because of wide differences in therapy, it is difficult to assess the effects of nutrition alone. However, in children suffering from PCM without intercurrent illness, adequate nutrition will restore normal immune function. Data on adults are less conclusive. However, in a recent study of patients with inoperable oesophageal carcinoma, restoration of delayed hypersensitivity was achieved using intravenous nutrition as the only form of therapy[40]. Other authors have demonstrated restoration of defects in humoral immunity and CMI in patients suffering from burns and severe trauma[25,33]. In both series, improvement correlated positively with survival. On the basis of currently available data, it is justifiable to recommend an aggressive approach to nutritional therapy.

(4) Iatrogenic immunodeficiency

(a) Drug-induced immunodeficiency

The spectrum of immunodeficiency syndromes associated with the use of glucocorticoids and antineoplastic drugs is well-reviewed in major texts and will not be discussed here. Suffice to say that the effects of these agents should be borne in mind. However, a great variety of agents used in routine clinical practice are associated with immunodepression. These will be reviewed in more detail.

(b) Antibacterial agents

Numerous chemotherapeutic agents can alter host immunocompetence. Raeburn[41] pointed out that chloramphenicol was capable of depressing humoral immunity. More recent work has demonstrated a depressant effect of topical sulphonamides (silver sulphadiazine, sodium sulphadiazine and sulphamylon) on humoral immunity[42]. PHA induced blastogenesis has been shown to be depressed by sulphonamides, tetracyclines and chloramphenicol[43]. However, in the above series, no depression was noted with gentamicin, penicillin, carbenicillin, clindamycin or cephalosporins. It should be noted that the agents capable of consistently affecting immune function are bacteriostatic rather than bactericidal. Organisms exposed to bacteriostatic agents are inhibited from multiplying rather than killed outright; processing of these organisms is still required by phagocytic cells. Consequently if one uses a bacteriostatic agent in severe infection, the depressant effect may be of significance. Furthermore if the choice of agent is inappropriate, the combination of an ineffective agent and drug-induced immunodeficiency may combine to do the patient more harm than good.

(c) Anaesthesia, operation, transfusion and radiation

In a general ICU, post-operative patients comprise a considerable proportion of referrals. It is therefore pertinent to discuss the effects of operation on immunity. Perhaps the most specific example associated with operative intervention is the post-splenectomy syndrome[44]. Its occurrence is difficult to predict: cases have been recorded as long as 25 years following splenectomy. In a classical case, the patient undergoes an acute deterioration. Fever, profound shock and non-specific gastrointestinal manifestations are the cardinal features. Disseminated intravascular coagulation can occur. In over 50% of cases *Str. pneumoniae* is the causative organism, but the syndrome has been associated with *N. meningitidis, E. coli, H.*

41

influenzae and *Staph. aureus*. Both long-term prophylactic penicillin and pneumococcal vaccine have successfully reduced the incidence of the syndrome, but problems with patient compliance and the availability of pneumococcal vaccine have limited their usefulness. In the established case, high dose antibiotic therapy is life-saving.

Operative intervention *per se* is capable of depressing normal immunity. Disorders of cell mediated immunity have been demonstrated during donor nephrectomy in normal patients[45] and in association with surgery for malignant disease[46]. This phenomenon is, in part, related to anaesthetic agents. Fluothane has been shown to inhibit PHA induced blastogenesis, probably due to an effect on DNA synthetase[47]. Similar results have been found with nitrous oxide and barbiturates[48] but not with ketamine[49]. The vast majority of patients undergo elective surgery without any untoward risk of infection. However, in the compromised host, anaesthetic-associated immunosuppression may assume importance. In patients undergoing surgery for malignant disease and for other non-malignant conditions, the incidence of anergy has been shown to correlate with the duration of anaesthesia and the degree of blood loss. Again, anergy correlated closely with the incidence of infection.

Interestingly, blood transfusion appears to be protective. Anaesthetic-associated immunodepression can be prevented and reversed by blood transfusion[50-52]. The mechanism is probably related to non-specific stimulation by platelet and leukocyte antigens[53].

Artificial cooling in febrile states is widely practised. However, this may be harmful. Animal experiments demonstrate an increased survival from infection in the presence of pyrexia. Leukocyte proliferation and migration have been shown to be optimal at a temperature of 38.5–39 °C. In the light of these data, the rationale for artificial cooling in states of moderate pyrexia must be questioned. Furthermore, an additional reason is provided for maintaining a normal core temperature during anaesthesia.

CONCLUSION

Immunodeficiency states have been described in a wide variety of clinical situations. However, before accepting or dismissing such data and their implied clinical applications, it is necessary to consider the problem as a whole. Perhaps the most important factor is overall host competence. Countless numbers of patients undergo general anaesthesia, receive courses of antibiotics, cytotoxic drugs and corticosteroids and suffer no infectious complications. Equally large numbers of patients are rendered anergic by a variety of infectious and inflammatory disorders (Table 2.1). Again, recovery is the rule rather than the exception. However, patients admitted to an ICU suffer not one insult, but many. Immunocompetence is altered by a combination of drug therapy, operation, nutrition, and as part of the host response to injury. A logical hypothesis is that there exists a critical degree of immunodepression, beyond which infection becomes more likely. A patient may be rendered anergic by a single insult and recover, but should this be combined with a more severe insult, such as protein-calorie malnutrition, additive effects occur with a consequent increase in mortality. The problems await solution.

References

1. La Force, F. M. and Eickhoff, T. C. (1977). The role of infection in critical care. *Anaesthesiology*, **47**, 195
2. Larson, H. E., Price, A. B. and Honour P. (1978). *Clostridium difficile* and the aetiology of pseudomembranous colitis. *Lancet*, **1**, 1063
3. Maki, D. G., Goldman, D. A. and Rhame, F. S. (1973). Infection control in intravenous therapy. *Ann. Intern. Med.*, **79**, 867
4. Bjornsen, A. B. and Alexander, J. W. (1973). Opsonic activity of sera from patients after thermal injury. *Surg. Forum*, **24**, 44
5. Scovill, W. A., Saba, T. M., Kaplan, J. B., Bernard, H. and Powers, S. (1976). Deficit in reticuloendothelial humoral control in patients after trauma. *J. Trauma,* **16**, 898
6. Zweifach, B. W., Benacerraf, B. and Thomas L. (1957). The relationship between the vascular manifestations of shock produced by endotoxin, trauma and haemorrhage. II. The possible role of the reticuloendothelial system in resistance to each type of shock. *J. Exp. Med.*, **106**, 403
7. Alexander, J. W. and Wixson, D. (1970). Neutrophil dysfunction and sepsis in burn injury. *Surg., Gynecol. Obstet.*, **130**, 432
8. Van Epps, D. E., Palmer, D. L. and Williams, R. C. (1974). Characterisation of serum inhibitors of neutrophil chemotaxis associated with anergy. *J. Immunol.*, **113**, 189
9. Chambler, K. and Batchelor, J. R. (1969). Influence of defined incompatabilities and area of burn on skin – homograft survival in burned subjects. *Lancet*, **1**, 16
10. Nineman, J. L., Fisher, J. C. and Watchel, T. C. (1979). Thermal injury – associated immunosuppression: occurrence and *in vitro* blocking effect of post recovery serum. *J. Immunol.*, **122**, 1736
11. Bjornsen, A. B., Altemeier, M. A. and Bjornsen, H. S. (1976). Reduction in C3 conversion in patients with severe thermal injury. *J. Trauma*, **16**, 905
12. Till, G. and Ward, P. A. (1975). Two distinct chemotactic factor inactivators in human serum. *J. Immunol.* **114**, 843
13. Tripoldi, D., Parks, L. C. and Brugmans, J. (1973). Drugs induced restoration of cutaneous delayed hypersensitivity in patients with cancer. *N. Engl. J. Med.*, **289**, 354
14. Roberts-Thomson, I. C., Whittingham, S., Youngchaiyud, U. and Mackay,

I. R. (1974). Ageing, immune response and mortality. *Lancet*, **2**, 368

15. Kishimoto, S., Tomino, S, Mitsuya, H. and Pjuiwara, H. (1979). Age related changes in suppressor functions of human T-cells. *J. Immunol.*, **123**, 1586

16. Chandra, R. K. (1974). Rossette forming T-lymphocytes and cell-mediated immunity in malnutrition. *Br. Med. J.*, **3**, 608

17. Edelman, R., Suskind, R. and Olson, R. E. (1973). Mechanisms of defective delayed cutaneous hypersensitivity in children with protein-calorie malnutrition. *Lancet*, **1**, 506

18. Geefhuysen, J., Rosen, E. U., Katz J., Ipp, T. and Metz, J. (1971). Impaired cellular immunity in kwashirokor with improvement after therapy. *Br. Med. J.*, **4**, 527

19. Sirisinha, S., Suskind, R., Edelman, R., Charaupatana, C. and Olson, R. E. (1973). Complement and C3-proactivator levels in children with protein-calorie malnutrition. *Lancet*, **1**, 1016

20. Matthews, J. D., Whittingham, S., Mackay, I. R. and Malcolm, L. A. (1972). Protein supplementation and enhanced antibody-producing capacity in New Guinean school children. *Lancet*, **2**, 675

21. Law, D. K., Dudrick, S. S. and Abdou, N. I. (1973). Immunocompetence of patients with protein–calorie malnutrition: the effects of nutritional repletion. *Ann. Intern. Med.*, **79**, 545

22. Johnson, W. C., Ulrich, F., Meguid, M. M., Lepak, N., Bowe, P., Harris, P., Alberts, L. H. and Nabseth, D. C. (1979). Role of delayed hypersensitivity in predicting postoperative morbidity and mortality. *Am. J. Surg.*, **137**, 536

23. McLean, I. D., Meakins, J. L., Taguchi, K., Duignan, J. P., Dhillon, K. S., and Gordon, J. (1977). Host resistance in sepsis and trauma. *Ann. Surg.*, **180**, 207

24. Eilber, F. R. and Morton, D. L. (1970). Impaired immunologic reactivity and recurrence following cancer surgery. *Cancer*, **25**, 362

25. Copeland, E. M., MacFadyen, B. V. and Dudrick, S. J. (1974). Effect of intravenous hyperalimentation on established delayed hypersensitivity in the cancer patient. *Ann. Surg.*, **184**, 60

26. Ota, D. M., Copeland, E. M., Coriere, J. N. and Dudrick, S. J. (1979). The effects of nutrition and treatment of cancer on host immunocompetence. *Surg. Gynecol. Obstet.*, **148**, 104

27. Meakins, J. L., Pietsch, J. B., Bubenick, O., Kelly, R., Rode, H., Gordon, J. and McLean, L. D. (1977). Delayed hypersensitivity: indicator of acquired failure of host defences in sepsis and trauma. *Ann. Surg.*, **186**, 241

28. Dhillon, K. S., McLean, L. D. and Meakins, J. L. (1975). Neutrophil function in surgical patients. Correlation of neutrophil bactericidal function, serum albumin, and sepsis. *Surg. Forum*, **26**, 27

29. Holmes, B., Quie, P. G., Windhorst, D. B., and Good, R. A. (1966). Fatal granulomatous disease of childhood. An inborn abnormality of phagocytic function. *Lancet*, **1**, 1225

30. Alexander, J. W., and Meakins, J. L. (1972). A physiological basis for the development of opportunistic infections in man. *Ann. Surg.*, **176**, 273

31. Law, D. K., Dudrick, S. J. and Abdou, N. I. (1974). The effects of protein–calorie malnutrition on immune competence of the surgical patient. *Surg. Gynecol. Obstet.*, **139**, 257

32. Holborow, E. J. and Reeves, W. G. (eds.) (1977). *Immunology in Medicine: A Comprehensive Guide to Clinical Immunology.* (London: Academic Press)
33. Alexander, J. W. (1974). Emerging concepts in the control of surgical infections. *Surgery,* **75,** 934
34. Knochel, J. P. (1977). The pathophysiology and clinical characteristics of severe hypophosphataemia. *Arch. Intern. Med.,* **137,** 203
35. Lichtman, M. A. (1974). Hypoalimentation during hyperalimentation. *N. Engl. J. Med.,* **290,** 1432
36. Okada, A., Takagi, Y., Itakura, T., Santani, M., Manabe, H., Iida, Y., Tanigaki, T., Iwasaki, M. and Kasahara, N. (1976). Skin lesions during intravenous hyperalimentation: zinc deficiency. *Surgery,* **80,** 629
37. Golden, M. H. N., Golden, B. E., Harland, P. S. E. G. and Jackson, A. A. (1978). Zinc and immunocompetence in protein–energy malnutrition. *Lancet,* **1,** 1226
38. Blackwell, E. A., Leer, J., Hawson, G. A. T. and Bain, B. (1978). Acute pancytopenia due to megaloblastic arrest in association with co-trimoxazole. *Med. J. Austral.,* **2,** 38
39. Avery, G. S. (1976). *Drug Treatment,* p. 550. Australian Drug Information Service
40. Hafferjee, A. A., Angorn, I. B., Brian, P. P., Duursma, J. and Baker, L. W. (1978). Diminished cellular immunity due to impaired nutrition in oesophageal carcinoma. *Br. J. Surg.,* **65,** 480
41. Raeburn, J. A. (1972). Antibiotics and immunodeficiency. *Lancet,* **2,** 954
42. Warden, G. D., Mason, A. D., Pruitt, B. A. (1975). Suppression of leucocyte chemotaxis *in vitro* by chemotherapeutic agents used in the management of thermal injuries. *Ann. Surg.,* **181,** 363
43. Munster, A. M., Loadholot, C. B., Leary, A. G. and Barnes, M. A. (1977). The effect of antibiotics on cell mediated immunity. *Surgery,* **81,** 692
44. Krivit, W., Giebink, G. S. and Leonard, A. (1979). Overwhelming postsplenectomy infection. *Surg. Clin. N. Am.,* **59,** 223
45. Slade, M. S., Simmons, R. L., Yunis, E. and Greenberg, L. J. (1975). Immunodepression after major surgery in normal patients. *Surgery,* **78,** 363
46. Tarpley, J. L., Twomey, P. C., Catalona, W. J. and Chretien, P. B. (1976). Suppression of cellular immunity by anaesthesia and operation. *J. Surg. Res.,* **22,** 195
47. Bruce, D. L. (1972). Halothane inhibition of phytohaemagglutinin induced transformation of lymphocytes. *Anaesthesiology,* **36,** 201
48. Bruce, D. C. and Wingard, D. W. (1971). Anaesthesia and the immune response. *Anaesthesiology,* **34,** 271
49. Cullen, B. F. and Chretien, P. B. (1973). Ketamine and *in vitro* lymphocyte transformation. *Anaesth. Analg.,* **52,** 518
50. Jubert, A. V., Lee, E. T., Hersh, E. M. and McBride, C. M. (1973). Effects of surgery, anaesthesia and intraoperative blood loss on immunocompetence. *J. Surg. Res.,* **15,** 399
51. Roth, J. A., Golub, G. H., Grimm, B. A., Eilber, R. F. and Morton, D. L. (1976). Effects of operation on immune response in cancer patients: sequential evaluation of *in vitro* lymphocyte function. *Surgery,* **79,** 46
52. Hunt, P. S. and Trotter, S. (1976). Lymphocyte response after surgery and

blood transfusion. *J. Surg. Res.*, **21**, 57

53. Schechtor, G. P., Soehnlen, F. and McFarland, W. (1972). Lymphocyte response to blood transfusion in man. *N. Eng. J. Med.*, **287**, 1169

54. Roberts, N. J. (Jnr), and Sandberg, K. (1979). Hyperthermia and human function. II. Enhanced production of and response to leucocyte migration inhibition factor (LIF). *J. Immunol.*, **122**, 1990

3
Microbial infection

STEPHEN ATHERTON AND DAVID WHITE

Microbial infection is an important problem that frequently harms the intensive care patient. It provides the intensive care team with the most difficult of therapeutic challenges and despite the most devoted and expert management the patient often succumbs after a long illness. The problems fire the emotions of the staff, who all too often witness the tragic death of a patient who might otherwise have been expected to recover. A detailed understanding of the infection problem is therefore essential to any discussion of current therapy in intensive care.

Infection usually arises as a complication of the primary disease in a critically ill patient. This is seen following surgery, multiple trauma, burns or acute renal failure. The survival of the patient depends on many factors: the underlying disease, the severity of the infection, the skills of the nurses and doctors and the methods of therapy available. Assuming that the primary disease is curable, the treatment is correct and the skills of the staff are appropriate, then the severity of the microbial infection and the host response are the factors which determine survival. When microbial infection kills the patient it does so because of the development of multiple organ failure[1]. All types of micro-organisms may be implicated: viruses, as in influenzal pneumonia, encephalitis and hepatitis, bacteria, both gram-positive and gram-negative, and fungi. The commonest micro-organism causing disease in the ICU is the gram-negative bacillus. A list of the common gram-negative pathogens is shown in Table 3.1. These organisms are known as opportunistic pathogens, that is they are normally innocuous comensals or contaminants but have become able to multiply in tissues and cause disease[2]. There are several reasons why these organisms of low virulence become invasive and cause serious illness. The immune response is severely impaired in the traumatized patient (Chapter 2). Several procedures are carried out in the critically ill which repeatedly breach the mucous membranes and increase the likelihood of local infection[3]. Recognition of infecton can be difficult, since many of the classical features of infection, fever and leukocytosis, can also occur in the metabolic response to injury[4]. The treatment is often difficult because gram-negative bacteria are often resistent to antimicrobial agents. Finally, tissue damage by bacteria may occur without bacteraemia or an obvious focus of infection[5].

Table 3.1 Gram-negative bacilli encountered in the ICU

Enterobacteria	*E. coli*
	Klebsiella spp.
	Proteus spp.
	Enterobacter spp.
	Citrobacter spp.
	Seratia spp.
Pseudomonas	*Ps. aeruginosa*
Parvobacteria	*H. influenzae*
Bacteroides	*B. fragilis*

This chapter is devoted to the problem of opportunist infections, mainly gram-negative, that are seen in the ICU. It is based on 8 years experience gained in a general ICU which cares for 400 patients a year. Of these about 50 are infected with opportunist pathogens and a further 100 patients are considered to be at risk from developing infection. The information is divided into two parts, the pathophysiology of gram-negative infection and, secondly, the management.

(I) PATHOPHYSIOLOGY

(1) Source of gram-negative bacilli

The natural habitat of many gram-negative bacilli is the human gastrointestinal tract. Millions of bacteria live and multiply in the large bowel and terminal ilium but are rarely found in the proximal small bowel or stomach[6]. These colonic organisms include *Pseudomonads*, coliforms, *Proteus* spp., *Klebsiella* spp., *Enterobacter, Bacteroides* spp., *Clostridia* and anaerobic streptococci. The gram-negative bacteria that may colonize and subsequently infect the high risk patient may be classified as, cross-infection, exogenous and endogenous.

Cross-infection

Cross-infection is the transfer of a micro-organism from one human to another. This source may be another patient, a member of staff or a visitor[7,8]. In the early days of intensive care, when detailed bacteriological monitoring was not undertaken and prophylactic broad spectrum anti-biotics were the rule, cross-infection was thought to be very common. In the last decade increasing awareness of the problem, together with more rigorous measures to reduce cross-infection, has greatly reduced this as a mode of colonization. In this unit there has been no documented cross-infection for the last 2 years.

Exogenous infection

Environmental sources of infection have been well-described, the list

Table 3.2 Environmental sources of infection

Cross-infection	patients
	staff
Equipment	ventilators
	suction apparatus
	catheters
	infusion sets
	electrical thermometers
	cooling mattress
Bed, mattress and linen	
Sinks, taps and overflows	
Intravenous solutions and drugs	
Nasogastric feed	
Antiseptic solutions	
Lubricating jelly	

seemingly endless (Table 3.2). The source may be from the fixtures and fittings of the immediate environment or the equipment used to treat the patient[8,9]. The source of exogenous infection is often difficult to determine and may be impossible. An example serves to illustrate this point. In the early 1970s a severe outbreak of *Pseudomonas* infection occurred at St Thomas's Hospital, London. After many months of detailed investigation the source of the *Pseudomonas* was traced to the water sprayed on to the bottles that had been prepared in the hospital sterilization plant. On leaving the plant the screw capped bottles were hot and had been sprayed with water to cool them rapidly. This cooling water had carried the *Pseudomonas* and subsequently infected many of the patients. As a result of this outbreak the Department of Health and Social Security made recommendations regarding the preparation and sterilization of intravenous fluids within the hospital pharmacy[10]. These regulations are now in force throughout the United Kingdom and, together with improved methods of mixing additives with intravenous fluids (the use of laminar flow cabinets), have markedly reduced the incidence of contamination.

Endogenous infection

The recognition of the significance of the environment and other patients as sources of infection encouraged the development of methods to reduce the incidence of infection to an absolute minimum. The wearing of sterile masks and gowns by attendant staff and relatives[11], the use of clean disposable gloves and sterile suction catheters during the care of the artificial airway[12], sterilization of intensive care equipment such as ventilators, suction machines and humidifiers[13], and the use of heated traps in the sink waste pipe[3], all these approaches have been shown to greatly reduce the incidence of bacterial colonization. Despite these endeavours the incidence of infection remains alarmingly high. The reason for this depressing failure lies with the patient, who is at the greatest risk from his own intestinal flora. The transmission of such colonization and infection is easily understood in patients with primary gastrointestinal disease, such as postoperative wound infection, subphrenic or pelvic abscess, peritonitis, an infected fistula, Crohn's disease and ascending cholangitis. In other cases the method of infection is less well understood. The clinical features of bacterial toxaemia develop without an obvious focus of infection or the bronchial tree may become colonized by colonic flora. How the colonic organisms reach the lungs has only recently been satisfactorily explained. In a few cases bacteria spread directly from the peritoneal cavity to the lung by passing through the diaphragm. The use of rectal thermometers has been incriminated[3], but this could not explain the majority of cases. Recently we have demonstrated an alternative pathway. In our original paper on patients undergoing prolonged IPPV, the stomach was shown to act as the source of the gram-negative bacteria colonizing the lungs[14]. The study was continued and the results on 24 patients are summarized in Table 3.3. In 11 patients the stomach was identified as the source of gram-negative bacteria colonizing the lungs. We have now demonstrated the route by which the majority of gram-negative bacilli reach the respiratory tree during IPPV. It is important to note that bacterial colonization of the gastric contents occurred very early in the course of the illness (mean 4.25 days ± SEM 0.79). The ventilated patient is nursed supine and a nasogastric tube is usually necessary. Reflux of gastric contents occurs, leading to colonization of the oesophagus, oropharynx and finally the tracheostomy site. It is then only a matter of time before the organisms find their way into the bronchial tree, since a cuffed endotracheal tube or tracheostomy tube does not provide complete protection[15].

Table 3.3 The stomach as a source of bacteria during IPPV; 24 patients studied

Bacteria isolated	Number of patients		
	Tracheal aspirate	Gastric aspirate (same bacteria)	Stomach before trachea
Klebsiella spp.	6	6	3
Proteus spp.	4	3	2
E. coli	4	3	3
Ps. aeruginosa	4	2	2
Str. faecalis	1	1	1
Total	19	15	11

There remain a few patients who develop bacterial toxaemia without evidence of gram-negative bacterial colonization. One possible explanation is that bacteria multiply in the bowel and liberate endotoxin into the portal circulation. The reticuloendothelial system, mainly the liver, is unable to detoxify the circulating endotoxin. This failure of detoxification may be due to an earlier period of hepatic hypoxia, itself secondary to hypovolaemic shock[16]. The endotoxin continues to enter the systemic circulation in quantities sufficient to produce the syndrome of bacterial toxaemia. Whilst this sequence has been demonstrated in the animal model, it has yet to be shown to occur in man.

(2) Host susceptibility

During the last 40 years increasing numbers of patients with compromised defence mechanisms have been admitted to hospital where the risk of infection is greatly increased. Patients admitted to the ICU form a small but clearly defined group whose antimicrobial defence mechanisms are severely impaired and yet have to be subjected to invasive procedures[3]. It is not surprising therefore, that opportunistic infections readily occur and are the most important single factor determining the outcome[17].

The body defence mechanism depends on the integrity of the skin and mucous membranes. If a micro-organism should breach this barrier then it must be recognized as foreign, the host defences must be mobilized, to localize and prevent the spread of infection and ultimately destroy and remove the infecting agent. The defences include identification of the antigen by macrophages and their destruction by phagocytosis, humoral antibodies and cell mediated immunity[18]. The skin and mucous membranes are usually breached by a variety of manipulations: urethral catherization, intravenous cannulation, endotracheal intubation or tracheostomy[3].

The metabolic response to injury depresses all aspects of the immune response to infection[19-21]. The more severe the injury, the greater the impairment of the immunological defences. The injuries most commonly associated with depressed immunity are burns[22,23], major trauma and surgery[17,19]. The immune system is depressed further when infection complicates any of these catabolic states. There are other diseases with depressed immunity which may require intensive therapy. These include hepatic failure[24], respiratory failure requiring IPPV[4], malnutrition from any cause[25], acute pancreatitis[26], severe inflammatory bowel disease[27], renal failure[28], diabetic ketosis[29], and diseases treated by immunosuppression[30].

(3) Patterns of infection

The recognition of infection can be one of the most difficult aspects of management of the intensive care patient. Clinical signs such as fever and leukocytosis often occur, without infection, as a feature of the metabolic response to injury[4]. The signs may also be seen in acute pancreatitis and inflammatory bowel disease. Isolation of bacteria from sites normally considered to be bacteria free, such as the tracheal aspirate, do not necessarily imply infection. This colonization of such sites by bacteria is almost the rule, particularly in the patient with an artificial airway[3].

The importance of early recognition of infection cannot be overemphasized. Bacterial infection has been incriminated as the cause of multiple organ failure in 70% of cases[1]. The onset is insidious, the first 2 or 3 days after injury is deceptively trouble-free. But oliguria, jaundice, transient respiratory insufficiency and circulatory failure progress in remorseless fashion. The clinician may initially attribute some of these disturbances to the metabolic response to injury and only in retrospect is bacterial infection incriminated.

In a classical paper Price and Sleigh[31] demonstrated that the withdrawal of prophylactic antibiotics in a neurosurgical unit virtually eliminated infections due to *Klebsiella* spp., with a corresponding increase in the survival rate. There are numerous other publications condemning the indiscriminate use of antibiotics[32,33]. Prophylaxis with antibiotics eliminates the normal body flora thus paving the way for superinfection with resistant opportunist pathogens such as gram-negative bacilli and fungi. Most ICUs have developed their own antibiotic policies, depending on the type of patient treated and the bacteria most commonly encountered. Our own policy was designed in 1973 and is based on clinical, laboratory and radiological signs, which can be made quickly and without recourse to specialist techniques[4]. The policy was designed because four patients died from infection due to gram-negative bacilli with bacterial toxaemia and multiple organ failure. All four patients had suffered multiple injuries and required IPPV because of an unstable chest wall. Antibiotics were started when the patient showed signs of bacterial toxaemia but were ineffective. Retrospective analysis showed that a rapid rise in core temperature, white cell count and blood glucose preceded the clinical features of bacterial toxaemia by 48 hours. The mean values for these parameters were a core temperature of 38.5°C, a

Table 3.4 An antibiotic policy for bacterial toxaemia when the pathogen is unknown

---

Indications

(1)   Gram-negative bacilli in stained films of the tracheal aspirate together with radiological evidence of collapse or consolidation

   or

(2)   Two of the following:
   a Core temperature of 38.5 °C or above.
   b White blood cell count of $11.0 \times 10^9/1$ or above.
   c Blood glucose of 12 mmol/1 or above; if 50% dextrose is being infused then greater than 22 mmol/1.

Antibiotics: all given intravenously

Gentamicin	(7.5 mg/kg body weight)/day in three doses
Benzylpenicillin	2 mega units 4 hourly
Metronidazole	500 mg 8 hourly

---

white cell count of $11 \times 10^9/1$ and a blood glucose of 11.2 mmol/1. The antibiotic policy was based on these signs together with additional criteria, namely radiological signs of consolidation or collapse together with gram-negative bacilli in stained films of the tracheal aspirate. This policy was tested out over 2 years on 16 patients with thoracic injuries. Six patients died, two from bacterial infection and toxaemia. Although the trial was uncontrolled, we felt that these results were beneficial. This policy remains in use with the modifications shown in Table 3.4.

The syndrome of bacterial toxaemia consists of the features, shown in Table 3.5. Bacterial toxaemia may occur with or without bacteraemia. When bacteraemia occurs the syndrome is much more responsive to antibiotics. It is bacterial toxaemia without bacteraemia that proves so resistant to treatment with antimicrobial agents. It is generally assumed that endotoxin is responsible for the pathophysiology of bacterial toxaemia; the evidence, however, remains circumstantial and controversial.

Table 3.5 Features associated with bacterial toxaemia

Warm hypotension
     Increased cardiac output, reduced peripheral resistance, raised blood lactate
Cold hypotension
     Reduced cardiac output, increased peripheral resistance, raised blood lactate
Adult respiratory distress syndrome
     Hypoxaemia, hypocapnoea, alkalosis, interstitial pulmonary oedema on radiograph
Bleeding tendency
     Disseminated intravascular coagulation
Acute reversible renal failure
     Uraemia and oliguria
Paralytic ileus
Jaundice
Pyrexia
Impaired conscious level

---

(4) Toxaemia

The concept that endotoxin is the mediator by which gram-negative organisms damage tissues has become widely accepted. It has been claimed that there are 2000 deaths a year due to endotoxaemia[34], and there is an abundance of literature to support this claim, but it remains unproven. Many studies have used animals and extrapolation of these results to man is not strictly justifiable. Endotoxin forms part of the cell wall of a bacterium and is liberated following the death of the bacteria, although endotoxin may also be released during active growth. It consists of a complex of phospho-lipid–polysaccharide–protein macromolecules, of which the lipopoly-saccharide (LPS) is the important constituent. The LPS of gram-negative organisms has three distinct components. These are a core polysaccharide, which is common to most gram-negative bacilli, an O specific poly-saccharide which determines the seriological specificity and virulence of the organisms, and a lipid A fraction which is responsible for toxicity[35,36]. In healthy persons endotoxin is produced in the gastrointestinal tract, mainly in the terminal ilium and colon, which are the sites of maximum bacterial growth. A continuous absorption of endotoxin occurs, reaching the liver via the portal system where it is detoxified by the Kupffer cells[36].

Toxic phenomena due to LPS certainly occur and can be reproduced in the animal by the intravenous injection of lipopolysaccharide. The phenomena include: (i) shock due to peripheral vasodilation[36] and depression of cardiac function[37]; (ii) increased capillary permeability leading to a loss of protein-rich fluid from the intravascular com-partments[16], thus exacerbating the hypotension and producing pulmonary oedema; (iii) activation of complement and kinin release, which is associated with activation of the coagulation cascade leading to dis-seminated intravascular coagulation[38]; (iv) endotoxin is pyrogenic, man being particularly sensitive. A dose of $0.002\,\mu g/mg$ of body weight is suf-ficient to produce fever by release of pyrogen from macrophages and poly-morphs[36]; (v) acute renal failure has also been caused by endotoxaemia[39]. Endotoxin has direct metabolic effects at cellular level. It increases mito-chondrial permeability to potassium, leading to mitochondrial swelling and membrane damage with the result that the production of ATP is inhibited[40]. Patients suffering from the ravages of gram-negative infection show many of these features and so the concept developed that endotoxin is responsible for the pathophysiology.

In 1968 Levin and Bang[41] developed the *Limulus* amoebocyte lysate assay (LALA), an extremely sensitive test capable of detecting plasma levels of less than a nanogram of endotoxin[42]. The same authors also demonstrated circulating endotoxin in patients suffering from gram-negative infection. Reinhold and Fine subsequently quantified the LALA test[43]. Since then there have been many reports incriminating endotoxin as the mediator of bacterial toxaemia. In 1972 Caridis *et al.*[5] demonstrated that the LALA test was positive both in patients with a known infective focus due to gram-negative bacilli and in certain patients without such an obvious focus. If the infected focus was removed then the signs of toxaemia rapidly disappeared and recovery was the rule; these patients often had a bacteraemia. In the second group of patients endotoxaemia persisted and the clinical features of toxaemia persisted, often without a bacteraemia. Most of the patients did not respond to antibiotics and intensive supportive therapy and many died.

Using a rabbit model, Caridis *et al.* demonstrated that the gastrointestinal tract was the source of endotoxin. A group pre-treated with oral kanamycin was compared with a control. A minimum lethal dose of LPS was injected into both groups. In the control group endotoxaemia occurred and persisted, causing death within 12 hours. In the kanamycin treated group shock did not develop, endotoxaemia did not persist and the animals recovered. These results suggested that persistent endotoxaemia had its origin in the gastrointestinal tract. In irreversible haemorrhagic shock, the absorption of endotoxin from the gut increases dramatically. It has also been shown that, in the laboratory animal, endotoxin and viable intestinal flora can move transmurally. This occurs in ischaemia of the intestine and in bacterial and chemical peritonitis, so that endotoxin gains access to the systemic circulation. Liver injury from any cause results in the failure of the Kupffer cells to detoxify endotoxin. This injury may be due to shock or chronic liver dysfunction[16,44]. We have now demonstrated that bacterial overgrowth within the gastrointestinal tract, particularly the stomach, is a common finding in the critically ill requiring IPPV[14] thus increasing the potential source of endotoxin. These arguments are strongly persuasive that endotoxin from the gut is the important cause of irreversible bacterial toxaemia. The theory is as follows. Endotoxin can reproduce the clinical features of bacterial toxaemia. Bacterial overgrowth in the gut readily occurs in the critically ill producing an excess of endotoxin. In the shocked patient without a demonstrable infective focus, the gut is the major source of endotoxin and this, together with depression of the reticuloendothelial system which follows stress, can lead to persistent endotoxaemia.

This theory has been challenged by several workers on the following grounds: (i) false positive reactions may occur with the LALA, (ii) extrapolation from animal experiments to the human clinical situation may not be valid, (iii) further experimental studies have produced conflicting results, (iv) certain gram-negative infections are not associated with endotoxaemia. The specificity of the LALA in detecting gram-negative lipopolysaccharide has been questioned. Elin *et al.*[45] obtained a positive LALA in only 12 out of 29 patients with bacteraemia (23 due to gram-negative bacteria), and 15 patients with gram-negative bacteraemia had a negative test. Two patients without any features of infection had a positive LALA. Unfortunately they did not attempt to correlate the features of bacterial toxaemia and outcome with the results of the LALA. Levin[42] showed that a positive LALA was associated with an increase in the severity of shock and mortality but Stumacher[46] and Elin were unable to confirm this. Stumacher found a positive LALA in 8 out of 22 cases of gram-positive bacteraemia. If one doubts the role of endotoxin in bacterial toxaemia, then alternative pathways must be involved. It has been suggested that plasma effector systems may be responsible for the circulatory and haemostatic changes observed in bacterial toxaemia[35]. The essential feature appears to be activation of the Hageman factor during the early stages of a bacteraemia. This activation triggers a sequence of reactions leading to activation of the coagulation cascade, kinin release; e.g. bradykinin, kallikrein and slow re-acting substance, complement activation, and increase in fibrinolysis. The physiological effect of such activation may result in the circulatory changes previously described. However, despite some evidence to the contrary, the majority of studies suggest that endotoxin is the chief mediator in the pathophysiology of bacterial toxaemia occurring in gram-negative infections. Whether it acts alone or in conjunction with vasoactive kinins and complement activation remains to be determined. The main difficulty lies in the lack of definite evidence in the human disease and caution must be maintained in interpreting animal studies. The role of endotoxin will only definitely be known when prospective studies are made which prevent or protect against endotoxaemia. The future holds exciting prospects for all concerned with infection in the ICU.

(II) ASSESSMENT

Infection is the most important single factor which determines the outcome of the intensive care patient. All patients must be considered to be at risk from infection for the reasons already given. It is essential that this fact is recognized by the therapeutic team so that steps to prevent bacterial colonization can commence on admission. We have found it valuable to adopt standardized procedures which are made familiar to all grades of staff and are then rigidly applied. Such standardization avoids omissions and errors, facilitates continuity and allows continuing assessment of a particular treatment. Our scheme has evolved during 20 years of intensive care but is adapted to changing circumstances and advances in knowledge. The methods are constantly under review and are examined critically by both experienced medical and nursing staff. The first essential for success is co-operation between all members of the team: the nurses, the clinician, the microbiologist and the technical staff responsible for the maintenance, servicing and sterilization of the equipment.

(1) Bacterial monitoring

If antibiotics are to be effective they must be given as soon as infection is recognized but before bacterial toxaemia develops. In practice this means that antibiotics are often used before the offending bacteria are identified and their sensitivities known. Such a dilemma demands blunderbuss therapy and is far from satisfactory. Careful monitoring of the patient's microbial flora can provide early warning of impending infection and so aid the clinician to choose an antibiotic. The bacterial monitoring chart used in

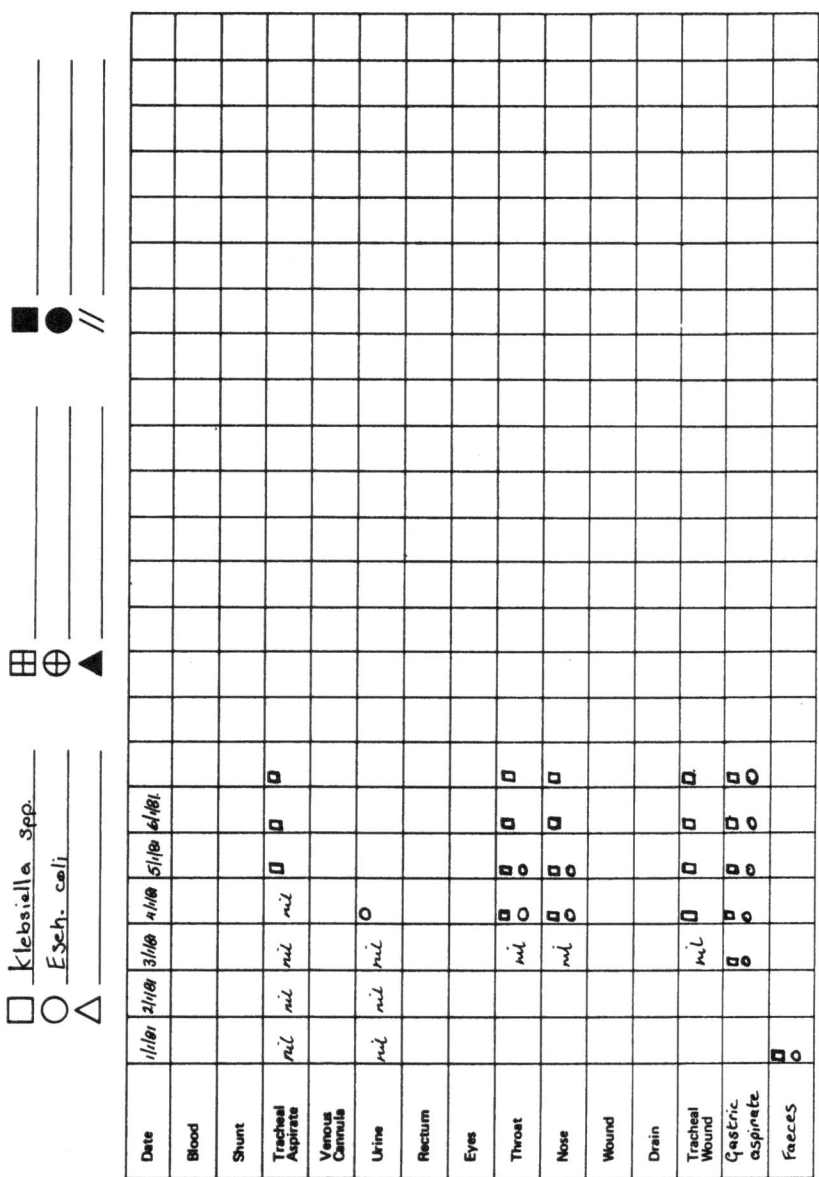

Figure 3.1 Bacterial monitoring chart

our ICU is shown in Figure 3.1. This was designed 10 years ago and has proved to be a valuable aid in the management of microbial infection. The drawback is the additional work for the bacteriology department. We are convinced that daily cultures are essential from certain sites, which include: (i) sites where the continuity of the skin or mucous membranes has been breached by invasive manipulations such as intravenous cannulae, tracheostomy, chest and abdominal drains, and Schribner shunts, (ii) urine and secretions aspirated from the stomach and trachea, (iii) oropharynx – since microbes descending into the bronchial tree are usually found in this site 2 or 3 days before their appearance in the tracheal aspirate. Daily blood cultures are unnecessary, but are mandatory when the core temperature rises rapidly or signs of bacterial toxaemia develop. The resident intestinal flora should be established as soon as possible after admission to the ICU. A specimen of faeces is cultured on the first day and then at weekly intervals. A fresh specimen should be collected into a sterile container, sent to the laboratory within one hour of collection and cultured for aerobic and anaerobic micro-organisms and fungi.

(2) Assessing the risk

All patients are at risk, some more than others. A definitive list of such diseases is not possible because of the inevitable variations between centres

Table 3.6 High risk patients common to this ICU

Respiratory failure needing IPPV
            asthma
            poisoning
            pulmonary burns
            adult respiratory distress
Major trauma
Acute reversible renal failure
Chronic renal failure
Peritonitis
Acute pancreatitis
Inflammatory bowel disease
Upper gastrointestinal haemorrhage
Hepatic failure
Diabetic ketoacidosis
Obstetric problems
            pre-eclampsia and eclampsia
            disseminated intravascular coagulation
Post-operative

            arterial surgery
            major abdominal surgery
            surgery for cancer of the head and neck

and the different patient populations. There are three major reasons for such variations; firstly the admission policy and particular interests of the unit; secondly the amount of major trauma and finally the presence or absence of other specialized units in the hospital, such as cardiothoracic, renal or burns. Table 3.6 lists the common high risk patients seen in this ICU.

(III) PREVENTION OF COLONIZATION

The prevention of bacterial colonization of sites, normally bacteria free, contributes more to the successful management of the critically ill than any other single measure. The source of the bacteria may be from the immediate environment (exogenous) or from the host (endogenous). The methods of prevention developed during the last two decades. Our policy is as follows. (i) All invasive procedures are carried out under aseptic conditions. (ii) Subsequent care and handling of the mucosal breach is a clean procedure, incorporating a face mask, hand wash and clean disposable plastic gloves. (iii) Sterile gowns are worn continuously by the visitors and all nursing and medical staff. The hands are washed on entering and leaving each patient area and masks and gowns are changed between patients. (iv) Whenever possible nurses do not cross over from patient to patient, so reducing the possibility of cross-infection. The exceptions to this rule are the unit rounds and when the nurse–patient ratio is less than ideal. (v) All the equipment is sterile and the disposable software is changed daily. Urinary catheters are changed weekly. The bladder is irrigated with 100 ml 2.5% noxythiolin every 12 hours. The non-disposable hardware, ventilators, suction machines and the haemodialysis machines, are sterilized before use by ethylene oxide or formaldehyde. The ventilators are fitted with bacterial filters, thus ensuring sterile gas for ventilation. (vi) The patient environment is made as bacteria free as possible. Mattresses and bedding are sterilized by ethylene oxide or autoclave. The sink traps are soaked in phenol and heated to 60 °C for 20 minutes twice a day. After the patient has left the ICU the bed, floor and walls are cleaned with glutaraldehyde or phenol. (vii) The final, but equally important aspect of prevention concerns the endogenous flora of the host. In our series of 24 patients host enteric gram-negative bacilli were responsible for 75% of all tracheal colonists. We were able to demonstrate that the stomach acted both as the source and a reservoir for continuing or recurring colonization of the respiratory tract. In fact, this route was responsible for colonization in 50% of patients requiring IPPV. Prevention of the gastric overgrowth is another matter altogether. Complete eradication of the intestinal bacteria has been shown to be impossible, but reducing the bacterial content of the gut may reduce the incidence of gram-negative colonization of the trachea during IPPV; it may also reduce the production of endotoxin.

(IV) ANTIMICROBIAL THERAPY

The correct use of antibiotics is a craft which unfortunately seems to be beyond the scope of many clinicians, who lack the appropriate knowledge and attitudes necessary for good prescribing. Antibiotics remain a most powerful weapon against infection and if used correctly can be of great benefit to the seriously ill patient. To achieve maximum benefit from anti-biotics infection must be recognized before bacterial toxaemia develops; the sensitivity pattern of the likely pathogens should be known; the antibiotic given in adequate dosage and titrated to maintain effective plasma levels. To overcome the pitfalls and obtain the desired result antibiotic policies are essential. Clear guidelines must be laid down and rigidly enforced.

(1) Prophylactic antibiotics

Few subjects are more contentious than the use, more often the abuse, of antibiotics for prophylaxis. The concept of 'sterilizing' the patient is attractive but mistaken[32]! Sterilization cannot be achieved and antibiotics used prophylactically often increase rather than decrease the incidence of infection[31,32]. Furthermore, when infection does develop in patients receiving prophylactic antibiotics, it may be due to an antibiotic resistant organism, making therapy extremely difficult. There are, however, occasions when prophylaxis has been proved to be of value. In the intensive care patient there are only a few indications but it is vital that they be clearly recognized; failure to do so may have disastrous consequences. The indications for prophylaxis are as follows. (i) Major trauma, particularly when the blood supply to the soft tissues has been compromised. Such patients are at risk from anaerobic (e.g. clostridia) infection[47]. A 5 day course of benzylpenicillin (10–12 mega units/day) is recommended. (ii) Vascular surgery on the lower limbs carries a similar hazard of clostridial infections and warrants a course of penicillin[33]. (iii) Colorectal, appendi-cular and gynaecological surgery. The lower gastrointestinal tract harbours both aerobic and anaerobic gram-negative bacilli. Post-operative infection, peritonitis and abscess formation are all too common. Only recently has the role of the anaerobes (especially *Bacteroides* spp.) been appreciated. There are many reports of the success of a regime combining a non-absorbable antibiotic such as kanamycin, with one active against *Bacteroides* spp[48,49]. Attention has recently centred on the use of metronidazole (suppository, 1 g 6 hourly), as the sole prophylactic agent. The theory is that elimination of the anaerobes may be as effective as a combined attack against the aerobic and anaerobic gram-negative bacilli[50]. At the present time we recommend the use of metronidazole 1 g 6 hourly rectally as the sole prophylaxis in patients undergoing gynaecological operations[51]. For colorectal and appendicular surgery we give gentamicin 160 mg and metronidazole 500 mg intravenously 1 hour preoperatively. (iv) Open heart surgery remains a controversial subject. The use of prophylactic antibiotics stems from the early days of valve replacement surgery when an infection rate of 20% was commonplace. Many antibiotic regimes have been tried over the last 20 years. The consensus of opinion is to give a 2 to 3 day course of β-lactam antibiotics. The results from the Papworth group are impressive: cloxacillin, benzylpenicillin and gentamicin are given preoperatively and for 48 hours postoperatively. During a 4 year period 800 open heart operations were performed without any cases of early (within 6 months) prosthetic valve endocarditis[52]. A cautionary remark by Herxheimer[53] is however worth noting before unbridled enthusiasm develops. 'Controlled trials of such prophylaxis is meaningless because the incidence of postoperative infections depends more on the surgical team than on the antibiotics'. (v) Endocarditis remains a problem for many general intensive care patients, who frequently undergo invasive procedures which can cause a bacteraemia. Examples are operations on the urinary and lower alimentary tract and indwelling pulmonary artery and right atrial catheters. No controlled trial of prophylactic antibiotics in man has reduced the incidence of bacterial endocarditis, although their value has been accepted from numerous animal studies[33]. The antibiotic used should be selected on a prior knowledge of the patient's own resident flora, the type of surgery and the pathogenic bacteria prevalent in the ICU.

Although they are not antibiotics, antiseptics have an important role to play in prophylaxis against microbial infection. It is appropriate that they be considered within the context of general prophylaxis. Indwelling urethral or venous catheters are an important source of microbial infection and antibiotics are useless as prophylactic agents (Chapter 12). Antiseptics, particularly povidone-iodine, have been shown to provide bactericidal and fungicidal protection in venous cannulation, arteriovenous shunts and urethral catheters[54,55].

In conclusion it must be remembered that, whilst prevention is the keystone of modern medical practice, there are very few indications for the use of antibiotics in such a manner. The incorrect use of these potent drugs is not only unjustified, but it is positively dangerous.

(2) Therapeutic antibiotics

The rationale choice of an antibiotic is only occasionally straightforward. To take one example: the evidence favours respiratory infection rather than colonization. There are classical signs: fever, tachycardia, pulmonary consolidation, and a leukocytosis; a bacterium has been isolated from the sputum and the antibiotic sensitivities are known. All that remains in such a case is to prescribe adequate doses of an antibiotic and perhaps monitor the plasma levels. Unfortunately such situations are rare. The more usual situation is for infection to be suspected but not proven, the responsible organism may or may not have been isolated and its sensitivity pattern not yet determined. In the latter situation the antibiotics have to be prescribed 'blind', and to have any chance of success the clinician needs a detailed knowledge of the likely causative pathogens, together with a bacterial 'profile' of the patient. Help from a microbiologist is invaluable at this stage in the management of the patient. Table 3.7 summarizes the pathogens found in various sites of the body together with the appropriate blind antibiotic. A brief description now follows of those antibiotics of most value in intensive care.

Table 3.7 Antibiotic therapy depending on the site of infection

Site	Likely pathogen	Antibiotic
Skin local	*Staph. aureus*	Flucloxacillin
cellulitis	*Str. pyogenes*	Benzylpenicillin
Intravenous line	*Staph. aureus*	Flucloxacillin
Brain abscess	Aerobes	Chloramphenicol
	Anaerobes (*Bacteroides* spp)	Metronidazole
Meningitis	*N. meningitidis* ⎫	Benzylpenicillin
	Str. pneumoniae ⎭	
	H. influenzae	Chloramphenicol
Urinary tract ⎫	Enterobacteria	Gentamicin
Genital tract ⎬		
Lower GIT ⎭	Enterobacteria	Gentamicin
Biliary tract	*Bacteroides* spp.	Metronidazole
Lung	*Str. pneumoniae*	Benzylpenicillin
	H. influenzae	Ampicillin

Aminoglycosides

Aminoglycosides are a group of antibiotics produced either by *Streptomyces* spp. or *Micromonospora* spp. The most important and widely used member of the group is gentamicin, which was the first aminoglycoside to be produced from *Micromonospora purpurae* and became available in 1966[56]. Gentamicin is the first choice antibiotic in life-threatening infections due to the enteric bacilli (*E. coli, Klebsiella, Enterobacter* and *Proteus*) and pseudomonads. Amikacin should be held in reserve for instances of gentamicin resistance. Aminoglycosides are distributed throughout the extracellular fluid compartment but the concentration is only one quarter to one half that of the serum. However, aminoglycosides penetrate poorly into the CSF, even when the meninges are inflamed. Ototoxicity and nephrotoxicity are common to all the aminoglycosides, the degree of toxicity varying with the compound. Gentamicin certainly causes vestibular damage but the evidence for its role as a nephrotoxic agent is controversial; invariably other factors are present, such as shock or bacterial toxaemia. However, there is evidence of nephrotoxic synergy when cephalosporins have been used in conjunction with an aminoglycoside. In this unit gentamicin has been the aminoglycoside of choice in cases of gram-negative infection for the last 10 years and has been used in more than 500 cases. There have been two cases of vestibular damage, both reversible on withdrawing the drug, but we have been unable to incriminate gentamicin as an aetiological factor in any case of renal failure. The aminoglycosides appear to prevent synthesis of bacterial proteins and this makes them rapidly bactericidal. The speed with which organisms are killed is species dependent, pseudomonads taking considerably longer than other gram-negative bacilli.

Bacterial resistance to aminoglycosides is plasmid borne and therefore transmissable from species to species. The important fact to remember is that the plasmids carry the resistance to several antibiotics, and the inappropriate use of ampicillin can induce gentamicin resistance in several enteric bacilli. This serves to emphasize the folly of using drugs like ampicillin, tetracyclines or cephalosporins in the intensive care patient, who may well develop a gram-negative infection at some stage of the illness. If the clinician fails to practice this self-discipline in dealing with the intensive care patient, then he must be prepared for the consequences: a patient dying from gram-negative infection for which there is no effective antibiotic. It is a temptation we must refuse!

Antibiotic interactions are complex and ill-understood. As well as nephrotoxic synergy with cephalosporins, aminoglycosides interact with carbenicillin to produce bactericidal synergy against many strains of gram-negative bacilli[57]. Paradoxically, gentamicin is inactivated by carbenicillin when both are mixed *in vitro* and the two drugs should not be infused together. Synergy between penicillin and aminoglycosides can be exploited in the treatment of enterococcal endocarditis[58,59].

Antimicrobial therapy with gentamicin (or other aminoglycosides) can be expected to have a marked beneficial effect on the course of the illness. The response is usually pronounced, with signs of improvement within 2 to 3 days of starting the antibiotic. On other occasions the anticipated response fails to occur. The patient deteriorates, with the features of continuing bacterial toxaemia; multiple organ failure develops and becomes irreversible, leading to death. In our experience the major problem with gentamicin is the misuse of the drug (indiscriminate prophylaxis or unproven infection) and the prescribing of sub-therapeutic doses. The results are a complete failure to kill the organisms and the rapid emergence of resistant strains. Such problems usually occur outside the ICU. The therapeutic and toxic plasma levels of gentamicin are very close; the therapeutic index is low. This induces undue caution in many doctors. In an attempt to overcome this problem nomograms have been designed which give the starting and maintenance doses. The best nomogram available at present is probably that of Mawer *et al*.[60], which almost guarantees an adequate initial dosage. The nomogram is based on age, sex, body weight and serum creatinine concentration, and gives the starting dose, maintenance dose and the frequency of administration. Although useful, a few exceptions occur which preclude the use of this nomogram in the high risk patient. For example, patients in acute renal failure requiring daily haemodialysis have required gentamicin in dosages of 6 mg/kg body weight daily, which would have been appropriate with normal renal function. A particular case involved a young woman with an *E.coli* bacteraemia secondary to pyelonephritis. In order to maintain an adequate peak serum level of gentamicin (8–10 μg/ml) the dose required was 12 mg/kg body weight daily (200 mg t.d.s.).

As a result of these discrepancies our policy has been to decide the dosage by monitoring the serum concentration. A microbiological assay is used and its accuracy maintained by a National Quality Control[61]. The initial doses are calculated on the basis of body weight (7.5 mg/kg body weight each day in three divided doses) irrespective of renal function. After the first 24 hours the doses are adjusted accordingly to the peak and trough estimations made on alternative days. The one exception to this rule is the patient on daily haemodialysis. Gentamicin is then administered once after dialysis and the serum levels measured ½ hour after injection (peak) and immediately before the next dialysis (trough). The optimum serum levels are shown in Table 3.8. This scheme has been in operation for 2 years, during which 110 patients have been treated with gentamicin for 5 days or longer (range 5–21

Table 3.8 Gentamicin: ideal serum levels

Enterobacteria

peak	8–12	μg/ml
trough	0–3	μg/ml

Pseudomonas

peak	10–15	μg/ml
trough	0–3	μg/ml

Peak levels: half an hour after intravenous injection
Trough levels: half an hour before intravenous injection

days). Optimum serum levels were obtained in all cases and in only two instances did gentamicin resistance develop during therapy; in both instances the organism was *Pseudomonas aeruginosa*. In view of this excellent record we feel that routine serum assay is the only practical way of ensuring an adequate therapeutic level in the intensive care patient.

Penicillins

Although penicillin was discovered in 1929[62], it was not until the 1940s that its widespread clinical use ushered in the modern era of antibiotics. The next chapter in the penicillin story was the isolation of penicillin nucleus, 6-amino penicillanic acid (6APA) in 1959[63].

This allowed the development of various side chains at the 6-amino position from which a series of semi-synthetic penicillins were produced. The first of these was ampicillin, an amino substitution at the α-position of the side chain of benzylpenicillin.

Since 1959 many other substitutions have been developed. (i) *Carboxy group at the α-position*[64]. These compounds include carbenicillin and ticarcillin which are particularly active against *Pseudomonas aeruginosa*. Unfortunately làrge doses of the sodium salt are required, which result in a massive sodium load which is often retained, causing oedema. Also resistance can readily develop. (ii) *Amino group at the α-position (ampicillin)*. This was one of the earlier semi-synthetic penicillins to have activity against gram-negative bacilli. Its activity is inferior to the aminoglycosides and resistance readily develops. A more significant increase in activity was obtained when the α-amino group of ampicillin itself was substituted. These are the ureido penicillins and include pirbenicillin, mezlocillin and azlocillin[64]. Pirbenicillin has marked antipseudomonal activity, being eight times more active than carbenicillin and also more stable in serum[65].

Resistance is R factor mediated and carbenicillinase producing strains of *Pseudomonas* are resistant to pirbenicillin as well as carbenicillin. Mezlocillin and azlocillin have a spectrum similar to carbenicillin but their activity is enhanced, particularly against *Pseudomonas, Bacteroides* spp. and *Klebsiella* spp. Organisms producing β-lactamase and one third of coliforms are resistant[66]. (iii) *Amidino group at the 6-amino position of 6APA (mecillinam)*. These were the first penicillins without acylation of the 6-amino position of 6APA found to have an appreciable antibacterial activity[67]. They are active against most gram-negative bacilli (especially coliforms, *Klebsiella, Proteus, Enterobacter* and *Salmonella*) but not pseudomonads or β-lactamase producing organisms[68]. Resistance to mecillinam occurs when long courses are used against *Salmonella*, but short courses do not induce bacterial resistance in host faecal flora[69]. (iv) *Penicillinase resistant penicillins (flucloxacillin)*. These resulted from the discovery that a change in the side chain of penicillin could protect the central β-lactam ring from the action of penicillinase, without losing antibacterial activity[70]. The most widly used antibiotics of this group are cloxacillin and its derivative flucloxacillin. They have become the antibiotics of first choice for staphylococcal pneumonia and bacteraemia[71,72]

Cephalosporins

Cephalosporins were discovered during investigations into the antibacterial activity of sewage discharged into the sea off the coast of Sardinia[73]. They are derived from 7-amino-cephalosporanic acid, the cephalosporin nucleus, which is structurally and chemically related to 6APA.

Many cephalosporin derivatives are now available but a full description of their antibacterial properties and indications is beyond the scope of this chapter. For a detailed account the interested reader is referred to a review by O'Callaghan[74]. The cephalosporins can be placed into three categories[75]: (i) susceptible to most β-lactamases, cephalothin, cephaloridine, and cephazolin, (ii) resistant to some β-lactamases, cephalexin, cephradine, and cephamandole, (iii) resistant to most β-lactamases, cefoxitin, cefuroxime, and cefotaxime.

For intensive care the only cephalosporins worth further consideration are those in the third category, namely cefoxitin, cefuroxime and cefotaxime. They have been extensively tried in serious gram-negative infections and have been shown to be effective against most enteric gram-negative organisms, both aerobic and anaerobic. A high cure rate[76-79] was obtained in most studies with the exception of infections by *Pseudomonas* spp., where a failure rate of more than 75% was recorded[77,80]. Toxic effects are minimal and appear to be reversible on stopping the antibiotic; they include a transient rise in hepatic transaminases and a positive direct Coombs test but without haemolysis[81,82]. These new cephalosporins, whilst not replacing the aminoglycosides as first choice antimicrobials, have proved to be a useful addition to the antibiotic armoury of the intensive care clinician.

Chemotherapy of anaerobic infections

Both gram-positive and negative anaerobes can be encountered in intensive care. The gram-positive anaerobic bacilli, *Clostridia* spp., are always very sensitive to benzylpenicillin and this remains the antibiotic of choice for such infections. Gram-negative anaerobic bacilli, *Bacteroides* spp., are normal inhabitants of the lower gastrointestinal tract. They are commonly incriminated in pelvic and abdominal sepsis, brain abscesses and chronic pulmonary infections. The antimicrobials most effective against such organisms are clindamycin, lincomycin and metronidazole[83-85]. Clindamycin and lincomycin, whilst being very effective suffer from one major drawback; they can produce pseudomembranous colitis[86], a disease which may be fatal. This complication excludes the use of these antibiotics in the ICU. Metronidazole has no such toxic effects and so has become the antimicrobial agent of choice for gram-negative anaerobic infections. Metronidazole was first tested as an antitrichomonal agent in 1958[87], and its value in anaerobic infections was reported by Shinn in 1962[88], who found it effective in treating acute ulcerative gingivitis. It acts solely against obligate anaerobes, facultative anaerobes being resistant[83]. All obligate anaerobes of clinical significance are sensitive to metronidazole whose action is consistently bactericidal[85]. The drug acts by inhibiting nucleic acid synthesis; oxidation of thiamine pyrophosphate is prevented and thus no energy is released for nucleic acid synthesis[89]. In clinical studies it has proved highly effective as a prophylactic agent against anaerobic pelvic sepsis[51] and as a therapeutic agent in cases of *Bacteroides* bacteraemia[86,90]. Toxic effects are rare but nausea and vomiting, aplastic anaemia, and more rarely peripheral neuropathy and epileptiform seizures have been reported. In animals there is a suggestion of carcinogenicity following prolonged therapy[87]. Short courses of 7–10 days have not as yet been associated with side effects. It would appear that metronidazole (intravenous, oral or rectally) is highly effective in gram-negative anaerobic infections and without serious toxicity. It must therefore be regarded as the antimicrobial agent of choice for such infections.

Antifungal agents

Fungal infections occur in patients previously treated with broad spectrum antibiotics, corticosteroids or immunosuppressives[91], therapy often used in the intensive care patient. The diagnosis of fungal infections is notoriously difficult despite the use of special culture media. The lesions are often inaccessible and blood cultures frequently negative[92]. To complicate matters further, therapy is fraught with dangerous toxic effects, as no effective but non-toxic antifungal has yet been produced[92]. The first antifungal was potassium iodide which was shown to be effective against sporotrichosis as long ago as 1903. Nystatin, the first polyene antifungal became available in 1950[91]. The other agents developed since then are: amphotericin B, 5-flucytosine and the imidazole derivatives[93,94]. Each of these antifungal agents has its place in the therapy of fungal infections within the ICU. The sites of infection and appropriate agent are shown in Table 3.9. The systemic antifungals, amphotericin B and 5-flucytosine, can be life saving but are extremely toxic and must therefore be used most judiciously. Amphotericin B may cause fever, rigors, venous thrombosis and a potassium-losing nephritis; whereas 5-flucytosine is toxic to the bone marrow causing thrombocytopenia and leukopenia[92].

Table 3.9 Fungal infections

Site	Antifungal agent
Oropharynx	Amphotericin B lozenges
Lung	Nystatin suspension – nebulized
Gastrointestinal	Nystatin suspension – intragastric
Meningeal	Miconazole – intrathecal
Fungaemia	Amphotericin B ⎫ intravenous Flucytosine ⎭
Fungaemia with renal failure	Flucytosine ⎫ intravenous Miconazole ⎭

(V) ADDITIONAL THERAPY

The intensive care patient with bacterial infection or toxaemia invariably requires more than treatment with antimicrobials. This additional therapy can be grouped under three headings.

(1) Intensive supportive therapy

We rely on an approach similar to that of Ledingham et al.[95]. In the established syndrome of bacterial infection or toxaemia this includes the following: (i) oxygen therapy and the early use of IPPV, (ii) circulatory resuscitation with blood or colloid solution, to maintain a normal right atrial or pulmonary artery wedge pressure. If shock continues despite normal atrial pressures then inotropic and vasodilator agents are used (Chapter 5), (iii) antibiotics, prescribed in accordance with our own rigid antibiotic policy (Table 3.4), (iv) correction of a metabolic derangement and then maintaining metabolism, usually by intravenous feeding (Chapter 1), (v) early treatment of acute renal failure by frequent haemodialysis when the blood urea reaches 30 mmol/l, (vi) disseminated intravascular coagulation treated by replacement therapy and sometimes heparin as described in Chapter 4, (vii) surgical drainage of an abscess, (viii) the principles of prevention of bacterial colonization already described are rigidly adhered to in all high risk patients, with or without bacterial infection.

(2) Corticosteroid therapy

Large dose steroid therapy, 'the big shot'[96] (30 mg methylprednisolone/kg body weight) has been used in the treatment of shock for 10 years. The evidence in favour is based on theoretical considerations and animal experiments. Large dose steroids stabilize lysosomes, increase peripheral perfusion by counteracting circulating pressor substances and increase coronary blood flow and cardiac output, probably by depressing various cardioinhibitory factors. They may accelerate the clearance of circulating endotoxin by protecting the function of the reticuloendothelial system[96,97]. When steroids are given before or immediately after the induction of bacterial toxaemia in the dog, then survival is increased[98]. There are few adequate clinical trials in man[99] but claims have been made for a reduction in mortality of the order of three times the control group as opposed to the steroid treated group[100].

There is considerable evidence against the efficacy of steroids. The dog model has been criticized on the grounds that it is a poor model of bacterial toxaemia in man[99]. In a primate model the pathological changes were similar to the human disease but steroids neither prevented the histological changes nor improved the survival rate[101,102]. In a prospective double blind study methylprednisolone did not improve patient survival[103]. Methylprednisolone in large doses causes a transient fall in the heart rate and temperature which can be interpreted as an improvement in the condition of the patient[104].

In summary, there is no doubt that in certain animal models pre-treatment with large doses of a steroid reduces the death rate from bacterial infection and toxaemia. However, there is no conclusive evidence that steroid therapy benefits established bacterial toxaemia in man[105]. Our own practice is never to use steroids.

(3) Enhancing immunity and neutralizing endotoxin

Gram-negative bacterial infections stimulate a humoral antibody response resulting in the production of a wide variety of antibodies against capsular and O-specific antigens and lipopolysaccharide[35]. Stimulation of the humoral antibody system by vaccination was recommended for bacterial infections as long ago as 1939[106]. From animal experiments the treatment suggested was a combination of sulphapyridine and vaccine. With the development of powerful antibiotics this therapy was soon forgotten by the medical and pharmaceutical professions. The problem with gram-negative bacilli is the enormous variety of antigens that are produced between species. Thus immunization against each antigen would be extremely difficult, if not impossible. Fortunately only two antigens seem to be clinically important, namely O-specific and cross-reactive. Cross-reactive antigen appears to be an antigen shared by most gram-negative organisms. Antibodies against these two antigens can protect against lethal doses of endotoxin. If resistance can be enhanced by immunization against this cross-reactive antigen, then real protection against the harmful effects of endotoxin may result[35].

Noxythiolin (oxymethylone methylthiourea) decomposes in solution, to liberate free formaldehyde[107]. It is used mainly as a lavage into body cavities, such as the bladder and peritoneal cavity, to prevent or treat gram-negative infections[107,108]. The liberated formaldehyde inactivates endotoxin. Taurolin is closely related to noxythiolin and has a linked ring structure combining two molecules of taurine with three of formaldehyde[109]. The formaldehyde is released on contact with bacteria or endotoxin[110] and is then effective against all faecal pathogens, both aerobic and anaerobic[109]. The main advantage of taurolin over noxythiolin is its lack of toxic effects and it can be administered intravenously, so neutralizing circulating endotoxin[111]. In the mouse and rabbit, intravenous taurolin gave significant protection against the pyrexic and lethal effects of endotoxin derived from *E. coli* and *Bacteroides fragilis*[111,112]. This new approach to the treatment of endotoxaemia warrants further investigation regarding its toxicity and possible role in the management of bacterial toxaemia in man.

We are confident that attempts to maintain and increase host immunity and reduce the production of endotoxin in the gut together with the development of agents to neutralize circulating endotoxin, hold the key to reducing the dreadful mortality of gram-negative bacterial toxaemia.

References

1. Eisman, B., Beart, R. and Norton, L. (1977). Multiple organ failure. *Surg. Gynecol. Obstet.*, **44**, 323
2. Spaulding, E. H. (1974). Introduction. In Prier, J. E. and Friedman, H. (eds.). *Opportunistic Pathogens*. p. 8. (Baltimore: University Park Press)
3. Stoddart, J. C. (1978). The management of infection: infection and the ITU. In Hanson, G. C. and Wright, P. L. (eds.). *Medical Management of the Critically Ill*. p. 477. (London: Academic Press)
4. Atherton, S. T., Wright, D. M., White. J. D. and Jones. E. S. (1977). An antibiotic policy for bacterial infections after thoracic and other injuries. *Thorax*, **32**, 596
5. Caridis, D. T., Reinhold, R. B., Woodruff, P. W. H. and Fine, J. (1972). Endotoxaemia in man *Lancet*, **1**, 1381
6. Drasar, B. D. and Hill, M. J. (1974). The distribution of bacterial flora in the intestine. In *Human Intestinal Flora*. Chap. 3. (London: Academic Press)
7. Casewell, M. and Phillips, I. (1977). Hands as route of transmission for *Klebsiella* species. *Br. Med. J.*, **2**, 1315
8. Bagshawe, K. D., Blowers, R. and Lidwell, O. M. (1978) Isolating patients in hospital to control infection. I. Sources and routes of infection. *Br. Med. J.*, **2**, 609
9. Robertson, M. H., Hoy, G. and Peterkin, I. M. (1980). Antistatic mattress as reservoir of pseudomonas infection. *Br. Med. J.*, **1**, 831
10. Department of Health and Social Security (1977). *Guide to Good Pharmaceutical Manufacturing Practice*, p. 41. (London: HMSO)
11. Bagshawe, K. D., Blowers, R. and Lidwell, O. M. (1978). Isolating patients in hospital to control infection. IV. Nursing procedures. *Br. Med. J.*, **2**, 808
12. Crampton Smith, A. (1967). Intensive care of the surgical thoracic patient: Discussion. *Postgrad. Med. J.*, **43**, 278
13. Lumley, J. (1976). Decontamination of anaesthetic equipment and ventilators. *Br. J. Anaesth.*, **48**, 3
14. Atherton, S. T. and White, D. J. (1978). Stomach as a source of bacteria colonising respiratory tract during artificial ventilation. *Lancet*, **2**, 963
15. Mehta, S. (1972). The risk of aspiration in presence of cuffed endotracheal tubes. *Br. J. Anaesth.*, **44**, 601
16. Nolan, J. P. (1975). The role of endotoxin in liver injury. *Gastroenterology*, **69**, 1346

17. British Medical Journal (1977). Crush injuries. *Br. Med J.*, **2**, 1244
18. Maudgil, G. C. and Wade, A. G. (1976). Anaesthesia and immunocompetence. *Br. J. Anaesth.*, **48**, 31
19. Schimpff, S. C., Miller, R. M., Polakavetz, S. and Horrick, R. B. (1974). Infection in the severely traumatized patient. *Ann. Surg.*, **179**, 352
20. Alexander, J. W. (1968). Neutrophil function in selected surgical disorders. *Ann. Surg.*, **168**, 447
21. Miller, R. W., Polakavetz, S., Horrick, R. B. and Cowley, R. A. (1973). Analysis of infections acquired by the severely injured patient. *Surg. Gynecol. Obstet.*, **1**, 7
22. MacMillan, B. G. (1981). The control of burn wound sepsis. *Int. Care Med.*, **7**, 63
23. Bjorrison, A. B., Alteimer, W. A., Bjorrison, S., Tang, T. and Isorson, M. L. (1978). Host defense against opportunist micro organisms following trauma. I. Studies to determine the association between changes in humoral components of host defense and septicaemia in burned patients. *Ann. Surg.*, **188**, 93
24. Triger, D. R., Boyer, T. D. and Levin, J. (1978). Portal and systemic bacteraemia and endotoxaemia in liver disease. *Gut*, **19**, 935
25. Lee, H. A. (1975). Intravenous nutrition. *Ann. R. Coll. Surg.*, **56**, 59
26. Jacobs, M. L., Daggett, W. M., Civetta, J. M., Vasu, M. A., Lawson, D. W., Warshaw, A. L., Nardi, G. L. and Bartlett, M. (1977). Acute pancreatitis: analysis of factors influencing survival. *Ann. Surg.*, **185**, 43
27. Palmer, K. R., Duerdon, B. I. and Holdsworth, C. D. (1980). Bacteriological and endotoxin studies in cases of ulverative colitis submitted to surgery. *Gut*, **21**, 851
28. Lindsay, R. M. (1974). The prognosis of acute renal failure. In Flynn, C. T. (ed.). *Acute Renal Failure*. p. 110. (Lancaster: MTP Press)
29. Oakley, W. G., Pyke, D. A. and Taylor, K. W. (1978). *Diabetes and its Management*. Chap. 9. (Oxford: Blackwell Scientific Publications)
30. Mims, C. A. (1976). *The Pathogenesis of Infectious Disease*. p. 26. (London: Academic Press)
31. Price, D. A. and Sleigh, J. D. (1970) Control of infection due to *Klebsiella aerogenes* in a neurosurgical unit by withdrawal of antibiotics. *Lancet*, **2**, 1213
32. Lancet (1970). Prophylactic antibiotics. *Lancet*, **2**, 1231
33. Brumfitt, W. and Hamilton-Miller, J. M. T. (1975). The place of antibiotic prophylaxis in medicine. *J. Antimicrob. Chemother.*, **1**, 163
34. Wardle, E. N. (1978). Septic shock. *Lancet*, **1**, 1360
35. Craven, D. E., Bruins, S., and McGabe, W. R. (1977). Sepsis due to Gram negative bacilli: epidemiology, pathogenesis and immunologic aspects. In Ledingham, I. McA. (ed.). *Recent Advances in Intensive Therapy*. Chap. 13. (London: Churchill Livingstone)
36. Mims, C. A. (1976). Mechanisms of cell and tissue damage. In *The Pathogenesis of Infectious Disease*. pp. 146–7. (London: Academic Press)
37. Alican, F., Dalton, M. L. and Hardy, D. J. (1962). Experimental endotoxin shock. Circulatory changes with emphasis on cardiac function. *Am. J. Surg.*, **103**, 702
38. Levin, J. (1973). Endotoxin and endotoxaemia. *N. Engl. J. Med.*, **288**, 1297
39. Wardle, E. N. (1975). Endotoxinaemia and the pathogenesis of acute renal

failure. *Q. J. Med.*, **44**, 389

40. Nicholas, G. G., Mela, L. M. and Miller, L. D. (1974). Early alterations in mitochondrial membrane transport during endotoxaemia. *J. Surg. Res.*, **16**, 375

41. Levin, J. and Bang, F. B. (1968). Clottable protein in Limulus: Its localization and kinetics of its coagulation by endotoxin. *Thromb. Diath. Haemorrh.*, **19**, 186

42. Levin, J., Poore, T. E. and Young, N. S. (1972). Gram negative sepsis: detection of endotoxaemia with the limulus test: with studies of associated changes in blood coagulation, serum lipids and complement. *Ann. Intern. Med.*, **76**, 1

43. Reinhold, R. B. and Fine, J. (1971). A technique for quantative measurement of endotoxin in human plasma. *Proc. Soc. Exp. Biol. Med.*, **137**, 334

44. Hershey, S. G. and Altura, B. M. (1969). Function of the reticulo endothelial system in experimental shock and combined injury. *Anaesthesiology*, **30**, 138

45. Elin, R. J., Robinson, R. A., Levine, A. S. and Wolff, S. M. (1975). Lack of clinical usefulness of the limulus test in the diagnosis of endotoxaemia. *N. Engl. J. Med.*, **293**, 521

46. Stumacher, R. J., Kovnot, M. J. and McCabe, W. R. (1973). Limitations of the usefulness of the limulus assay for endotoxin. *N. Engl. J. Med.*, **288**, 1261

47. Chisholm, G. D. (1976). Preventing casualty wound infection. *J. Antimicrobial Chemother.*, **2**, 109

48. Feathers, R. S., Lewis, A. A. M., Sagar, G. R., Amirak, I. D. and Noone, P. (1977). Prophylactic systemic antibiotics in colorectal surgery. *Lancet*, **2**, 4

49. Lancet. (1978). Bowel preparation for surgery. *Lancet*, **2**, 1132

50. Lancet. (1980). Bacterial synergy in mixed aerobic/anaerobic infections. *Lancet*, **1**, 405

51. Seligman, S. A. (1978). Metronidazole in obstetrics and gynaecology. *J. Antimicrobial Chemother.*, **4** (Suppl. C), 51

52. Newsom, S. W. B. (1978). Antibiotic prophylaxis for open-heart surgery. *J. Antimicrobial Chemother.*, **4**, 389

53. Herxheimer, A. (1977). Cephalothin prophylaxis in open-heart surgery and other uncontrolled studies. *J. Antimicrobial Chemother.*, **3**, 621

54. Hugo, W. B. (1978). Early studies in the evaluation of disinfectants. *J. Antimicrobial Chemother.*, **4**, 489

55. Rotter, M., Koller, W. and Wewalka, G. (1980). Povidone iodine and chlorhexidine gluconate containing detergents for disinfection of hands. *J. Hosp. Infect.*, **1**, 149

56. Finland, M. (1974). Gentamicin: Foreword *Review and Commentary on selected world literature*, p. vi. (USA: Schering Corp.)

57. Farrel, W., Wilks, M. and Drasar, F. A. (1979). Synergy between aminoglycosides and semi synthetic penicillins against gentamicin resistant gram negative rods. *J. Antimicrobial Chemother.*, **5**, 23

58. Noone, P. (1978). Use of antibiotics; aminoglycosides 1. *Br. Med. J.*, **2**, 549

59. Noone, P. (1978). Use of antibiotics; aminoglycosides 2. *Br. Med. J.*, **2**, 613

60. Mawer, G. E., Ahamed, R., Dobbs, S. M., McGough, J. G., Lucas, C. B. and Tooth, J. A. (1974). Prescribing aids for gentamicin. *Br. J. Clin. Pharmacol.*, **1**, 45

61. Reeves, D. S. and Bywater, M. J. (1975). Quality control of serum gentamicin assays - experience of national surveys. *J. Antimicrobial Chemother.*, **1**, 103

62. Fleming, A. (1929). On the antibacterial action of cultures of a penicillin, with special reference to their use in the isolation of *B. influenza*. *Br. J. Exp. Pathol.*, **10**, 226

63. Batchelor, F. R., Doyle, F. P., Naylor, J. H. C. and Robinson, G. N. (1959). Synthesis of penicillin: 6-aminopenicillanic acid in penicillin fermentation. *Nature (London)*, **183**, 257

64. Wise, R. (1977). Substituted ampicillins. *J. Antimicrobial Chemother.*, **3**, 289.

65. Wise, R., Andrews, J. M. and Bedford, K. A. (1977). Pirbenicillin - a semi synthetic penicillin with anti pseudomonal activity. *J. Antimicrobial Chemother.*, **3**, 175

66. Ellis, C. J., Geddes, A. M., Davey, P. G., Wise, R., Andrews, J. M. and Grimely, R. P. (1979). Mezlocillin and azlocillin: an evaluation of two new B-lactam antibiotics. *J. Antimicrobial Chemother.*, **5**, 517

67. Lund, J. and Tybring, L. (1972). B-amidinopenicillin acids - a new group of antibiotics. *Nature New Biol.*, **236**, 135

68. Reeves, D. S. (1977). Antibacterial activity of mecillinam. *J. Antimicrobial Chemother.*, **3** (Suppl. B), 5

69. Anderson, J. D. (1977). Mecillinam resistance in clinical practice - a review. *J. Antimicrobial Chemother.*, **3** (Suppl. B), 89

70. Garrod, L. P., Lambert, H. P. and O'Grady, F. (1973). *Antibiotic and Chemotherapy*. 4th Edn., p. 71. (London: Churchill Livingstone)

71. Bagg, R. (1978). Antibiotic treatment of staphylococcal pneumonia in adults. *J. Antimicrobial Chemother.*, **4**, 297

72. Noone, P. (1982). *A Clinician's Guide to Antibiotic Therapy*. p. 11. (Oxford: Blackwell Scientific Publications)

73. Garrod, L. P., Lambert, H. P. and O'Grady, F. (1973). Cephalosporins. In *Antibiotic and Chemotherapy*. 4th Edn., p. 87. (London: Churchill Livingstone)

74. O'Callaghan, C. H. (1979). Description and classification of the newer cephalosporins and their relationships with the established compounds. *J. Antimicrobial Chemother.*, **5**, 635

75. Williams, J. D. (1978). Which cephalosporins? *J. Antimicrobial Chemother.*, **4**, 109

76. Diakes, G. K., Kesmidis, J. C., Stathakis, C. and Giamarellou, H. (1977). Cefuroxime: antimicrobial activity, human pharmacokinetics and therapeutic efficacy. *J. Antimicrobial Chemother.*, **3**, 555

77. Mashimo, K. (1978). Clinical experience with cefoxitin sodium. *J. Antimicrobial Chemother.*, **4** (Suppl. B), 113

78. Tally, F. P., Miaer, P. V. W., O'Keefe, J. P. and Garbach, S. L. (1979). Cefoxitin therapy of anaerobic and aerobic infections. *J. Antimicrobial Chemother.*, **5**, 101

79. Shah, P. M. and Bender, H. (1978). Bactericidal activity of cefoxitin and cefuroxime. *J. Antimicrobial Chemother.*, **4**, 163

80. Ramachandran Nair, S. and Cherubin, C. E. (1978). Use of cefoxitin sodium in difficult to treat infections. *J. Antimicrobial Chemother.*, **4** (Suppl. B), 167

81. Norrby, R., Foord, R. D. and Hedlund, P. (1977). Clinical and pharma-

cokinetic studies on cefuroxime. *J. Antimicrobial Chemother.*, **3**, 355

82. Reeves, D. S., Birt, A. J., Molt, H. A. and Stocks, P. J. (1978). Cefoxitin sodium: a clinical and pharmacological study. *J. Antimicrobial Chemother.*, **4** (Suppl. B), 155

83. Percival, A. and Cumberland, N. (1978). Antimicrobial susceptibilities of gram negative anaerobes. *J. Antimicrobial Chemother.*, **4** (Suppl. C), 3

84. Tracy, C., Gordon, A. M., Moran, F., Love, W. C. and McKenzie, P. (1972). Lincommycins in the treatment of bacteroides infections. *Br. Med. J.*, **1**, 280

85. McLosky, R. V. (1979). The treatment of anaerobic infections. *J. Infect.*, **1** (Suppl. 1), 73

86. Noone, P., Abeysundare, R. and Bradley, J. M. (1978). Bacteraemia. *J. Antimicrobial Chemother.* **4** (Suppl. C), 83

87. Roe, F. J. C. (1977). Metronidazole: review of uses and toxicity. *J. Antimicrobial Chemother.*, **3**, 205

88. Shinn, D. L. S. (1962). Metronidazole in acute ulcerative gingivitis. *Lancet*, **1**, 1191

89. Ingham, H. R., Selkin, J. B. and Hale, J. H. (1975). The antibacterial activity of metronidazole. *J. Antimicrobial Chemother.*, **1**, 355

90. Eykyn, S. J. and Philips, I. (1978). Metronidazole in surgical infections. *J. Antimicrobial Chemother.*, **4** (Suppl. C), 75

91. Cartwright, R. Y. (1975). Antifungal drugs. *J. Antimicrobial Chemother.*, **1**, 141

92. Br. Med. J. (1980). Treating fungal infections. *Br. Med. J.*, **1**, 688

93. Medoff, G. and Kobayashi, G. S. (1980). Strategies in the treatment of systemic fungal infections. *N. Engl. J. Med.*, **302**, 145

94. Grunberg, E., Titsworth, E. and Bennett, M. (1963). Chemotherapeutic activity of 5-flurocytosine. *Antimicrob. Agents Chemother.*, **3**, 566

95. Ledingham, I. McA and McCardle, C. S. (1978). Prospective study of the treatment of septic shock. *Lancet.* **1**, 1194

96. Lancet (1977). The Big Shot. *Lancet*, **1**, 633

97. Hanson, G. C. (1978). Shock and infection. In Hanson, G. C. and Wright, P. L. (eds.). *Medical Management of the Critically Ill.* p. 368. (London: Academic Press)

98. Emerson, T. E. and Raymond, R. M. (1979). Methylprednisolone in the prevention of cerebral haemodynamic and metabolic disorders during endotoxin shock in the dog. *Surg. Gynecol. Obstet.*, **148**, 361

99. Smith, J. A. R. and Norman, J. N. (1979). Use of glucocorticoids in refractory shock. *Surg. Gynecol. Obstet.*, **149**, 369

100. Weil, M. H., Shubin, H. and Nishijima, H. (1974). Corticosteroid therapy in circulatory shock. *Int. Surg.*, **59**, 589

101. Coalson, J. J., Benjamin, B. A., Archer, L. T., Kefler, B. K., Spaet, R. H. and Hinshaw, L. B. (1978). A pathologic study of Escherichia coli shock in the baboon and the response to adrenocorticosteroid treatment. *Surg. Gynecol. Obstet.*, **147**, 726

102. Hinshaw, L. B., Coalson, J. J., Benjamin, B. A., Archer, L. T., Beller, B. K., Kling, O. R., Hasser, E. M. and Phillips R. W. (1978). Escherichia coli shock in the baboon and the response to adrenocorticosteroid treatment. *Surg. Gynecol. Obstet.*, **147**, 545

103. Leigh Thompson, W. (1977). Dopamine in the management of shock. *Proc. R. Soc. Med.*, **70** (Suppl. 2), 25
104. Gill, W. and Long, W. B. (1979). Multiple organ failure. In *Shock Trauma Manual*. p. 76. (Baltimore: Williams & Wilkins)
105. Percival, A. (1978). Microbial infections. In Jones, E. Sherwood (ed.). *Essential Intensive Care*. p. 228. (Lancaster: MTP Press)
106. MacClean, I. H., Rogers, K. B. and Fleming, A. (1939). M and B and pneumococci. *Lancet*, **1**, 562
107. Browne, M. K. and Stoller, J. L. (1970). Intraperitoneal noxythiolin in faecal peritonitis. *Br. J. Surg.*, **57**, 525
108. Browne, M. K., Leslie, G. B. and Pfirrman, R. W. (1978). A comparison of noxythiolin and povidone iodine in experimentally induced peritoneal infection in mice. *Br. J. Surg.*, **65**, 601
109. Browne, M. K., MacKenzie, M. and Doyle, P. J. (1978). A controlled trial of taurolin in established bacterial peritonitis. *Surg. Gynecol. Obstet.*, **146**, 721
110. Browne, M K., Leslie, G. B. and Pfirrman, R. W. (1976). Taurolin, a new chemotherapeutic agent. *J. App. Bacteriol.*, **41**, 363
111. Pfirrman, R. W. and Leslie, G. B. (1979). The anti-endotoxic activity of taurolin in experimental animals. *J. Appl. Bacteriol.*, **46**, 97
112. Browne, M. K., Leslie, G. B. and Pfirrman, R. W. (1976). Taurolin, a new *in vitro* and *in vivo* activity of taurolin against anaerobic organisms. *Surg. Gynecol. Obstet.*, **145**, 842

4
Coagulopathies

BARBARA BAIN

Haematological perturbations are almost universal in critically ill patients and can aggravate the primary disease and complicate management. Shock, infection, and renal and hepatic failure are common in critically ill and injured patients; some of their deleterious effects are mediated through the haemopoietic system, and in turn haematological dysfunction may contribute to shock, infection and failure of one or more organs. Since almost every haematological disorder is seen at some time during intensive care, it is not practicable to deal with all aspects. The coagulopathies are described in this chapter and blood transfusion in Chapter 6. Blood coagulation abnormalities and their management are of major importance in critically ill patients, who frequently suffer from abnormal bleeding, thromboembolism, or both. Depression of erythropoiesis is usual in critically ill patients but there is no effective management beyond the maintenance of adequate nutrition, which is described in Chapter 1. Megaloblastic arrest can be of vital importance and is dealt with together with other causes of thrombocytopenia. This chapter is based on my experience as the haematologist associated with a busy ICU in the Princess Alexandra Hospital, Brisbane. This unit admits 700 patients per year, and detailed coagulation studies were performed on many of these patients. Where management is controversial, I have made this clear.

The coagulation factors of the intrinsic and extrinsic coagulation systems are shown in Figure 4.1. It is probable that factor VIII is produced by reticuloendothelial cells, particularly those of the liver, while most, if not all,

Table 4.1 Basic laboratory tests for diagnosis of coagulopathy

Test	Function tested
Platelet count	
Bleeding time	platelet number and function
Prothrombin time (PT)	extrinsic and common pathways
Activated partial thromboplastin time (aPTT)	intrinsic and common pathways
Thrombin clotting time (TCT)	the conversion of fibrinogen to fibrin, and therefore the level and function of fibrinogen, the presence of heparin and the presence of other antithrombins such as fibrin/fibrinogen degradation products
Fibrinogen level	
Fibrin/fibrinogen degradation products (FDPs)	lysis of either fibrin or fibrinogen
Clot observation	excessive fibrinolysis

of the other coagulation factors are produced by hepatic parenchymal cells. Table 4.1 shows the basic laboratory tests required for diagnosis of a coagulopathy, together with standard abbreviations. More detailed tests, including assays of specific factors and studies of fibrinolysis have contributed to our understanding of underlying mechanisms, but these tests are not often available in an emergency. It is important that the ICU should provide the laboratory with an appropriate blood sample, since activation of coagulation during a difficult venepuncture may produce abnormal laboratory tests simulating those of disseminated intravascular coagulation (DIC). Unless the blood sample is added to the correct volume of trisodium citrate, factitious prolongation of test results will occur. If DIC is suspected, a blood sample should also be taken into a tube containing thrombin plus an inhibitor of fibrinolysis, for the estimation of fibrin/fibrinogen degradation products (FDPs). If this estimation is done on a sample which has not been mixed with a fibrinolysis inhibitor then fibrinolysis *in vitro* may cause factitious elevation of FDPs. The blood sample should be free of contaminating heparin; samples taken in conjunction with an arterial sample for blood gas estimations are not infrequently contaminated with heparin, and heparin may also be in use for

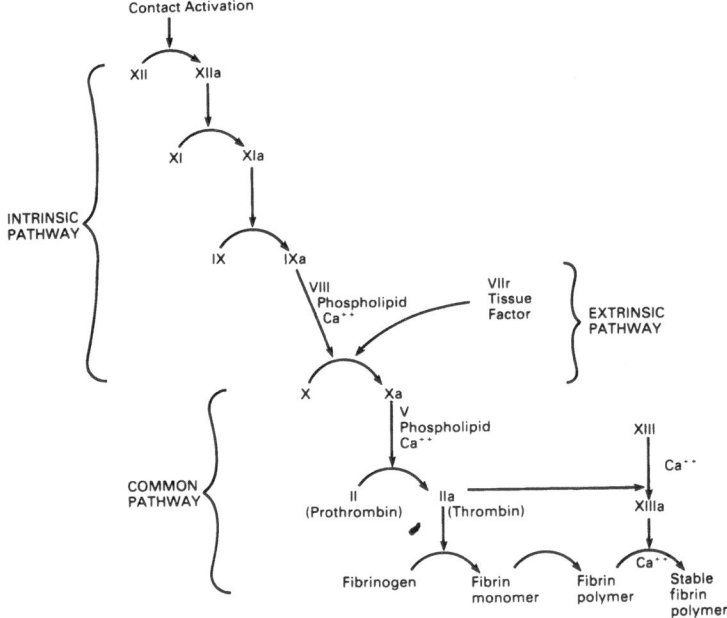

Figure 4.1 The coagulation cascade; the pathway initiated by contact activation of factor XII is designated the intrinsic pathway; the pathway initiated by the interaction of factor VII and tissue factor is designated the extrinsic pathway

maintaining the patency of catheters and cannulae, or during peritoneal dialysis.

(I) CHANGES IN COAGULATION IN THE INTENSIVE CARE PATIENT

(1) Clotting factors

After trauma, major surgery, burns and shock, a characteristic pattern of changes in coagulation factors and the fibrinolytic system is seen. Similar changes can be seen during any severe acute illness. The usual response to trauma and haemorrhage is a hypercoagulable state which may be a defence mechanism against exsanguination. Wessler and Yin[1] have defined a hypercoagulable state as 'an altered state of circulating blood that requires a smaller quantity of a clot initiating substance to induce intravascular coagulation than is required in the normal state'. It is not certain whether a hypercoagulable state is produced by increased levels of coagulation factors alone or whether the presence of coagulation activators and decreased levels of inhibitors are also required. The increased tendency to thrombosis in pregnancy, and in women taking oral contraceptives may indicate that high levels of clotting factors do play a part. William Hewson in 1772 made the classical observation that when sheep were exsanguinated or patients were subjected to blood letting 'the blood which issued last coagulated first'[2]. More recently Turpini and Stefanini[3] found that when rabbits were bled there was a prompt rise in the platelet count and acceleration of *in vitro* thromboplastin generation. The latter was due to a factor present in serum and an additional factor present in absorbed plasma. Turnover studies in dogs indicate that production of fibrinogen and platelets is markedly increased following trauma[4]. In man the whole blood clotting time often shortens after injury but returns to normal or is even prolonged within a few hours[5]. Other global tests of the intrinsic pathway – the silicone clotting time[6] and the recalcification time[7,8] may be similarly shortened. The PT[7] and the aPTT may also be shortened. The acceleration of various clotting tests may be due to the elevation of levels of clotting factors or the presence of activated clotting factors. Fibrinogen, factor VIII and factor V may rise[9]. An elevation of the platelet count can be seen within hours of trauma[6,10], and platelet adhesiveness can be increased[11]. An apparent elevation of factor VIII when a one-stage factor VIII assay is used may indicate either a raised level or the presence of activated factor VIII; a two-stage assay shows that a true rise often occurs. Increased production of clotting factors and platelets can also be present in patients with normal plasma levels, because increased consumption is balanced by increased production. Slichter[12] found platelet and fibrinogen turnover to be increased up to fivefold following elective surgery. The hypercoagulable state is mediated partly by catecholamines and partly by adrenal corticosteroids. A noradrenaline infusion in dogs rapidly shortens the clotting time[13]. Catecholamines lead to increased levels of factor VIII and an increased platelet count[14]. Fibrinogen production is increased by cortisone[15]. Some of the hypercoagulable state following trauma may be due to the mobilization of free fatty acids which can cause platelet aggregation and activation of factor XII[16] and can also inhibit fibrinolysis[17].

(2) Fibrinolysis

The fibrinolytic system shows striking changes after injury or surgery. The earliest response to trauma is an enhanced fibrinolytic potential, which may be mediated by catecholamines and to a lesser extent by corticosteroids. Fear alone can increase fibrinolysis. Hypotension, ischaemia and hypoxia are potent inducers. The initial enhancement of fibrinolysis is due to a release of plasminogen activator from the vascular endothelium.

Plasminogen activator can then convert plasminogen to plasmin within a blood clot or this can occur, sometimes, in the circulating blood.

To study fibrinolysis it is necessary to reduce the effect of antiplasmins, which retard the lysis of clots formed *in vitro*; the fibrinolytic potential of blood is then revealed. This may be done by diluting the blood (the dilute blood lysis time, devised by Fearnley[18]) or by extracting the euglobulin fraction which contains 90% of the plasminogen of plasma, but less of the antiplasmins. Both the dilute blood lysis time[5] and the euglobulin clot lysis time (ECLT)[11,19] are accelerated soon after injury or surgery. The shortening of the ECLT correlates with the severity of the injury, the presence of shock and with hypoxaemia[8]. Fibrinolysis may also be quantified by lysis of a fibrin plate. In a heated fibrin plate assay, the plasminogen is destroyed, so that the zone of lysis quantifies plasmin. In contrast, an unheated fibrin plate allows quantification of the combined effect of plasminogen activator and free plasmin. Following trauma or surgery free plasmin is rarely present, but plasminogen activator is increased for several hours[19,20]. During cardiopulmonary bypass free plasmin can appear as well as an increase in plasminogen activator[21]. Plasminogen can be assayed by a caseinolytic assay, by radioimmune assay, or by the streptokinase activated lysis time of dilute blood. Following trauma, plasminogen falls due to an increased consumption, particularly in those with DIC[19,22].

The early increase of fibrinolytic potential is followed by depression, which may be profound, particularly in those with adult respiratory distress syndrome or the fat embolism syndrome[23]. Impaired fibrinolysis is associated with an inhibitor, an antiplasminogen activator[4,5], which appears to be α_2-plasmin inhibitor[24]. However, not all observers agree that an inhibitor is responsible for the post-traumatic inhibition of fibrinolysis[25].

(3) The platelets

Thrombocytosis or thrombocytopenia are both common in critically ill patients.

(a) Thrombocytosis is common after haemorrhage, trauma, surgery and burns, usually appearing several days after the injury. Thrombocytosis is also a common response to sepsis and tissue necrosis. Platelet counts are usually of the order of $500-1000 \times 10^9/1$. Patients who have suffered trauma or been submitted to major surgery and have required splenectomy may have a much more marked thrombocytosis, with counts of the order of $1000-3000 \times 10^9/1$. Such marked rises of the platelet count may contribute to a hypercoagulable state. The use of aspirin (acetylsalicylic acid) to inhibit platelet aggregation is indicated in patients with extreme elevation of the platelet count; in the ICU patient this is most conveniently given by rectal suppository once daily. Dipyridamole will potentiate aspirin.

(b) Thrombocytopenia may be defined as a platelet count below 140 $\times$ $10^9/1$ but abnormal bleeding does not usually occur until the platelet count falls below 60 $\times$ $10^9/1$. When platelet function is abnormal, or if there is extensive tissue damage, a lesser degree of thrombocytopenia can cause bleeding. Thrombocytopenia can be seen in DIC, following massive transfusion of stored blood, following cardiopulmonary bypass, as an idiosyncratic reaction to heparin, and following charcoal perfusion; these topics are discussed in Sections II and III. Other causes of thrombocytopenia are megaloblastic arrest, alcohol abuse and drugs. Viral infection is an uncommon cause of thrombocytopenia in the intensive care patient.

Idiosyncratic drug reaction is an uncommon cause of acute thrombocytopenia. In the ICU sulphonamides and their derivatives are the drugs most often responsible. Thrombocytopenia has been observed in burnt patients following the topical application of a sulphonamide. Management is withdrawal of the drug with or without a brief course of corticosteroids. Platelet transfusions should only be given if serious haemorrhage occurs as the drug-antibody complexes will bind to the donor platelets, shortening their lifespan and reducing their efficacy. Alcohol induced thrombocytopenia is not uncommon in ICU patients. Toxic effects of alcohol include thrombocytopenia, usually without haemorrhage, and this will correct within a week of withdrawal. A poor granulocyte response to infection may also be seen. Because alcoholics have an increased incidence of folic acid deficiency, those with a cytopenia should be given folic acid.

The management of thrombocytopenia depends on the aetiology. Replacement therapy is more likely to be of benefit when there is a failure of platelet production or when thrombocytopenia follows massive transfusion rather than when excessive destruction of platelets is occurring. For example, platelets transfused into patients with megaloblastic arrest are likely to have a normal life span and maintain adequate haemostasis until bone marrow recovery occurs; whereas platelet transfusion is of little use in drug induced thrombocytopenia as drug–antibody complexes become bound to the donor platelets and cause their premature destruction. The most rapidly effective therapy for thrombocytopenia is the transfusion of platelet concentrates. Concentrates from 6–8 blood donations is usually effective but in patients with extensive tissue damage 8–10 concentrates are recommended. Platelet concentrates can be of the same ABO group as the recipient, or O platelets may be used in recipients of other blood groups. If no ABO compatible platelets are available, then ABO incompatible platelets can be given and appear to be only slightly less efficacious. Male patients and postmenopausal women may be given platelet concentrates without regard to the Rh group, but young girls and women in the reproductive age range who are Rh negative should not be given Rh positive platelets. Although there are no Rh antigens on platelets, the contaminating red cells may cause Rh immunization. If only Rh positive platelets are available, then 50 μg of anti D should be given within 24 hours. Platelet concentrates have a shelf life of up to 48 hours if stored at 22 °C with constant gentle mixing, rather than at 4 °C. Since this allows the ready availability of platelets at weekends, these storage conditions are now used by most blood transfusion services. Platelets so stored have good post-transfusion survival, but may not regain full function for several hours after transfusion.

When platelet concentrates are not available, then fresh blood (24–less than 48 hours old) or fresh platelet rich red cells can be used to correct thrombocytopenia. Since approximately 30% of platelets are lost on preparation of concentrates, and since there is further loss of viable platelets with storage, one unit of whole blood can be regarded as equivalent to two platelet concentrates. It will be seen that the possibility of volume overload renders whole blood or platelet rich red cells less than ideal for the correction of thrombocytopenia, except when a blood transfusion is needed. Nevertheless, if platelet concentrates are not available for treating haemorrhage then fresh blood, used if necessary, with a partial exchange technique, can be efficacious.

Megaloblastic arrest due to folic acid deficiency is an important cause of thrombocytopenia. Because of the acuteness of the process, and because the production of red cells may virtually cease, there can be a precipitous fall in the platelet and white cell counts without accompanying macrocytosis. This makes diagnosis difficult unless there is a high index of suspicion and the bone marrow is examined. In the ICU megaloblastic arrest has been recognized in patients with malnutrition and those with increased folate needs due to trauma, surgery and infection. Pregnancy may be a predisposing factor and alcohol infusions[26] and weak antifolate drugs such as co-trimoxazole[26,27] can precipitate its development. Peritoneal or haemodialysis will remove folate and can aggravate the process[28].

Megaloblastic arrest due to acute folate deficiency can be prevented by the prophylactic administration of folic acid, which should be routinely administered to acutely ill patients having parenteral nutrition (Chapter 1). A dose of 5 mg daily is quite adequate. In patients over 50 years of age it is prudent to give prophylactic vitamin B_{12} together with folic acid because of the possibility of undiagnosed pernicious anaemia. If megaloblastic arrest does occur, the patient should be given intravenous folic acid and if haemorrhage occurs, then fresh blood or platelet transfusions are given. Megaloblastosis can also occur in patients exposed to nitrous oxide. It has been reported in patients ventilated with nitrous oxide and oxygen, either following cardiac surgery, or as part of the management of tetanus[29,30]. An exposure of 5–6 hours can be enough to induce a megaloblastic change and an abnormal dU suppression test[29,31]; the mechanism is inactivation of the methylcobalamin form of vitamin B_{12}. Patients who are ventilated for more than 24 hours with nitrous oxide should have daily blood counts. Those who develop a cytopenia should have the nitrous oxide discontinued, since it has been observed that the administration of B_{12} fails to prevent the metabolic abnormality[29] or correct the cytopenia once this has occurred[30]. Recovery may not occur for several days after withdrawal of nitrous oxide and platelet or granulocyte concentrates can be required during this time.

(c) Defective platelet function may occur with or without thrombocytopenia and can cause pathological bleeding at a platelet count which would otherwise be safe. The quickest way to assess platelet function is to measure bleeding time, but extra information can be obtained by studying platelet adhesion and platelet aggregation *in vitro*. The most accurate method of measuring the bleeding time is the Ivy technique, using the forearm. The Duke technique, using the ear lobe, is less accurate. It is also unsuited for repeated observations, since a prolonged bleeding time is often associated with considerable bleeding into the ear lobe.

Defective platelet function occurs in DIC (Section II) due to inhibition by FDPs. If DIC is arrested by removal of the precipitant or by heparin therapy, then FDPs will be cleared within 12–24 hours, with a restoration of platelet function. Therapy with streptokinase or urokinase will also generate FDPs which will inhibit platelet function. Platelet transfusions are often less efficacious in patients with elevated FDPs; the number of concentrates required to stop bleeding or bring the bleeding time towards normal is often greater than would be predicted from the degree of thrombocytopenia. Defective platelet function usually follows cardiopulmonary bypass, when platelets which have been damaged in the extracorporeal circulation remain in the blood stream for many hours (Section III). Abnormal platelet function commonly follows charcoal perfusion (Section III). Other causes of defective platelet function are described in this section. Decreased platelet adhesiveness has been reported in patients with stress ulceration following trauma or infection[37]. Since these patients commonly have multiple defects of haemostasis, it is difficult to isolate the effect of 'stress'. Poor adhesiveness sometimes responds to fresh frozen plasma but may require fresh blood. Uraemia is a common cause of defective platelet function in critically ill patients. Defective function is due to a plasma factor and will improve with adequate dialysis. Donor platelets transfused into a uraemic patient are less effective than in a non-uraemic patient and a larger number of concentrates is necessary to treat haemorrhage. Dextrans interfere with the factor VIII – Von Willebrand's molecule – and thereby with platelet function. If abnormal bleeding is observed together with a long bleeding time, the dextran should be stopped (Section III). Acetylsalicylic acid has a potent effect on platelet function due to an inhibition of prostaglandin synthesis. In some patients aspirin can have a valuable antithrombotic effect, but in the others, abnormal bleeding can occur. When bleeding occurs the drug is stopped. Platelets which have been acetylated by aspirin continue to function poorly for the rest of their life span (7 days), but transfused platelets will restore haemostasis. Other anti-inflammatory drugs which inhibit prostaglandin synthesis have a much less marked effect on platelet function and I have not seen them cause haemorrhage. Sodium nitroprusside can inhibit platelet function in clinical dosage; platelet aggregation is inhibited and blood loss can increase[36]. Penicillins in high dosage interfere with platelet function, causing a marked prolongation of the bleeding time[32-34] and larger doses can have a heparin-like effect. Such disorders have been seen most often in patients with renal failure but may also occur in those with normal renal function. Adverse effects have been caused by different penicillins. Protamine is said to reverse the bleeding diathesis[33]. Defective platelet function persists for several days after stopping the drug[32]. Cephalothin appears to have the same effect as the penicillins[35].

(II) DISSEMINATED INTRAVASCULAR COAGULATION (DIC)

(1) Definitions

Disseminated or diffuse intravascular coagulation (DIC) is a syndrome in which thrombin is generated and fibrin thrombi form within blood vessels, particularly within the microcirculation. When the coagulation cascade is activated, there is a simultaneous activation of the fibrinolytic, complement and kinin systems. The clinical signs which follow are determined by the rate of thrombin generation and by the degree of activation of the fibrinolytic system. At one extreme, when there is rapid thrombin generation and very active fibrinolysis, coagulation factors are quickly depleted causing haemorrhage, but as thrombi are rapidly lysed, then tissue damage is not a major feature. This variant, which is seen typically following amniotic fluid embolism, is also designated the defibrination syndrome, or consumption coagulopathy. At the other extreme is a chronic DIC seen in association with metastatic malignancy, in which fibrinolysis is less active; microthrombi form in the capillaries of many organs and a microangiopathic haemolytic anaemia occurs, as red cells are damaged by fibrin strands. In chronic DIC the consumption of coagulation factors is compensated for by a marked overproduction, so that depletion of factors is uncommon and the terms defibrination syndrome and consumption coagulopathy are less appropriate. In the ICU patient chronic compensated DIC is rarely seen; subacute and acute DIC are common, although these do not always produce clinical manifestations.

(2) Pathogenesis

In broad terms DIC can be due to activation of the intrinsic pathway of coagulation (Figure 4.1) or to extrinsic activation when thromboplastic substances reach the circulating blood in sufficient quantities to overwhelm the inhibitors of coagulation and thus generate thrombin. If a hypercoagulable state exists then smaller quantities of such thromboplastic substances are necessary. An intact reticuloendothelial system, capable of removing activated clotting factors, is important in the defence against DIC. In the ICU patient thromboplastins are generated when there is tissue damage by trauma, shock, hypoxia, burns and sepsis. The same patients often have a hypercoagulable state and reticuloendothelial impairment (Chapter 2) so that the action of thromboplastins is potentiated.

The pathogenesis of DIC following major surgery and trauma with or without shock illustrates the mechanisms which operate. DIC can be triggered by the release of tissue thromboplastin into the circulation. Experimentally, the intravenous injection of either thromboplastin or tissue homogenate can trigger consumption of platelets and fibrinogen, or even frank DIC[38,39]. Damaged tissue entering the circulation during surgery or trauma may act similarly. DIC is more likely to occur with extensive soft tissue damage than with penetrating injury. The finding of bone marrow emboli in the lungs of traumatized patients indicates that damaged tissue does enter the circulation, and a thromboplastic effect of damaged tissue is further supported by the frequent coexistence of DIC and fat embolism[11,40]. The rapid accumulation of labelled fibrinogen in the lungs when fractures are manipulated and particularly when a prosthesis is driven into the marrow cavity provides evidence of this mechanism[41]. It has been suggested that in head injury, damaged brain tissue can enter the circulation and act as a thromboplastin[42].

At the site of injury the extrinsic system is activated by thromboplastin released from damaged tissues; the intrinsic system is activated by exposure to collagen; platelets are activated by exposure to collagen, by ADP released from damaged cells and by traces of thrombin released during activation of the coagulation cascade. The coagulation factors activated at traumatized and hypoxic sites together with platelet aggregates can then enter the general circulation. The pre-existing hypercoagulable state makes the triggering of DIC very likely. If the patient is shocked, venous stasis and acidosis further aggravate the process. The occurrence of DIC following the restoration of the circulation to a previously ischaemic tissue (e.g. bowel infarcted by intussusception) and the development of pulmonary microvascular thrombosis after the release of an arterial clamp used during vascular surgery, are examples of this mechanism[11]. In addition, thromboplastic substances are released into the general circulation during the period of hypoxia. Following experimental trauma without significant blood loss, platelet aggregates from the site of injury reach the lungs and occasionally the systemic circulation[43,44] and can induce DIC[45]. Conversely, haemorrhagic shock or even normotensive hypovolaemia without trauma will cause microembolism of the lungs by fibrin strands and platelet aggregates[3,46]. When shock and tissue damage coexist many potent factors interact to cause DIC. Simmons *et al.*[7] in studying combat casualties in Vietnam found that hypotension, increased levels of lactic acid, and acidosis correlated with coagulation abnormalities. Blood volume estimations made immediately post-operatively in 22 patients showed that a volume deficit of greater than 15% was associated with coagulation anomalies, although the relationship was not statistically significant.

Hypoxia, hypothermia and acidosis aggravate endothelial cell and other tissue damage. A pH of less than 7.2 accelerates the clotting of both native and heparinized blood and increases the consumption of prothrombin *in vitro*[13]. In experimental animals lactic acidosis alone can induce DIC[71]. Experimentally, DIC in haemorrhagic shock is much reduced by buffering with sodium bicarbonate or TRIS buffer[13]. Catecholamines may cause DIC[47] and their release will aggravate the situation. Reticuloendothelial (RE) blockade with defective clearance of activated clotting factors and fibrin microthrombi, is a further adverse factor. The protective effect of the RE system can be seen in experimental animals, when shunting blood from ischaemic tissue through the liver prevents death from pulmonary microembolism. Trauma and other forms of stress also lead to the mobilization of fatty acids which can cause platelet aggregation and activation of the intrinsic system[16].

In bacterial infection or toxaemia, additional mechanisms operate (III, 1) and DIC is common. DIC can follow burns (III, 2) and can be caused by the initial tissue damage or by superimposed infection. It is likely that autotransfusion of shed blood (III, 4) can both induce and aggravate DIC by the reinfusion of activated coagulation factors produced by exposure of the blood to air and damaged tissues. A large pulmonary embolus can lead to DIC; the mechanism is not clear. Transient DIC occurs following cardiac arrest[48]; the likely mechanism is endothelial damage due to hypoxia. In rabbits, a sharp fall of factor XII during cardiac arrest occurs indicating its activation[49]. Severe intravascular haemolysis will cause DIC both in man and in experimental animals, the red cell stroma[50,51] acting as a thromboplastin. The experimental animal will suffer only transient DIC unless there is coexisting shock when severe DIC can occur[50]. There have been occasional reports of DIC in drowned patients[52] but significant haemolysis is rare even in fresh water[53] drowning, and the DIC is probably due to hypoxia. Incompatible blood transfusion is an uncommon cause of DIC but in the anaesthetized or paralysed patient widespread haemorrhage from DIC may be the first sign of incompatible transfusion. DIC can also be seen in acute pancreatitis when trypsin appears to be a mediator[54]. DIC can follow insertion of a Le Veen shunt, when thromboplastic substances in ascitic fluid enter the blood stream, and can also result from snake bite. DIC can occur following cardiopulmonary bypass, but in this situation increased fibrinolysis is a prominent feature, and the evidence is conflicting as to whether DIC or primary fibrinolysis is the major pathological process (III, 5). Thus DIC may be triggered by various mechanisms, many of which are common in critically ill and injured patients.

The incidence of DIC following injury or surgery is variably reported. Effeney et al.[55] found evidence of severe or moderate DIC in 77% of patients following trauma or major surgery. Other studies suggest DIC is uncommon after trauma. Counts et al.[56] found DIC in 3 out of 27 patients who had been massively transfused, mainly following trauma and of 21 battle casualties requiring massive transfusion, only one was considered to have DIC[57]. Since criteria for the diagnosis of DIC were not precisely defined in the latter two studies, it is likely that the different estimates of the frequency of DIC are consequent on different criteria as well as different patient populations. In my experience, using the haematological criteria given below, DIC is common following trauma or major surgery in which hypotension and poor tissue perfusion have been features. DIC is also common in patients with severe bacterial infection, particularly if septic shock has occurred.

DIC may cause tissue damage by a number of mechanisms additional to vascular obstruction. Fibrinopeptides A and B have constrictive effects on the pulmonary vasculature[65]; fibrinopeptide B is chemotactic for neutrophils and monocytes; fibrin fragments D and E are chemotactic for monocytes[66]; FDPs increase capillary permeability[67]; serotonin released from platelets constricts bronchi and precapillary arterioles[68]. Serotonin may be responsible for decreased lung compliance, since this is blocked by serotonin antagonists[69]. It has been demonstrated in experimental animals that DIC can itself cause shock, which can be prevented by heparinization[11,70]. There is an association between DIC which immediately follows injury and subsequent infection[55]; an aetiological relationship mediated by impaired reticuloendothelial function can be postulated.

(3) Criteria for diagnosis

(a) Clinical criteria

The clinical manifestations of acute DIC are two in number, occurring singly or together. They are haemorrhage and microvascular thrombosis, causing failure of one or more organs; the first sign is more dependable than the second. Haemorrhage is characteristically generalized from venepuncture sites, wounds, and tracheostomy and operative sites. The bleeding occurs diffusely from capillaries. Purpura is common, and less often petechial haemorrhage may be seen. Petechiae may result from severe thrombocytopenia or from leaking capillaries which were previously obstructed by microthrombi. In severe consumption coagulopathy when fibrinogen has been virtually totally removed, the clinician may note that the shed blood fails to clot. Unexplained venous or arterial gangrene or multiple infarcts of the skin should also alert the clinician to the likelihood of DIC and the laboratory tests should be carried out without delay.

The organ failure characteristic of DIC is most commonly renal, hepatic and respiratory. Siegal et al.[58] in a survey of 118 patients, in whom a diagnosis of DIC was made, found that 64% had abnormal bleeding, 25% renal failure, 19% hepatic dysfunction and 16% respiratory failure. He found hepatic and renal failure to occur particularly with post-infective DIC and respiratory failure with post-traumatic DIC. In a number of studies specifically on injured patients the occurrence of DIC, diagnosed on laboratory criteria, correlated with clinical features of adult respiratory distress syndrome (ARDS)[8,22,55]. Clinical features of ARDS also correlated with microemboli found at autopsy[59]. Thus DIC should be suspected and appropriate laboratory tests performed whenever there is pathological bleeding, particularly diffuse bleeding, and whenever there is unexplained failure of the lungs, kidney or liver. Hypoxaemic, respiratory failure or radiological changes suggesting ARDS (Chapter 8) call for urgent consultation with the haematologist. Unfortunately, determining the cause of respiratory or renal failure in the ICU patient is often difficult and can be impossible with present techniques. Following trauma or surgery organ failure can be due to DIC alone or bacterial infection or toxaemia which themselves trigger off DIC. It is important to restate here that bacterial toxaemia can occur without clinical signs of infection or bacteraemia (Chapter 3).

(b) Haematological criteria

The laboratory criteria for the diagnosis of DIC are not straightforward and criteria which apply in all situations cannot be laid down. It is necessary to recognize patterns of laboratory results in an appropriate clinical setting. Interpretation should also take into consideration the effects of coexisting fibrinolysis, increased production of coagulation factors and the transfusion of stored blood. DIC may be diagnosed by demonstration of consumption of platelets and coagulation factors with evidence of fibrin breakdown, by turnover studies on platelets and fibrinogen, and by the response to heparin therapy.

(i) Consumption of clotting factors in DIC results in a prolongation of the PT and aPTT and reduction of specific clotting factors. In a recent analysis of 346 patients Spero *et al.*[62] found factors VII, X, II and V to be those most commonly reduced and the PT was more frequently prolonged than the aPTT. Factor VIII was reduced in only 9% of patients[62]. Reduction of factor VIII and fibrinogen is very significant when found but neither is a very sensitive indicator of DIC. This is because both are acute phase reactants whose synthesis is increased in many of the conditions in which DIC is found. Occasionally in DIC, coagulation tests (PT, aPTT and WBCT) are shortened rather than lengthened, due to activated clotting factors in the circulating blood. In severe consumption coagulopathy a gross prolongation of the PT, aPTT, TCT and WBCT may be found and the blood is virtually incoagulable. If heparin administration or contamination is excluded, these findings are virtually pathognomonic of DIC, and urgent fibrinogen and FDP estimation should be carried out. Thrombocytopenia is common in DIC, and was found by Spero to be a sensitive indicator[62]. The bleeding time is usually prolonged due to both thrombocytopenia and the inhibition of platelet function by FDPs. DIC is accompanied by the simultaneous activation of other systems, so that plasminogen, kininogen and complement fall. The generation of thrombin leads to the consumption of antithrombin III; Spero *et al.*[62] found a reduction to be a sensitive indicator of DIC.

Because fibrinolysis is commonly activated simultaneously with coagulation, fibrin degradation products (FDPs) are usually present in the serum in DIC; occasionally when fibrinolysis is inactive the levels may be low despite proven DIC. The TCT is a useful test in DIC since it is prolonged by a very low fibrinogen (less than 0.5 g/1) and/or by a significant elevation of FDPs. A direct estimation of FDPs may be readily performed by an immunological technique. The measurement should be performed whenever DIC is suspected, since an FDP titre of 40–80 μg/1 compatible with low grade DIC, causes only a slight prolongation of the TCT; a higher level will prolong it markedly.

(ii) Fibrinogen and platelet turnover studies using radioisotopic labels give reliable evidence of the markedly increased production and consumption which occur after injury, but do not distinguish appropriate consumption at the site of injury, from inappropriate DIC. If turnover is not reduced by heparin, as in some patients with uncomplicated burns, it can reasonably be inferred that DIC is absent[96]. If radioactive labelling is followed by surface counting over the lungs or other organs distant from the site of injury then the deposition of fibrinogen and platelets in these organs can be demonstrated[11,41]. These studies may also show the rapid dissolution of microemboli which is usually brought about by the fibrinolytic mechanisms[41]. Fibrinogen and platelet turnover studies have clearly demonstrated a striking overproduction which occurs following injury and have explained how patients can have DIC without a lowering of clotting factors.

(iii) It is important to distinguish DIC from primary fibrinogenolysis (usually referred to as primary fibrinolysis) which can be caused by liver disease, snake bite or cardiopulmonary bypass. In primary fibrinogenolysis all the coagulation factors which are consumed in DIC may be destroyed by proteolysis. Platelets, however, are not affected and thrombocytopenia suggests DIC rather than primary fibrinogenolysis. Unfortunately, the standard immunological tests for FDPs do not distinguish the degradation products of fibrin from those of fibrinogen. Tests for fibrin monomer have a theoretical advantage over tests for FDPs, since fibrin monomer is generated by the action of thrombin on fibrinogen. Unfortunately, many laboratories find these tests unhelpful. The ethanol gelation test commonly gives false negative results and the protamine paracoagulation test may give false positive results. Cryofibrinogen may be produced in DIC, but it is commonly absent. Tests for fibrinopeptide A (split off from fibrinogen by the action of thrombin) are useful in giving firm evidence of DIC, but unfortunately the tests are unsuitable for routine diagnosis purposes. Tests for D-dimer, a degradation product of cross-linked fibrin, have not yet been made sufficiently specific. The occurrence of a micro-angiopathic haemolytic anaemia (consequent on red cell damage by fibrin strands) occurs in DIC but not in primary fibrinolysis; however, it is only present in a minority of patients with DIC. The distinction between DIC with associated fibrinolysis, and primary fibrinolysis (strictly fibrinogenolysis) is of more than theoretical importance, since fibrinolytic inhibitors may be harmful in the former but are indicated in the latter. The relative frequency of DIC and primary fibrinolysis following cardiopulmonary bypass remains uncertain and controversial (III, 5), but in other clinical situations laboratory and clinical evidence now suggest that primary fibrinolysis is rare, and even patients in whom fibrinolysis appears dominant may also have DIC. Patients who were thought to have primary fibrinolysis have sometimes recovered with heparin therapy[63] and others have suffered tissue damage from microthrombi following the administration of epsilon-amino-caproic acid (EACA), an inhibitor of fibrinolysis[63,64]. EACA does not cause thrombosis when given to experimental animals in large doses and it appears likely that patients who have suffered from its administration have had DIC plus fibrinolysis rather than primary fibrinolysis.

(iv) The effects of massive transfusion of stored blood on coagulation tests must be considered. Stored blood is low in factors V and VIII and lacks viable platelets. Consequently patients who virtually have had an exchange transfusion will have a prolonged PT and aPTT and thrombo-cytopenia. However, if there is a prolongation of the TCT or a reduction of fibrinogen, factor II, or other stable factors, these findings suggest a complicating DIC. In this situation it is very useful to do a rapid fibrinogen assay. When coagulation tests show a further deterioration after the completion of transfusion this is good evidence of increased consumption.

(v) The ultimate validation of a diagnosis of DIC during life is the response to heparin. If stable or deteriorating laboratory tests are corrected by heparin therapy then the diagnosis is confirmed. Correction of laboratory parameters is often accompanied by the cessation of bleeding.

To summarize, the usual laboratory findings in DIC are: a reduction in the platelet count to less than $100 \times 10^9/l$; prolongation of the PT, aPTT and usually the TCT; a reduction in the fibrinogen level to 0.5–1.5 g/l or less; and elevation of the FDP level, usually to 20–80 mg/l or higher. Low levels of plasminogen and antithrombin III are usual. A rapid deterioration of the platelet count or fibrinogen level suggests DIC, since normally both have long half lives. Since no single laboratory test is always abnormal, strict criteria cannot be laid down and tests must be interpreted in the light of the usual findings in the underlying disease. Specific factor assays, other than a fibrinogen estimation, are often not immediately available but are not essential for a diagnosis. Knowledge of low levels of plasminogen and antithrombin III will often be available only in retrospect.

(c) Histological diagnosis

The histological diagnosis of DIC has mainly been of use in autopsy surveys, but occasionally it has been useful in confirming the diagnosis in living patients from a biopsy of skin lesions or kidney[61]. Histological diagnosis of DIC is made difficult by the simultaneous occurrence of increased fibrinolysis. The activation of Hageman Factor (factor XII) not only activates the coagulation cascade but also the fibrinolytic, complement and kinin systems. When fibrinolysis is very active the histological diagnosis of DIC may be difficult. Specific fibrin stains or even electron microscopy may be necessary to demonstrate fibrin[11]. It has been pointed out[11,20] that in experimental animals given thrombin or endotoxin, DIC severe enough to cause death but preventable by heparin can occur, yet at autopsy no thrombi are seen on light microscopy; electron microscopy, however, shows diffuse fibrin strands. Fibrin thrombi which have been present during life may have been lysed by the time death occurs[60]. Saldeen et al.[40] found fibrin in pulmonary vessels by the second day after injury, but it was rarely present for more than 10 days.

(4) Treatment

Treatment of DIC is indicated when there is evidence that either haemorrhage or microvascular obstruction are harming the patient. One or more of four treatments are possible.

(a) Prevention or removal of the precipitating factor

The most important factor in the management of DIC is the prevention or alleviation of the precipitating factors. Thus hypotension, hypovolaemia, hypothermia and acidosis should be prevented or alleviated. Manipulation of fractured and damaged limbs should be minimized but devitalized tissue should be removed. Infection should be treated. If the stimulus which initiated DIC has been removed and if there is no bleeding, then therapy is unnecessary. If the stimulus has been removed but the patient has haemorrhage or severe coagulation factor deficiencies, then replacement therapy is indicated. This is the case in patients who have suffered an episode of shock but have been resuscitated. If there is a continuing stimulus to DIC or evidence of associated pulmonary or renal dysfunction then replacement of coagulation factors and heparin are indicated.

(b) Coagulation factors

Coagulation factors are best replaced with fresh frozen plasma (FFP) and platelet concentrates. If haemorrhage requires transfusion, then fresh whole blood is given. The use of platelet concentrates has been discussed (I, 3b). FFP may be of either group AB or of the same group as the patient. FFP from Rh positive donors should not be given to Rh negative girls or women in the reproductive age range, as small amounts of contaminating red cell stroma can cause Rh immunization. Apart from this consideration, FFP may be given regardless of Rh group. The transfusion of FFP not only replaces deficient clotting factors, but also replaces antithrombin III which is consumed during DIC: low levels make further thrombosis more likely. Antithrombin III is also necessary for the action of heparin. A patient with DIC of sufficient severity to cause bleeding will usually require a minimum of two units of FFP and eight platelet concentrates. The use of fibrinogen is inadvisable as there have been reports of deterioration (probably due to thrombosis of renal vessels) after its administration[72]; it also has a high risk of transmission of hepatitis B and for this reason is no longer available in the USA. Fibrinogen is only indicated when there is exsanguinating haemorrhage together with gross hypofibrinogenaemia which is not corrected by FFP or fresh blood. Fibrinogen may also be replaced by infusing cryoprecipitate which contains factor VIII and about a third of the fibrinogen from the plasma. Because cryoprecipitate is obtained from a smaller number of donors the risk of hepatitis is less. During the first hour after major surgery or trauma fibrinolysis is active and replacement of clotting factors may be all that is required. Thereafter, a combination of DIC and inhibition of fibrinolysis makes tissue injury increasingly likely and heparin should be considered.

(c) Heparin

The use of heparin is controversial. Experimental evidence clearly indicates its efficacy. When given prior to the stimulus to DIC, heparin will prevent both consumption of coagulation factors and organ damage; its role once DIC is established is less clear cut. There is anecdotal evidence that heparin therapy will correct DIC and arrest haemorrhage with or without replacement of deficient factors[60,73-75] but there have been no controlled trials. The theoretical reasons for giving heparin are particularly strong in those patients who already have evidence of organ damage. The existence of a micro-angiopathic haemolytic anaemia indicates that microthrombi are not being rapidly lysed, so that organ damage is likely and heparin is therefore indicated. In my experience, heparin will often arrest a consumption coagulopathy and can be given with reasonable safety in injured and postoperative patients provided that it is given as a continuous infusion and controlled by laboratory tests. The dose required is that which will control the process; the lower end of the usual therapeutic range[76] is often satisfactory. Markedly thrombocytopenic patients tolerate less heparin than other patients. On the other hand, patients with enhanced coagulation may be heparin resistant. Suitable laboratory tests for the control of heparin therapy include the WBCT and the aPTT. The WBCT should be prolonged to two to three times the mean normal, since this range has been established by animal experiments[76]. The degree of prolongation of the aPTT required depends on the sensitivity to heparin of the individual reagent, and varies from 1.3 to 1.8 times the mean normal for an insensitive reagent to 2.0–3.5 for a sensitive reagent[76]; it follows that each laboratory must know the sensitivity of its aPTT reagent and must establish the therapeutic range accordingly. Some laboratories successfully use the TCT for heparin control, but many consider that its exponential lengthening with increasing heparin level makes it unsuitable. Heparin level may be used, but in general it does not appear to have any advantages over the simpler and less expensive aPTT. It may, in fact, be preferable to use a test which assesses the effect of heparin on a patient's coagulation status rather than the heparin level. In the patient with DIC a problem may arise if the test used for heparin control is grossly prolonged prior to therapy because of the depletion of coagulation factors. In this circumstance it is possible to distinguish an undesirable prolongation due to factor depletion from a desirable prolongation due to heparin by the fact that the latter is reversed by the addition of protamine sulphate or toluidine blue to the sample. The determination of heparin level is also useful in this specific circumstance, a level of approximately 0.2–0.6 units/ml being desirable. The most practical procedure is to start with an infusion rate of 750–1000 units/hour and increase the dose if DIC is not corrected and if heparin effect is not shown in laboratory tests. Laboratory tests should be used to prevent excessive dosage; if tests are below the usual therapeutic range the dose should be increased if DIC is continuing, but if a beneficial effect has been seen, no dosage change is necessary.

Successful therapy results in a rise of fibrinogen and platelets and a fall of the FDP titre. The PT, aPTT and TCT are less helpful, since they are usually prolonged by the heparin. FDP titres usually fall within 12–24 hours and fibrinogen rises towards normal in the same period; the platelet count may take several days to return to normal. Laboratory tests are not straightforward in the patient receiving heparin for DIC. It is important that the fibrinogen method is one which is not affected by heparin and that the specimen for FDP testing has been thoroughly clotted. The addition of reptilase to the FDP tube is much more reliable in achieving adequate clotting than the addition of thrombin.

(d) Fibrinolytic inhibitors

Infusion of inhibitors of fibrinolysis (EACA or tranexamic acid) is contraindicated in DIC. In experimental animals they are clearly detrimental, increasing tissue damage[77] and mortality[11]. Conversely, plasmin decreases the mortality of DIC in experimental animals[11]. In man, the administration of EACA has been associated with glomerular thrombosis and renal cortical necrosis[63] and may aggravate the respiratory distress syndrome[59]. The use of EACA might be justified when life-threatening haemorrhage due to DIC cannot be controlled by any other measures.

(III) SPECIFIC PROBLEMS

(1) Bacterial infection and toxaemia

These can cause a hypercoagulable state of the blood. Fibrinogen and factors V and VIII are both acute phase reactants and are commonly elevated not only in bacteraemia[78] but also in focal infections such as acute cholecystitis[79]. The clotting time may be shortened[80], thrombocytosis may occur[81] and platelet adhesiveness may be increased[79]. In addition to provoking a hypercoagulable state, infection or toxaemia can trigger DIC. DIC is seen in both gram-negative and gram-positive infections but the pathogenesis is more clearly understood in gram-negative infections. Injection of purified endotoxin in man causes a fall of platelets and factors V and VIII [82]. Endotoxin may directly activate factor XII [72] thereby also activating the kinin and complement systems. The fall of factor VII in dogs given endotoxin and the partial protection by factor VII deficiency, indicates that coagulation is induced, at least in part, through the extrinsic pathway. The necessary tissue factor activity could originate from damaged endothelial cells or leukocytes[83]. Exposure of monocytes to endotoxin[84] or to C3b and immune complexes[85] stimulates coagulant activity which is identical to tissue factor on several criteria. Endotoxin, bacterial cell walls and antigen–antibody complexes all cause endothelial cell damage[86]. Antigen-antibody complexes with an excess of antigen can shorten the silicone clotting time, the effect being mediated through cellular elements[13]. Endotoxin induces platelet aggregation in rabbits and rats; this does not occur with human platelets, but a release reaction may be induced[87,88]. In 'septic shock', stasis and acidosis are further potent stimuli to coagulation; there is a strong association between septic shock and DIC[78,89]. Release of catecholamines and histamine are further aggravating factors, as is blockade of the reticuloendothelial system (RES).

Septic shock with DIC may be the primary reason for admission to an ICU. More commonly, infection complicates injury, burns or surgery. Following trauma, DIC may herald subsequent infection[55]. Indeed DIC, by inducing RES blockade may be a causative factor. In addition, infection in a traumatized or burnt patient is a common cause of a second episode of DIC. In addition to specific treatment of the infection, correction of hypotension and acidosis are important. Corticosteroids in one or two large bolus doses (e.g. methylprednisolone 15 mg/kg) may be beneficial by limiting endothelial damage. In patients with gram-negative sepsis, it is logical to administer the drug at the same time as commencing antibiotics. In this way the damaging effects of endotoxin may be reduced. However, in man the value of steroid therapy in septic shock remains controversial and although advocated by Schumer (Chapter 5) others remain sceptical. Likewise, the use of heparin remains controversial. Heparin is indicated when DIC persists after treating the causative factors and when there is organ failure, and is given with replacement factors when there is life-threatening haemorrhage. If infection persists it can be difficult to prevent DIC with heparin.

(2) Burns

A large consumption of coagulation factors and platelets occurs in the burnt areas, and coagulation factors also diffuse into the burn with the other plasma proteins. Thrombocytopenia occurs early and parallel changes occur in factors I, V and VIII[90]. A hypercoagulable state exists. In rats the PT aPTT and TCT shorten significantly[91]. Platelet aggregates occur[90] and thromboplastic substances released from burnt tissues lead to DIC. Microthrombi can be found in tissues remote from the burn, including the skin and lung[92,93] and extensive pulmonary microembolism can cause a fatal respiratory failure similar to the respiratory distress syndrome[94]. Cerebral dysfunction may also result from microembolism. If infection occurs the consumption coagulopathy is worsened[90] and the platelet count falls further. McManus et al.[93] found clinically significant DIC in five out of 274 patients and all five had infection. Changes in fibrinolysis are similar to those which follow trauma. Initially, there is a hyperactive fibrinolysis with rapid destruction of [^{125}I]plasminogen[62]. Subsequently, plasminogen is severely depressed[95]. Platelet and fibrinogen production are increased up to threefold[96]. During the phase when consumption is greater than production, the platelet count and the levels of clotting factors rise with a risk of thromboembolism. Heparin is indicated in burnt patients who develop DIC, particularly when there is respiratory or renal failure. Heparin has only slight beneficial effects on the overall consumption of platelets and fibrinogen[96].

(3) Massive transfusion of stored blood

A definition of massive transfusion is arbitrary, but this term is commonly used when 5 litres or 1.0–1.5 times the patient's estimated blood volume have been transfused during 24 hours. When more than 48 hours old, stored blood has few viable platelets. There is a progressive fall in labile coagulation factors; factor VIII falls exponentially to approximately 15% at 7 days and to 9% at 3 weeks; factor V falls more slowly to approximately 60% at 1 week and 35% at 3 weeks[56]. Massive transfusion with stored blood could therefore be expected to cause a reduction in both platelets and factors V and VIII. However, this reduction is ameliorated by an increased production of factor VIII and of platelets which commences soon after injury and during an acute illness. There is a weak correlation between the levels of factors V and VIII and the number of units transfused[56,97]. Thus patients transfused more than 10 units of blood in 24 hours can have factor VIII levels of three times normal. A fall of platelets is more common[7, 56, 57, 97] and does correlate with the number of units transfused[56]. However, the fall is less than would be expected if platelet production were unchanged[57]; in one study the platelet count was infrequently lowered by transfusions large enough to replace the blood volume[10]. Abnormal platelet function can follow massive transfusion[97]. Following massive transfusions there is often an element of DIC, in addition to dilution of the clotting factors. The coagulation defects are related to both the size of the transfusion and to the presence or absence of shock. Thus Wilson et al.[98] found that the coagulation defects correlated better with the presence of shock than with the volume of blood transfused. Harke and Rahman[99] compared five groups of patients who had been transfused 11–14 litres of blood, but in whom the duration of shock varied from 0 to 5 hours. They found that following transient shock, factor V activity was increased and the aPTT was shortened. When shock was prolonged there was prolongation of the aPTT, the clotting factors and platelets were reduced and platelet function was impaired. A finding of a low fibrinogen is good evidence of DIC in the massively transfused patient, since fibrinogen is stable in stored blood.

In the absence of DIC, pathological bleeding due to the dilutional effect only occurs when 15–20 units have been transfused[56,57]. When more than 5 l are given in 1–2 hours pathological bleeding due to dilution can be prevented by including some 'fresh blood' (blood less than 24–48 hours old). This policy will mean that some patients will be given fresh blood who would not have developed pathological bleeding despite marked laboratory abnormalities. If supplies allow, this preventive approach is preferable. An alternative policy is to reserve fresh blood or platelet concentrates for those who develop pathological bleeding. Some centres have used 'fresh warm blood'[100] but it is not clear that this has any advantages over blood less than 24 hours old. Replacement of platelets is more important than replacement of coagulation factors, as bleeding often stops with platelet concentrate alone, whereas fresh frozen plasma alone is usually ineffective[57,97]. In postoperative or traumatized patients a platelet count of $100 \times 10^9/1$ may be necessary to stop pathological bleeding where in non-traumatized patients $60 \times 10^9/1$ or even less is adequate.

(4) Blood salvage and intraoperative autotransfusion

Intraoperative autotransfusion has the potential advantage of transfusing fresh warm blood which has adequate platelets and labile coagulation factors. This advantage may be offset when activated clotting factors are present and it has even been suggested that autotransfusion may cause a coagulopathy. It is difficult to be certain of this since the conditions in which autotransfusion are used often cause consumption coagulopathy. The likelihood of infusing tissue thromboplastin and activated clotting factors should be reduced to a minimum by collecting blood only when there is free flow. If washed cells rather than whole blood are infused the risks are less, but dilution of coagulation factors may then occur. Patients admitted to the ICU following intraoperative autotransfusion are likely to develop the same range of coagulation defects as do injured patients and should be treated similarly.

(5) Cardiopulmonary bypass

Coagulation anomalies are common after cardiopulmonary bypass. Detailed coagulation studies are necessary in order to decide whether haemorrhage is surgical or due to coagulopathy and then determine the type of defect and also to indicate that reoperation is needed when no coagulation defect of sufficient severity to cause pathological bleeding is found.

(a) Excessive heparin effect

This may be due either to a failure to neutralize heparin adequately or to heparin 'rebound'. Both cause prolongation of the WBCT, which is reversed by protamine. A protamine titration test will determine the dose of protamine required for adequate reversal. Heparin rebound is seen 2–8 hours after the initial protamine neutralization[101,102] and is probably caused by protamine being metabolized more rapidly than heparin. It is less likely to occur when protamine chloride, which is more slowly metabolized than the sulphate, is used[101]. Heparin rebound is less common when large doses of protamine are used[101]. Excessive heparin effect and heparin rebound are less likely when heparin dosage is kept low by intraoperative monitoring by tests such as the protamine titration test, celite activated clotting time, whole blood activated recalcification time (BART) or activated clotting time (ACT)[103]. Heparin rebound may or may not cause recurrent haemorrhage[101]. Excessive heparin effect may be seen during prolonged hypothermic bypass[104]. Excess protamine dosage does not cause a clinically significant coagulation defect[105]; there is a transient and slight increase in the WBCT.

(b) DIC and activation of fibrinolysis

These are common after cardiopulmonary bypass, a consequence of contact of the blood with artificial surfaces and gases. There is a fall of platelets and factor V and a smaller reduction in fibrinogen and factor VIII. Fibrin monomer may be detected and FDPs can increase. When heparinization is inadequate, consumption of coagulation factors is more marked. Following protamine neutralization the underlying hypercoagulable state may be revealed. The WBCT, aPTT and TCT are shortened and a fall of platelets and fibrinogen may occur[106,107]. Overt DIC may complicate a profound fall of cardiac output after bypass[73]. Fibrinolysis is activated prior to bypass or early during bypass; the ECLT shortens, plasminogen activator increases, free plasmin appears, and plasminogen falls. In some studies fibrinolysis was no longer excessive at the end of the bypass[21,109] but in others it remained excessive and even persisted for 60–90 minutes after bypass[110,111]. It is difficult to determine how much of the coagulopathy is attributable to primary fibrinolysis, and how much to DIC with secondary fibrinolysis. The failure to detect fibrin monomer in some studies[110] and the normal, or near normal, antithrombin III levels favour primary fibrinolysis. A coagulation defect, which is less when larger doses of heparin are used[112]; the further fall in fibrinogen and platelets which can follow protamine neutralization, and the shortening of coagulation times all point to DIC. It is likely that the degree of activation of fibrinolysis, and the relative contributions of DIC and primary fibrinolysis vary considerably according to the perfusion techniques and equipment used.

DIC will usually correct spontaneously, but, when severe, heparin and replacement of coagulation factors are necessary. Inhibitors of fibrinolysis should not be given blindly since they can be harmful in those with DIC and their empirical use may have increased rather than decreased the blood loss[110]. In one study there was no correlation between blood loss and either the intensity or duration of increased fibrinolysis[111]. However, should patients with pathological bleeding have increased fibrinolysis demonstrated by laboratory tests, then EACA is indicated.

(c) Defective platelet function

This is probably invariable at the end of bypass. The bleeding time is often prolonged out of proportion to the degree of thrombocytopenia. Platelet retention *in vitro* is reduced[21], clot retraction is defective[106]. ADP-induced-aggregation is defective[21,107,108] and aggregation induced by collagen or adrenaline can also be reduced[21,107]. Defective platelet function is due to platelet activation on artificial surfaces and to exposure to thromboplastic substances or ADP released from damaged leukocytes and red cells. The fall in platelets is less and platelet function is better in patients given dipyridamole[107]. Large platelets, which would be expected to be haemostatically most effective, disappear preferentially during bypass[113]. Damaged platelets may be temporarily sequestered in the liver[108]. Platelets provided by transfused blood are non-viable unless the blood is less than 48 hours old.

If haemorrhage occurs and the bleeding time is prolonged, then either fresh blood or platelet concentrates are infused. The collection of fresh autologous blood prior to bypass for reinfusion after bypass may help to circumvent this problem. Hallowell *et al.*[114] and Oschner *et al.*[115] used profound haemodilution and then infused fresh autologous blood; the transfusion requirements were then markedly reduced. In contrast, Pliam *et al.*[116] used bank blood during bypass thus avoiding extreme haemodilution and infused fresh autologous blood at the end of operation; the transfusion requirements were not affected. Intraoperative haemodilution may itself be beneficial, possibly due to improved microcirculation; Bø[117] found the fall of platelet count, reduction in platelet adhesiveness and the operative blood loss were improved during deliberate haemodilution.

(d) Impaired liver function

This causes prolongation of the prothrombin time and depression of factor V as well as the vitamin K dependent factors II, VII, IX, and X. Fresh frozen plasma is given for bleeding due to deficiency of these factors. A prolongation of the PT due to an inhibitor similar to PIVKA was noted by Bachmann *et al.*[106] but was not associated with bleeding.

(6) Adverse reactions to heparin

Heparinized patients may bleed from therapeutic doses, such bleeding being commoner in the injured, in the elderly (particularly elderly women) and in patients who have other factors adversely affecting haemostasis, such as uraemia or aspirin administration. Heparinized patients can also develop thrombocytopenia and, paradoxically, arterial thrombosis. This appears to have an immune basis, since the responsible factor is in the immunoglobulin fraction and the appearance of thrombocytopenia is accelerated on a second exposure[118]. It may occur with heparin of either bovine or porcine origin and with low doses given prophylactically as well as during full dose therapy[119]. The incidence of thrombocytopenia has been variously estimated between 2%[120] and 31%[121]; my own observations are more in accord with the former. The incidence of arterial thrombosis is a great deal less than that of thrombocytopenia. The thrombi are of the white type and may contain fibrin as well as platelets. Since thrombocytopenia is common in critically ill patients it is necessary to establish that the thrombocytopenia is due to heparin. This can be done by demonstrating a factor in the patient's serum which causes aggregation of normal platelets in the presence of heparin[118]. Recognition of this rare syndrome of thrombocytopenia with arterial thrombosis is important, as delay may lead to gangrene requiring amputation. Management is by the substitution of dextran and warfarin for heparin. Protamine has been advised since this may reverse platelet aggregation[122] but should not be given unless there is ischaemia.

(7) Dextrans and other plasma expanders

Dextrans can produce a coagulation defect which is more severe, the higher the molecular weight of the dextran or the larger the amount given. Platelet adhesiveness[4,123], aggregation[123], and platelet factor 3 availability[123] are all reduced and the bleeding time is prolonged[124]. The factor VIII molecule may be altered in such a way that an acquired von Willebrand's disease develops with a prolonged bleeding time and reduction in the following: platelet adhesiveness, factor VIII related antigen, factor VIII related-ristocetin-co-factor[125,126]. A haemorrhagic diathesis is rare after average infusions of dextrans of low or medium molecular weight, but a patient has been reported who developed acquired von Willebrand's disease following 500 ml of dextran 40, given 6 hourly[126]. With dextrans of high molecular weight there is good evidence that DIC can occur both in the experimental animal and in man[124,127]. Dextran infusions may add to other coagulation defects. The toxic effects of other plasma expanders have been reviewed by Rudowski[128]. Hydroxyethylstarch can coat platelets and cause a prolongation of the bleeding time, and decrease coagulation factors, thus prolonging the prothrombin time. Adverse effects have not been noted after the use of plasma substitutes derived from gelatine (Haemacel, Gelofusin).

(8) Coagulation changes following haemoperfusion

Haemoperfusion for the removal of drugs and other toxins may employ charcoal or exchange resins. Uncoated activated charcoal causes a profound loss of platelets and adsorption of coagulation factors. The loss of platelets and coagulation factors is much less when coated charcoal is used. Exchange resins may cause an even smaller reduction in platelets[129]. The use of prostacyclin in addition to heparin will markedly lessen the loss of platelets[130]. Prostacyclin is a potent inhibitor of platelet aggregation but its effects are rapidly reversible at the end of infusion; the drug is not yet generally available. Pathological bleeding following charcoal perfusion requires assessment for persisting heparin, platelet count and function, and the level of coagulation factors. If the PT and aPTT are essentially normal when protamine is added *in vitro* then coagulation factor levels are adequate. The treatment consists of protamine, transfusion of platelet concentrates or fresh frozen plasma, depending on the defect present.

(9) Thromboembolism

Because of the hypercoagulable state and immobilization, thromboembolism is a major risk in intensive care patients. In postoperative patients, prophylactic heparin, either sodium heparin or calcium heparin, in a dose of 5000 units subcutaneously, 8 or 12 hourly, has been found efficacious[131]. Heparin in this dose is effective if given prophylactically as it inhibits activated factor X (factor Xa) by potentiation of antithrombin III. If thrombosis has already occurred and thrombin has been generated, then much larger doses are required. In both traumatized and postoperative patients, it is logical to use prophylactic heparin from the time of admission to the ICU. However, it may be that in traumatized patients the stimulus to thrombosis is too great for prophylactic heparin to produce a useful reduction in thromboembolism[132]. Possible future approaches to the prophylaxis of pulmonary embolism and deep vein thrombosis are the combination of heparin with lignocaine or dihydroergotamine, or the infusion of antithrombin III when levels are reduced.

In established thromboembolic disease full dose heparin is required, and in the critically ill or injured patient is best given by a continuous infusion controlled by laboratory tests. A loading dose should be given, as otherwise it may take up to five half-lives of heparin for a stable state to be reached[133]. A larger dose is required in pulmonary embolism than in venous thrombosis[134]. Suitable loading doses in patients of average weight are 5000 units for venous thrombosis and 10 000 units for pulmonary embolism or 10–15 U/kg and 25 U/kg respectively. An infusion of 1000 units or more per hour is then started and after 3–4 hours a laboratory test is performed to determine whether enough is being given. The aPTT has been found to be a suitable test; the degree of anticoagulation required is that equivalent to a two to threefold prolongation of the whole blood clotting time[76]. When necessary the heparin dose should be progressively increased until the tests show that an adequate effect has been achieved. Intensive care patients often require very large doses, sometimes as much as 5000 U/h. The heparin requirements can vary from day to day so that laboratory tests need to be performed at least once daily. Variable effects are due to the presence of activated clotting factors, to variations in the levels of platelet factor 4 (which has an antiheparin effect) and to falling levels of antithrombin III (by which heparin mediates its effect). Heparin can be administered in normal saline, dextrose or any similar infusion fluid; fears that heparin was inactivated in weakly acidic solutions have not been substantiated. Heparin should be continued for 7 to 10 days, because this is the length of time required for a thrombus to become adherent to the vein wall. If the patient is in a stable state and further surgery is unlikely then the treatment should be converted to an oral anticoagulant. There should be an overlap of 2 or 3 days of oral anticoagulant and heparin to allow time for factors IX and X to fall before the heparin is stopped. During the first one to two days after commencing the oral anticoagulant, prolongation of the PT is due predominantly to lowering of factor VII. The antithrombotic effect of reducing factor VII is not as great as when factors IX and X are also reduced. During heparin therapy, antithrombin III levels fall significantly. This causes an increased risk of thrombosis immediately after stopping the heparin unless the clotting factors have been lowered.

(10) Renal failure

Acute renal failure is common in critically ill patients. The major effect of renal failure on coagulation is an inhibition of platelet function and a prolongation of the bleeding time by a factor in the plasma; dialysis may shorten the bleeding time although it does not do so consistently. Haemodialysis causes a temporary drop in the platelet count but this does not occur with peritoneal dialysis. Uraemic patients also have an increase of all factor VIII activities; factor VIII clotting activity and factor VIII antigen are increased more than Von Willebrand's factor activity; no clinical implications of these alterations are known. If uraemic patients are given penicillin in high doses further inhibition of platelet function occurs, and if blood levels of penicillin are sufficiently high, a heparin-like effect is seen, with inhibition of factor Xa and thrombin[33]. Protamine infusion will reverse the bleeding diathesis due to the heparin-like activity of the penicillins[33].

(11) Hepatic failure

Acute liver failure is not uncommon in critically ill patients. Chronic liver failure may also be seen in the ICU, particularly when patients with cirrhosis require admission because of uncontrolled bleeding. The coagulation derangements are similar in acute and chronic liver failure. All factors with the exception of factor VIII are likely to be reduced, but factor V followed by the vitamin K dependent factors (factors II, VII, IX and X) are often the first affected. The vitamin K dependent factors will also be reduced in patients with obstructive jaundice, and occasionally in malnourished patients who are on antibiotics. Fibrinogen is reduced to levels likely to cause bleeding only in very severe liver disease. An acquired dysfibrinogenaemia with prolongation of the TCT is common. An element of DIC may be present. In patients with cirrhosis, thrombocytopenia consequent on splenomegaly often coexists with coagulation factor deficiencies.

Patients with abnormal coagulation tests consequent on liver failure should be given vitamin K_1 10 mg slowly i.v. This frequently causes some improvement of coagulation tests, even when biliary obstruction or cholestasis do not appear to be features. If bleeding occurs, coagulation factors should be replaced with fresh frozen plasma. A concentrate of factors II, IX and X with or without factor VII is also available and may be used if fresh frozen plasma does not achieve significant correction. Such concentrates have caused abnormal clotting in patients with liver disease, a complication attributable to the presence of activated clotting factors and the defective clearing mechanisms of the patient with liver failure; these concentrates should be used with caution. In general fibrinogen is not indicated. Platelet concentrates are of little benefit in patients with portal hypertension and splenomegaly since many of the transfused platelets are trapped in the spleen. However, if there is thrombocytopenia, a prolonged bleeding time and pathological bleeding, then platelet concentrates are indicated and larger numbers will be required than in the patient without splenomegaly. In the bleeding patient with liver failure transfusion of stored blood can aggravate the clotting defect. When fresh blood is available then this should be given as part of the transfusion requirements.

CONCLUSION

The coagulation anomalies of the critically ill patient are complex. The haematologist and the director of the blood transfusion service are important colleagues of the ICU staff and a close working relationship may be vital to the welfare of the patient. The haematologist can only offer the best advice when fully informed of the clinical features and provided with suitable samples for laboratory study. Bedside consultation often increases the understanding of all concerned, to the ultimate benefit of the patient.

References

1. Wessler, S. and Yin, E. T. (1974). Role of animal models in thrombosis: a point of departure. *Thromb. Diath. Haemorrh.*, **59**, (Suppl.), 83
2. Gulliver, G. (1846). *The Works of William Hewson FRS*, p. 46. (London: Sydenham Society)
3. Turpini, R. and Stefanini, M. (1959). The nature and mechanism of the hemostatic breakdown in the course of experimental hemorrhagic shock. *J. Clin. Invest.*, **38**, 53
4. Bergentz, S. (1976). On bleeding and clotting problems in post-traumatic states. *Crit. Care Med.*, **4**, 41
5. Innes, D. and Sevitt, S. (1964). Coagulation and fibrinolysis in injured patients. *J. Clin. Pathol.*, **17**, 1
6. Scott, R. and Crosby, W. H. (1954). Changes in the coagulation mechanism following wounding and resuscitation with stored blood. A study of battle casualties in Korea. *Blood*, **9**, 609
7. Simmons, R. L., Collins, J. A., Heisterkamp, C. A., Mills, D. E., Andren, R. and Phillips, L. L. (1969). Coagulation disorders in combat casualties. I. Acute changes after wounding. II. Effects of massive transfusion. III. Post-resuscitative changes. *Ann. Surg.*, **169**, 455
8. Avikainen, V. (1977). Coagulation disorders in severely and critically injured patients. *Ann. Chir. Gynaecol.*, **66**, 269
9. Bradford, D. S., Foster, R. R. and Nossel, H. L. (1970). Coagulation alterations, hypoxaemia, and fat embolism in fracture patients. *J. Trauma*, **10**, 307
10. Crosby, W. H. and Howard, J. M. (1954). The hematologic response to wounding and resuscitation accomplished by large transfusions of stored blood. A study of battle casualties in Korea. *Blood*, **9**, 439

11. McKay, D. G. (1979). Trauma and disseminated intravascular coagulation. *J. Trauma*, **9**, 646

12. Slichter, S. J., Funk, D. D., Leandoer, L. E. and Harker, L. A. (1974). Kinetic evaluation of haemostasis during surgery and wound healing. *Br. J. Haematol.*, **27**, 115

13. Hardaway, R. M. (1966). *Syndromes of Disseminated Intravascular Coagulation*. (Springfield: Charles C. Thomas)

14. Ingram, G .I .C., Jones, R. V., Hershgold, E. J., Denson, K. W. E. and Perkins, J. R. (1977). Factor VIII activity and antigen, platelet count and biochemical changes after adrenocortical stimulation. *Br. J. Haematol.*, **35**, 81

15. Hardaway, R. M., Johnson, D. G., Houchin, D. N., Jenkins, E. B., Burns, J. W. and Jackson, D. R. (1964). Influence of stress on fibrinogen. *J. Trauma*, **4**, 673

16. Warner, W. A. (1969). Release of free fatty acids following trauma. *J. Trauma*, **9**, 692

17. Modig, J., Hedstrand, U., Fischer, J. and Lundstrom, J. (1976). Early recognition and treatment of post-traumatic pulmonary microembolism. *Crit. Care Med.*, **4**, 180

18. Fearnley, G. R. (1964). Measurement of spontaneous fibrinolytic activity. *J. Clin. Pathol.*, **17**, 316

19. Borowiecki, B. and Sharp, A. A. (1969). Trauma and fibrinolysis *J. Trauma*, **9**, 522

20. Attar, S., Hanashiro, P., Mansbergen, A., McLaughlin, J., Firminger, H. and Cowley, R. A. (1970). Intravascular coagulation – reality or myth. *Surgery*, **68**, 27

21. Moriau, M., Masure, R., Hurlet, A., Debeys, C., Chalant, C., Ponlot, R., Jaumain, P., Servaye-Kestens, Y., Ravaux, A., Louis, A. and Goenen, M. (1977). Hemostasis disorders in open heart surgery with extracorporeal circulation. Importance of the platelet function and heparin neutralization *Vox Sang.*, **32**, 41

22. String, T., Robinson, J. and Blaisdell, F. W. (1971). Massive trauma. Effect of intravascular coagulation on prognosis. *Arch. Surg.* **102**, 406

23. Lilienberg, G., Rammer, L., Saldeen, T., Thorin, L. and Uddströmer, L. (1970). Intravascular coagulation and inhibition of fibrinolysis and fat embolism. *Acta Chir. Scand.*, **136**, 87

24. Bagge, L. and Saldeen, S. (1978). The primary fibrinolysis inhibitor and trauma. *Thromb. Res.*, **13**, 1131

25. Kunz, F., Hortnagl, H., Kroesen, G. and Rumpl, E. (1978). Plasma lipids, coagulation factors and fibrin formation after severe multiple trauma, and in adult respiratory distress syndrome. *J. Trauma*, **18**, 115

26. Wardrop, C. A. J., Heatley, R. V., Tennant, G. B. and Hughes, L. E. (1975). Acute folate deficiency in surgical patients on amino acid/ethanol intravenous nutrition. *Lancet*, **2**, 640

27. Blackwell, E. A., Hawson, G. A. T., Leer, J. and Bain, B. J. (1978). Acute pancytopenia due to megaloblastic arrest in association with cotrimoxazole. *Med. J. Aust.* **2**, 38

28. Ibbotson, R. M., Colvin, B. T. and Colvin, M. P. (1975). Folic acid deficiency during intensive therapy. *Br. Med. J.,* **2**, 145

29. Amess, J. A. L., Burman, J. F., Rees, G. M., Nancekievill, D. G. and Mollin, D. G. (1978). Megaloblastic haemopoiesis in patients receiving nitrous oxide. *Lancet*, **2**, 339

30. Lassen, H. C. A., Henriksen, E., Neukirch, F. and Kristensen, H. S. (1956). Treatments of tetanus. Severe bone-marrow depression after prolonged nitrous oxide anaesthesia. *Lancet*, **1**, 527

31. Linnell, J. C., Quadros, E. V., Matthews, D. M., Jackson, B. and Hoffbrand, A. V. (1978). Nitrous oxide and megaloblastosis: biochemical mechanism. *Lancet*, **2**, 1372

32. Brown, C., Natelson, E., Bradshaw, M., Williams, T. and Alfrey, C. (1974). The hemostatic defect produced by carbenicillin. *N. Engl. J. Med.* **291**, 265

33. Andrassy, K., Weishchedel, E., Ritz, E. and Andrassy, T. (1976). Bleeding in uraemic patients after carbenicillin. *Thromb. Haemost.* **36**, 115

34. Andrassy, K., Ritz, E., Hasper, B., Scherz, M., Walter, E., Storch, H. and Vomel, W. (1976). Penicillin induced coagulation disorder. *Lancet*, **2**, 1039

35. Cazenave, J. P., Reimers, H. J., Senyi, A. F., Hirsh, J., Packham, M. A. and Mustard, J. F. (1976). Effects of penicillin G and cephalothin on platelet function *in vivo*. *Proc. Soc. Exp. Biol. Med.*, **152**, 641

36. Allen, F. B., Girson, J. I. and Davey, F. R. (1979). Platelet inhibition by nitroprusside and nitroglycerin. *Anesthesiology* **51** (Suppl.), 75

37. Atik, M. and Matini, K. (1972). Platelet dysfunction: an important factor in massive bleeding from stress ulcer. *J. Trauma*, **12**, 834

38. Bengmark, S., Hafstrom, L. O. and Korsan-Bengtsen, K. (1969). Effects on blood clotting and circulation of autologous connective tissue homogenate infusion in dogs. *J. Trauma*, **9**, 236

39. Saldeen, T. (1970). The importance of intravascular coagulation and inhibition of the fibrinolytic system in experimental fat embolism. *J. Trauma*, **10**, 287

40. Saldeen, T. (1970). Fat embolism and signs of intravascular coagulation in a post-traumatic autopsy material. *J. Trauma*, **10**, 273

41. Modig, J. (1977). Post-traumatic pulmonary microembolism. Pathophysiology and treatment. *Ann. Clin. Res.*, **9**, 164

42. Gamain, J., Bernard, F., Ossart, M., Legars, D. and Delcour, J. (1974). Consumption coagulopathy in cranial trauma. *N. Presse Med.*, **3**, 259

43. Berman, J. R., Smulson, M. E., Pattengale, P. and Schoenbach, S. F. (1971). Pulmonary microembolism after soft tissue injury in primates. *Surgery*, **70**, 246

44. Peer, R. M. and Schwartz, S. I. (1975). Development and treatment of post-traumatic pulmonary platelet trapping. *Ann. Surg.*, **181**, 447

45. Heideman, M., Kaijser, B. and Gelin, L. (1978). Complement activation and hematologic, hemodynamic and respiratory reactions early after soft tissue injury. *J. Trauma*, **18**, 696

46. Connell, R. S., Swank, R. L. and Webb, M. C. (1975). The development of pulmonary ultrastructural lesions during hemorrhagic shock. *J. Trauma*, **15**, 116

47. Whitaker, A. N., McKay, D. G. and Csavossy, J. (1969). Studies of catecholamine shock. I. Disseminated intravascular coagulation. *Am. J. Pathol.*, **56**, 153

48. Mehta, B., Briggs, D. K., Sommers, S. C. and Karpatkin, M. (1972).

Disseminated intravascular coagulation following cardiac arrest: a study of 15 patients. *Am. J. Med. Sci.*, **264**, 353

49. Latour, T. G., McKay, D. G. and Parrish, M. H. (1972). Activation of Hageman factor by cardiac arrest. *Throm. Diath. Haemorrh.*, **27**, 543
50. Hardaway, R. M., Johnson, D. G., Elovitz, M. J., Houchin, D. N., Jenkins, E. B., Burns, J. W. and Jackson, D. R. (1964). Influence of trauma and hemolysis on hemorrhage shock in dogs. *J. Trauma*, **4**, 624
51. Birndorf, N. I., Lopas, H. and Robboy, S. J. (1971). Disseminated intravascular coagulation and renal failure. Production in the monkey with autologous red blood cell stroma. *Lab. Invest.*, **25**, 314
52. Riedler, G., Frick, P. G. and Straub, P. W. (1968). The effect of acute intravascular haemolysis on coagulation and fibrinolysis. I. Near-drowning haemoglobinaemia. *Helv. Med. Acta*, **34**, 205
53. Golden, F. St. C. (1980). Problems of immersion. *Br. J. Hosp. Med.*, **23**, 371
54. Kwaan, H. C., Anderson, M. C. and Gramatica, L. (1971). A study of pancreatic enzymes as a factor in the pathogenesis of disseminated intravascular coagulation during acute pancreatitis. *Surgery*, **69**, 663
55. Effeney, D. J., Blaisdell, F. W., McIntyre, K. and Graziano, C. J. (1978). The relationship between sepsis and disseminated intravascular coagulation. *J. Trauma*, **78**, 689
56. Counts, R. B., Haish, C., Simon, T. L., Maxwell, N. G., Heinbach, D. M. and Carrico, C. J. (1979). Hemostasis in massively transfused trauma patients. *Ann. Surg.*, **190**, 91
57. Miller, R. D., Robbins, T. O., Tong, M. J. and Barton, S. L. (1971). Coagulation defects associated with massive blood transfusions. *Ann. Surg.*, **174**, 794
58. Siegal, T., Seligsohn, U., Aghai, E. and Moden, M. (1978). Clinical and laboratory aspects of disseminated intravascular coagulation (DIC): A study of 118 cases. *Thromb. Haemostas.*, **39**, 122
59. Lindquist, O., Rammer, L. and Saldeen, T. (1972). Pulmonary insufficiency, microembolism and fibrinolysis inhibition in a post-traumatic autopsy material. *Acta Chir. Scand.*, **138**, 545
60. Cafferata, H. T., Aggeler, P. M., Robinson, A. J. and Blaisdell, F. W. (1969). Intravascular coagulation in the surgical patient. Its significance and diagnosis. *Am. J. Surg.*, **118**, 281
61. Curreri, P. W., Katz, A. J., Dotin, L. N. and Pruitt, B. A. (1970). Coagulation abnormalities in the thermally injured patient. *Curr. Top. Surg. Res.*, **2**, 401
62. Spero, J. A., Lewis, J. H. and Hasiby, U. (1980). Disseminated intravascular coagulation. Findings in 346 patients. *Thromb. Haemostas.*, **43**, 28
63. Robboy, S., Colman, R. and Minna, J. (1969). Fibrinolysis vs disseminated intravascular coagulation. *N. Engl. J. Med.*, **281**, 222
64. Charytan, C. and Purtilo, D. (1969). Glomerular capillary thrombosis and acute renal failure after epsilon-aminocaproic acid therapy. *N. Engl. J. Med.*, **280**, 1102
65. Bayley, T., Clements, J. A. and Osbahr, A. J. (1967). Pulmonary and circulatory effects of fibrinopeptides *Circ. Res.*, **21**, 469
66. Richardson, D. L., Pepper, D. S. and Kay, A. B. (1976). Chemotaxis for

human monocytes by fibrinogen derived peptides. *Br. J. Haematol.*, **32**, 507

67. Gerdin, B. and Saldeen, T. (1978). Effect of fibrin degradation products on microvascular permeability. *Thromb. Res.*, **13**, 995

68. Comroe, J. H., Van Lingen, B. V., Stroud, R. C. and Roncoroni, A. (1953). Reflex and direct cardiopulmonary effects of 5-OH-tryptamine (Serotonin). *Am. J. Physiol.*, **173**, 379

69. Blaisdell, F. W., Lim, R. C. and Stallone, R. J. (1970). The mechanism of pulmonary damage following traumatic shock. *Surg. Gynecol. Obstet.*, **130**, 15

70. Hardaway, R. M. and McKay, D. G. (1959). Disseminated intravascular coagulation: a cause of shock. *Ann. Surg.*, **149**, 462

71. Broermsa, R. J., Bullemer, G. D. and Memmen, E. F. (1970). Acidosis induced disseminated intravascular microthrombosis and its dissolution by streptokinase. *Thromb. Diath. Haemorrh.*, **24**, 55

72. Rodriguez-Erdman, F. (1965). Bleeding due to increased intravascular blood coagulation. *N. Engl. J. Med.*, **273**, 1370

73. Boyd. A. D., Engleman, R. M., Beauder, R. L. and Lakner, H. (1972). Disseminated intravascular coagulation following extracorporeal circulation. *J. Thorac. Cardiovasc. Surg.*, **64**, 685

74. Colman, R. W., Robboy, S. J. and Minna, J. D. (1972). Disseminated intravascular coagulation: an approach. *Am. J. Med.*, **52**, 679

75. Hassman, G. C. and Keim, H. A. (1974). Disseminated intravascular coagulation (DIC) in orthopedic surgery. *Clin. Orthop.*, **103**, 118

76. Bain, B. J., Forster, T. H. and Sleigh, B. (1980). Heparin and the activated partial thromboplastin time (aPTT) – a difference between the *in vitro* and *in vivo* effect and implications for the therapeutic range. *Am. J. Clin. Pathol.*, **74**, 668

77. Arfors, K. E., Busch, C., Jakobson, S., Lindquist, O., Malmberg, P., Rammer, L. and Saldeen, T. (1972). Pulmonary insufficiency following intravenous infusion of thrombin and AMCA (tranexamic acid) in the dog. *Acta Chir. Scand.*, **138**, 445

78. Corrigan, J. J., Walker, L. R. and May, N. (1968). Changes in the blood coagulation system associated with septicaemia. *N. Engl. J. Med.*, **279**, 851

79. Isaacson, S. and Nilsson, J. M. (1972). Coagulation and fibrinolysis in acute cholecystitis. *Acta Chir. Scand.*, **138**, 179

80. Goodwin, N. M. (1976). Coagulation disorders in severe shock states. Presented at the *5th Annual Meeting of the Society of Critical Care Medicine*, Pittsburg

81. Goldenfarb, P. B., Zucker, S., Corrigan, J. J. and Cathey, M. H. (1970). The coagulation mechanism in acute bacterial infection. *Br. J. Haematol.*, **18**, 643

82. Beller, F. K. (1969). The role of endotoxin in disseminated intravascular coagulation. *Thromb. Diath. Haemorrh.*, **36** (Suppl.), 125

83. Garner, R. and Evenson, S. A. (1974). Endotoxin-induced intravascular coagulation and shock in dogs: the role of factor VII. *Br. J. Haematol.*, **27**, 655

84. Rivers, R. P. A., Hathaway, W. E. and Westen, W. L. (1975). The endotoxin induced coagulant activity of human monocytes. *Br. J. Haematol.*, **30**, 311

85. Prydz, H., Lyberg, T., Deteix, P. and Allison, A. C. (1979). *In vitro*

stimulation of tissue thromboplastin (factor III) activity in human monocytes by immune complexes and lectins. *Thromb. Res.*, **15**, 465

86. Coe, N. P. and Salzmann, E. W. (1976). Thrombosis and intravascular coagulation. *Surg. Clin. N. Am.*, **56**, 875
87. Hawiger, J., Hawiger, A., Steckley, S., Timmons, S. and Cheng, C. (1977). Membrane changes in human platelets induced by lipopolysaccharide endotoxin. *Br. J. Haematol.*, **35**, 285
88. Nagayama, M., Zucker, M. B. and Beller, F. K. (1971). Effects of a variety of endotoxins on human and rabbit platelet function. *Thromb. Diath. Haemorrh.*, **26**, 467
89. Mason, J. W., Kleeberg, U., Dolan, P. and Colman, R. W. (1970). Plasma kallikrein and Hageman factor in gram-negative bacteraemia. *Ann. Intern. Med.*, **73**, 545
90. Hergt. K. (1972). Blood levels of thrombocytes in burned patients. Observations on their behaviour in relation to the clinical condition of the patient. *J. Trauma*, **12**, 599
91. Curreri, P. W., Wilterdink, M. E. and Baxter, C. R. (1975). Coagulation dynamics following thermal injury. Effect of heparin and protamine sulphate. *Ann. Surg.*, **181**, 161
92. Blaisdell, F. W. (1973). Respiratory insufficiency syndrome. Clinical and pathological definition. *J. Trauma*, **13**, 195
93. McManus, W. F., Eurenius, K. and Pruitt, B. A. (1973). Disseminated intravascular coagulation in burned patients. *J. Trauma*, **13**, 416
94. Halleraker, B. (1972). Microcirculatory thrombosis as a cause of death in thermal burns. *Acta Chir. Scand.*, **138**, 731
95. Zuckerman, L., Caprini, J. A., Lipp, V. and Vagher, J. P. (1978). Disseminated intravascular multiple systems activation (DIMSA) following thermal injury. *J. Trauma*, **18**, 432
96. Simon, T. L., Curreri, P. W. and Harker, L. A. (1977). Kinetic characterization of hemostasis in thermal injury. *J. Lab. Clin. Med.*, **89**, 702
97. Lim, R. C., Olcott, C., Robinson, A. F. and Blaisdell, F. W. (1973). Platelet responses and coagulation changes following massive blood replacement. *J. Trauma*, **13**, 577
98. Wilson, R. F., Mammen, E. and Walt, A. J. (1971). Eight years of experience with massive transfusion. *J. Trauma*, **11**, 275
99. Harker, H. and Rakman, S. (1980). Haemostatic disorders during massive transfusion. *Bibl. Haematol.*, **46**, 179
100. Sheldon, G. F., Lim, R. C. and Blaisdell, F. W. (1975). The use of fresh warm blood in the treatment of critically injured patients. *J. Trauma*, **15**, 670
101. Ellison, N., Beatty, C. P., Blake, D. R., Wurzel, H. A. and Mac Vaugh, H. (1971). Heparin rebound. Studies in patients and volunteers. *J. Thorac. Cardiovasc. Surg.*, **67**, 723
102. Kaul, T. K., Crow, M. J., Rajak, S. M., Deverall, P. B. and Watson, D. A. (1979). Heparin administration during extracorporeal circulation. *J. Thorac. Cardiovasc. Surg.*, **78**, 95
103. Babka, R., Colby, C., El-Etr, A. and Piforre, R. (1977). Monitoring of intraoperative heparinization and blood loss following cardiopulmonary bypass surgery. *J. Thorac. Cardiovasc. Surg.*, **73**, 780

104. Entress, A., Estafanous, F. G. and Hoffman, G. C. (1979). Prolonged heparin activity during hypothermic cardiopulmonary bypass. *Anesthesiology*, **51** (Suppl.), 99

105. Ellison, N., Ominsky, A. J. and Wollman, H. (1971). Is protamine a clinically important anticoagulant. A negative answer. *Anesthesiology*, **35**, 621

106. Bachmann, F., McKenna, R., Cole, E. R. and Najafi, H. (1975). The hemostatic mechanism after open-heart surgery. *J. Thorac. Cardiovasc. Surg.*, **70**, 76

107. McKenna, R., Bachmann, F., Whittaker, B., Gilson J. R. and Weinberg, M. (1975). The hemostatic mechanism after open-heart surgery. II. Frequency of abnormal platelet functions during and after extracorpeal circulation. *J. Thorac. Cardiovasc. Surg.*, **70**, 298

108. Kalter, R. D., Saul, C. M., Wetstein, L., Soriano, C. and Reiss, R. F. (1979). Cardiopulmonary bypass. Associated hemostatic abnormalities. *J. Thorac. Cardiovasc. Surg.*, **77**, 427

109. Gralnick, H. R. and Fischer, R. D. (1971). The hemostatic response to open-heart operations. *J. Thorac. Cardiovasc. Surg.*, **61**, 909

110. Bick, R. L. (1976). Alterations in hemostasis associated with cardiopulmonary bypass. Pathophysiology, prevention, diagnosis and management. *Semin. Thromb. Haemostas.*, **3**, 59

111. Bentall, H. H. and Allwork, S. P. (1968). Fibrinolysis and bleeding in open-heart surgery. *Lancet*, **1**, 4

112. Rodvien, R. and Salzman, E. W. (1978). Thrombotic and hemorrhagic problems in surgery. *Thromb. Haemostas.*, **39**, 254

113. Laufer, N., Merin, G., Grover, B., Pessachowicz, B. and Borman, J. B. (1975). The influence of cardiopulmonary bypass on the size of human platelets. *J. Thorac. Cardiovasc. Surg.*, **70**, 727

114. Hallowell, P., Bland, J. H. L., Buckley, M. J. and Lowenstein, E. (1972). Transfusion of fresh autologous blood in open-heart surgery. *J. Thorac. Cardiovasc. Surg.*, **64**, 941

115. Oschner, J. L., Mills, N. L., Leonard, G. L. and Lawson, N. (1973). Fresh autologous blood transfusions with extracorporeal circulation. *Ann. Surg.*, **177**, 811

116. Pliam, M. B., McGoon, D. C. and Tarhan, S. (1975). Failure of transfusion of autologous whole blood to reduce banked blood requirements in open-heart surgical patients. *J. Thorac. Cardiovasc. Surg.*, **70**, 338

117. Bø G. (1977). What is the significance of 'blood sludge' today – cause or effect of disease. *Vox Sang.*, **32**, 251

118. Ansell, J., Slepchuk, N., Kumar, R., Lopez, A., Southard, L. and Deykin, D. (1980). Heparin induced thrombocytopenia. A prospective study. *Thromb. Haemostas.*, **43**, 6

119. Towne, J. B., Bernkard, V. M., Hussey, C. and Garancis, J. C. (1979). White clot syndrome. Peripheral vascular complications of herapin therapy. *Arch. Surg.*, **114**, 372

120. Powers, P. J., Cuthbert, D. and Hirsh, J. (1979). Thrombocytopenia found uncommonly during heparin therapy. *J. Am. Med. Assoc.*, **241**, 2396

121. Bell, W. R., Tomasulo, P. A., Alving, B. M. and Duffy, T. P. (1976). Thrombocytopenia occurring during the administration of heparin. A pro-

spective study in 52 patients. *Ann. Intern. Med.*, **85**, 155

122. Babcock, R. B., Dumper, C. W. and Scharfman, W. B. (1976). Heparin-induced thrombocytopenia. *N. Engl. J. Med.*, **295**, 237

123. Bygdeman, S. and Elisson, R. (1967). Effect of dextrans on platelet adhesiveness and aggregation. *Scand. J. Clin. Lab. Invest.*, **20**, 17

124. Nilsson, I. M. and Eiken, O. (1964). Further studies on the effect of dextran of various molecular weights on the coagulation mechanism. *Thromb. Diath. Haemorrh.*, **11**, 38

125. Åberg, M., Hedner, U. and Bergentz, S. (1979). Effect of dextran on factor VIII (antihemophilic factor) and platelet function. *Ann. Surg.*, **189**, 243

126. Brodman, R. F., Sarg, M., Veith, F. J. and Spaet, T. (1977). Dextran-40 induced coagulopathy confused with von Willebrand disease. *Arch. Surg.*, **112**, 321

127. Bergentz, S. E., Eiken, O. and Nilsson, I. M. (1961). The effect of dextran of various molecular weights on the coagulation in dogs. *Thromb. Diath. Haemorrh.*, **6**, 15

128. Rudowski, W. J. (1980). Evaluation of modern plasma expanders and blood substitutes. *Br. J. Hosp. Med.*, **23**, 389

129. Trafford, J. A. P., Jones, R. H., Evans, R., Sharp, P., Sharpstone, P. and Cook, J. (1977). Haemoperfusion with R-004 amberlite resin for treating acute poisoning. *Br. Med. J.*, **2**, 1453

130. Vane, J. R. (1979). Prostacyclin and the control of platelet function. *Thromb. Haemostas.*, **42**, 16

131. Multicentric Trial, (1977). Prevention of fatal postoperative pulmonary embolism by low doses of heparin. *Lancet*, **1**, 567

132. Blaisdell, F. W. (1978). Prevention of deep vein thrombosis. *Surgery*, **83**, 243

133. Goodman, T. L., Todd, M. E. and Goldsmith, E. I. (1976). Laboratory observations and clinical implications of monitoring the effect of heparin by bioassay. *Surg. Gynecol. Obstet.*, **142**, 678

134. Simon, T. L., Hyers, T. M., Gaston, J. P. and Harker, L. A. (1978). Heparin pharmacokinetics: increased requirements in pulmonary embolism. *Br. J. Haematol.*, **39**, 111

5
Shock

WILLIAM SCHUMER

Shock is defined as inadequate circulating blood volume producing decreased peripheral vascular perfusion and cellular metabolic derangements, first in the non-vital tissues – the gastrointestinal tract, muscle, connective tissue and skin, and later in the vital tissues – the brain, heart, lung, liver and kidneys. This inadequate microcirculatory perfusion is the common denominator of all types of shock.

(I) CLASSIFICATION

(1) Cardiogenic shock

Cardiogenic shock is caused by the heart's inability to maintain an effective circulating volume.

(2) Hypovolaemic shock

Hypovolaemic shock is caused by blood loss, either red cell mass, plasma, or plasma filtrate.

Endogenous hypovolaemic shock

(1)   Septic shock is caused by an immunological reaction secondary to endotoxin–antibody–complement complexing and leukocyte lyses which results in the production of histamine, serotonin, super radicals, lysosomal enzymes and kinins. These substances induce a marked capillary permeability and a third space loss leading to hypovolaemia.

(2)   Anaphylactic shock is caused by a severe antigen–antibody reaction with an instantaneous release of huge amounts of permeability factors, mainly histamine.

Exogenous hypovolaemic shock

This type is caused by haemorrhage, burns or gastrointestinal losses.

Distributive shock

Distributive shock is caused by a marked expansion of the vascular compartment that cannot be adequately perfused by the available blood volume.

Traumatic shock

Traumatic shock is not a definitive type but a combination of various forms of shock, primarily hypovolaemic, and/or septic, cardiogenic and distributive shocks.

(II) PATHOPHYSIOLOGY

(1) Hypovolaemia

Loss of blood volume, regardless of its cause, initiates metabolic and physiological reactions through the chemobarometric sensors which are sensitive to oxygen, carbon dioxide, and pressure. These sensors stimulate the pituitary gland. Pituitary hormones, including adrenocorticotropic hormone (ACTH), antidiuretic hormones (ADH), and aldosterone-stimulating hormone (ASH), are then released. ASH, the production of which is also stimulated by the juxtaglomerular apparatus in the kidney, induces the adrenal cortex to produce aldosterone. The main functions of aldosterone include the excretion of potassium and the retention of sodium chloride and water. ADH has a similar effect on water metabolism in the kidney, but it also causes the collecting tubules to absorb water, which decreases the urinary output. Therefore, aldosterone and ADH help to maintain blood volume (Figure 5.1)[1-4]. The medullary hormones of the adrenal gland (epinephrine) and norepinephrine sustain volume by promoting vasoconstriction in the capillaries. In small concentrations, these hormones increase flow through the vital and non-vital organs. This effect may be efficacious for a limited time, but during prolonged shock the vaso-constrictive action becomes so severe, that anaerobic metabolism develops

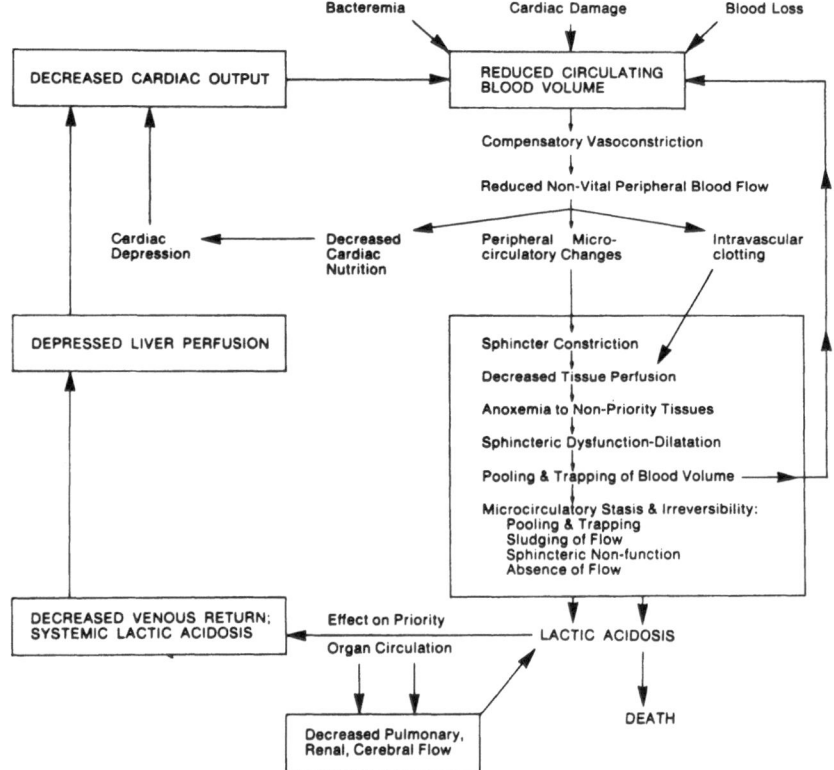

Figure 5.1 Feedback haemodynamic sequences in the progression of shock. (Reproduced from Schumer, W. (1976). The shock syndrome. *Compr. Ther.*, **2**, 18. Reproduced by permission of the American Society of Contemporary Medicine and Surgery)

in the peripheral tissue cells, producing large concentrations of metabolic acids[5,6].

As much as 20% loss of the total blood volume produces physiological change; however, greater loss results in vasoconstriction in the peripheral tissues, with the signs of pallor and cold, clammy skin. Skin moisture is due to the sympathetic stimulation of sweat glands. Weakness and lassitude result from the cellular energy deficit that impairs muscular function. As shock progresses, the vital organs are affected. Reduced perfusion of kidneys and marked antidiuresis cause oliguria. Acidosis forces the lung to compensate, first with dyspnoea and later with tachypnoea to augment carbon dioxide and hydrion excretion. With further volume loss, the central nervous system becomes involved, and the patient grows apprehensive and later comatose.

The cardiovascular system, especially the heart, is under stress, since the low venous return decreases output. The heart rate accelerates; but diastole necessarily grows shorter, and coronary perfusion is correspondingly reduced. Lowered output and reduced systolic pressure are manifested clinically in a weak, thready pulse. The peripherally produced metabolic acidosis further deteriorates cardiac function[1,2]. It should be noted that a decrease in blood pressure usually occurs late in the shock course, because of the body's efforts to maintain the systemic flow as long as possible. As shock progresses, symptoms of vital organ dysfunction appear; cardiac output continues to decrease, peripheral resistance may markedly increase, or there may be terminal peripheral vasodilation causing mottling of the skin. Underperfusion of the brain causes first somnolence and eventually coma.

How do these haemodynamic derangements occurring in the peripheral cell mass affect the gastrointestinal tract, muscle, skin and connective tissue? Moore stated that 'Shock is considered as the mechanism by which peripheral injury to non-vital organs (a leg, for example) is converted into vital organ damage and death'[7]. Shunting of blood from the periphery prevents oxygen and substrates from reaching the cells. The cells then function under anaerobic conditions and the end result is lactic acidosis. Lactic acid is the major and most harmful product of anaerobic metabolism. There are other metabolites supporting the acidotic state, such as free fatty acids and ketone bodies which are being released by lipolysis induced by epinephrine. Amino acids or protein breakdown releases sulphates and phosphates adding to the severity of the metabolic acidosis. Metabolic acidosis, the main acid–base imbalance, may appear as a respiratory alkalosis. This occurs when the body, in combating acidosis, increases carbon dioxide and water excretion, thus producing respiratory alkalosis. Ordinarily, a true metabolic acidotic state can be recognized by a low $PaCO_2$, a slightly raised pH, but the plasma bicarbonate is reduced below that predicted from the $PaCO_2$.

Shires reported that the body compensates for decreased capillary perfusion by interstitial space volume replenishment of the cellular mass and the vascular space[8]. The attendant cellular oedema is due to the fact that anaerobic metabolism produces a decrease in adenosine triphosphate (ATP). ATP depletion produces dysfunction of the sodium–potassium ATPase molecule so that sodium and water enter the cell and potassium leaves the cell producing hyperkalaemia.

In certain types of shock, a relative rather than absolute hypovolaemia occurs. For example, in cardiogenic shock the heart is unable to pump blood to non-vital tissues, therefore the non-vital tissues' microcirculation is underperfused. This relative hypovolaemia also occurs in distributive shock due to a marked expansion of the vascular volume rendering the available blood volume insufficient to perfuse these tissues.

(2) Sepsis (bacterial infection or toxaemia)

The sequence of events leading to septic shock begins with a bacterial invasion secondary to a major septic process, such as pneumonitis, subacute bacterial endocarditis, ruptured viscus peritonitis, and abdominal abscess. The precipitating agents, gram-negative and gram-positive bacteria, are opsonized, phagocytosed, releasing into the bloodstream fragments that contain either exotoxin, the intracellular content of bacteria, or endotoxin, a lipoprotein–polysaccharide (LPS) macromolecule of the cell membrane. This occurs because the phagocytic phagolysosomes degrade the cytoplasmic and membranous portions of the bacterial cell by the action of lysosomal enzymes and the myeloperoxidase hyaline system. The gram-negative, LPS or endotoxin, has been shown to be antigenic and contains the following three distinct antigens: an outer oligosaccharide antigen, an inner core known as the R antigen, and a lipid portion known as lipid A[9]. Lipid A is considered to be the toxic element of the endotoxin. When released in the blood, endotoxin initiates antibody formation and complement interactions, which promote opsonization of the endotoxin fragments so that the reticuloendothelial (RES) cells can absorb them for detoxification. However, if the infection is overwhelming, the RES cells are inundated with LPS, their function is depressed, and the serum complement endotoxin reaction is accelerated (Chapter 2). Anaphylotoxins created by this interaction release histamine and heparin from mast cells, the phagocytosis factor releases lysosomal enzymes and superoxide radicals from polymorphonuclear leukocytes, the myeloperoxidase system and the immune adherence factor releases serotonin from platelets. These substances produce marked capillary permeability and endothelial cell damage, which results in severe loss of plasma volume to the interstitial tissue throughout the capillary system[10]. Loss of effective circulating blood volume produces circulatory collapse and shock[11].

The haemodynamic pattern during this imunological reaction is a hyperdynamic phase characterized by decreased peripheral resistance, which is probably secondary to the release of histamine and serotonin, as well as an increase in cardiac output. With the loss of plasma volume, the circulatory response becomes similar to that of hypovolaemic shock. There is release of epinephrine and norepinephrine, producing increased peripheral resistance and cardiac rate. Cardiac output is depressed because of the decreased blood volume and venous return. This is known as the hypodynamic phase of septic shock. Depressed perfusion of non-vital tissue produces deranged cellular metabolism. The lack of oxygen results in the anaerobic metabolism of glucose with increased production of lactic acid, the main cause of metabolic acidosis in the hypodynamic phase of septic shock. Impaired function of the Krebs cycle depresses ATP, or energy production. This energy deficit probably aids in decreasing membrane ATP and function, allowing further loss of fluid through endothelial cells and resulting in the intracellular oedema of shock[11].

Recent work has indicated that endoxaemia interferes with the production of new glucose from alanine, glycerol and lactic acid. Apparently this is caused by depression of rate-limiting enzymes, specifically phosphoenolpyruvate kinase and fructose diphosphatase, as well as an energy defect, since ATP is necessary for converting gluconeogenic precursors into glucose[12]. Depressed gluconeogenesis may also cause the increase in lactic acid since it is not being used by the liver for new glucose production. Our studies in pigs, rats and mice have shown a positive correlation between serum endotoxin and lactate and a negative correlation between serum glucose and endotoxin. There was a positive correlation between blood pressure and the glucose–lactate ratio, indicating that the glucose–lactate ratio may be a useful prognostic and therapeutic monitor in septic shock[11]. New and important therapeutic concepts have been derived from studies of the immunology and molecular pathology of septic shock. *In vitro* studies of corticosteroids have shown that these agents have an anticomplementary effect. When administered *in vivo* they decreased the serum histamine and serotonin levels secondary to complement reaction. They also aided in the induction of gluconeogenic enzymes. Studies of the hypoglycaemia secondary to gluconeogenic inhibition have shown the need for an exogenous source of glucose. Therefore, glucose, insulin, and potassium solutions are now advocated as adjunctive resuscitative fluids. Although these studies were supported by noteworthy basic science and clinical data, further investigation is needed for the improvement of present therapeutic concepts and techniques to counteract the devastating effects of the complement reaction, the gluconeogenic block, and the membrane injury of sepsis[11].

(3) Anaphylaxis

Anaphylactic shock is another example of the relative hypovolaemic phase. These patients experience a severe cell-mediated antigen–antibody reaction, resulting from the complement complexing action on the cells of the vascular endothelium, which releases high concentrations of capillary permeability factors. (Mast cells and platelets release slow-reacting substance A, histamine and serotonin; and leukocytes release lysosomal enzymes). The plasma volume lost in the interstitial spaces causes oedema of the larynx, lungs, face, hands and feet. The patency of the pulmonary airway is most severely affected, and therefore maintenance of an adequate airway becomes the most important therapeutic priority in anaphylactic shock.

(III) INVESTIGATION AND MONITORING

Monitoring of the shock patient requires continuous evaluation of the status of the following: clinical signs, peripheral perfusion, vital organ function and volume requirements.

(1) Monitoring of clinical signs

The two most important aspects in clinical monitoring are observation of the skin and the sensorium. When the blood volume of the patient in hypo-volaemic shock is repleted and adequately perfuses the peripheral tissues, the skin becomes warm and dry and the colour changes from greyish-white to pink. During the hyperdynamic phase of septic shock, the skin may become reddened and moist, but this is easily differentiated from the warm, pink skin characteristic of a well-perfused periphery. Although the brain is the last vital organ to experience a reduced circulating blood volume, the effect on the sensorium is exhibited early in the shock state by the patient's irritability and restlessness. If the volume is not promptly replenished, coma may ensue.

(2) Monitoring of peripheral perfusion

If shock is to be overcome, peripheral tissue perfusion must be constantly monitored. Skin colour and temperature should be observed. Peripheral resistance, which is indicative of the status of perfusion rate, can be measured by dividing mean arterial blood pressure by cardiac output. A high peripheral resistance indicates shunting, while a normal peripheral resistance indicates adequate perfusion. Another way of determining peripheral perfusion rate is by measuring either lactate or the lactate–pyruvate ratio. High concentrations of lactate indicate increased anaerobiosis produced by decreased perfusion, and low concentrations signify improved or normal perfusion.

It is important to monitor peripheral cell function by measuring the arterio-venous oxygen difference (C(a-v)O_2) because the ability of the peripheral tissues to extract oxygen from the blood indicates their viability and also identifies the phase of septic shock. In hypovolaemic shock the peripheral cells extract oxygen at an increased rate until the cells are close to death. Once cell death occurs, oxygen extraction decreases. In the hyper-dynamic phase of septic shock, the peripheral cells have difficulty in extracting oxygen because of the mitochondrial injury secondary to sepsis or endotoxaemia. Later in the hypodynamic phase, oxygen extraction elevates the C(a-v)O_2, which is similar to what occurs in hypovolaemic shock. Measurement of pH and $PaCO_2$ monitors the acid–base alterations occurring secondary to anaerobic metabolism. These are indirect measurements, because the main component of anaerobic metabolic acidosis is lactic acid. Thus, lactic acid measurements provide more current and direct monitoring of peripheral perfusion. However, pH and $PaCO_2$ determinations monitor the acid–base compensations of blood buffer, respiration and kidney. A low pH and low $PaCO_2$ (metabolic acidosis) indicates severe metabolic alterations secondary to peripheral cell anaerobiosis. Contrari-wise, reparation of acid–base imbalance indicates improved perfusion.

(3) Monitoring of vital organ function

Heart

To monitor the heart, cardiac output, and either central venous pressure (CVP) or pulmonary artery wedge pressure (PAWP) should be measured via a CVP or pulmonary artery pressure (PAP) catheter, respectively. PAWP measurement is more accurate than CVP because the latter may be altered by pulmonary hypertension and severe shunting of blood from arteries to venules, so that these factors must be considered before using CVP as a function of left myocardial integrity. PAP catheter data is usually more current and accurate.

Lung

PaO_2 and $PaCO_2$ measurements differentiate the type and extent of injury inflicted by the shock state on the alveolar-vascular membrane. For

121

example, low PaO_2 measurement may indicate adult respiratory distress syndrome (ARDS) (Chapter 10) and high $PaCO_2$ and low pH measurements may indicate respiratory acidosis, probably representing an underlying massive atelectasis or ventilatory diffusion problems.

Liver

Serum glucose and lactate measurements (glucose–lactate ratio) determine the status of liver function. A glucose–lactate ratio of 10 or more indicates adequate liver function (gluconeogenesis and glycolysis); less than 10 falling to reversal of the ratio indicates inadequate liver function due to depressed perfusion and possible hepatocellular damage.

Kidney

Kidney function is monitored by measuring urinary output which is normally 30–70 ml/h with a urine osmolality of 600 mosmol/l. The kidney responds to depressed circulating volume by retaining water which increases urine osmolality (ADH effect). The glomerular filtration rate is also depressed causing oliguria – and as hypoperfusion progresses – nephron cell damage, inability to retain water and finally a salt-losing nephritis ensues. This effect is reflected in urinary water and salt losses.

(4) Monitoring of volume requirements

Volume is monitored by measuring PAP; the pulmonary vascular system blood volume is proportional to PAP, so that as PAP decreases so does volume. CVP determinations can be used to monitor young patients or those with moderate hypovolaemic shock. However, it should be noted that the CVP catheter is capable of monitoring blood volume changes so long as the left myocardium is functioning normally and there is no pulmonary hypertension and no severe shunting. Volume, being directly proportional to either urinary output or mean arterial pressure (MAP), can be indirectly monitored by measuring these two parameters. The pulse rate is inversely proportional to volume. Haematocrit – after transcapillary filling has occurred – is directly proportional to volume.

(IV) TREATMENT

(1) Objectives

There are four principal and equally important objectives in the treatment of shock: treatment of the aetiological condition, management of the hypovolaemic state, reparation of the metabolic acid–base imbalance, and correction of the nutritional deficit. There are no priorities; treatment must be rendered concomitantly and rapidly. In septic shock, it is essential that the septic and hypovolaemic processes be treated concomitantly since preventing the complexing of antigen–antibody and complement will deter vascular permeability and its consequent hypovolaemia. Prompt and adequate treatment of hypovolaemia prevents the development of attendant cellular metabolic derangements.

All shock patients should be admitted to the ICU. Shock is one of the most critical medical emergencies requiring specialized care by medical and paramedical staff trained in intensive care, and supported by appropriate monitoring equipment.

(2) Outline for therapy

(1) Cleanse and dress all wounds or drain abscesses, and maintain haemostasis.

(2) Provide respiratory care. (a) If the patient is not dyspnoeic or cyanotic, give 8–10 l/min of oxygen by a mask. (b) If there has been injury to the chest or if there is dyspnoea or cyanosis, then insert an endotracheal tube and attach it to either a 'T' tube or ventilator. (c) If acute respiratory failure is present then attach the endotracheal tube to a ventilator and treat as follows: the mechanical ventilator should promote increased tidal volume and driving pressure; and with a positive end-expiratory pressure (PEEP) of 5–10 cm, increase alveolar oxygen pressure and prevent alveolar collapse (Chapter 7). (d) Administer a diuretic such as frusemide (furosemide, USP) in 50 mg doses every 4 hours to maintain pulmonary artery pressure (PAP) at low normal levels. (e) Administer albumin if measured colloid osmotic pressure is below normal range. (f) Administer cardiotonic drugs to improve cardiac output if PAP or wedge pressure (PAWP) shows an abnormal increase. (g) Administer corticosteroids, either 30 mg/kg body weight of methylprednisolone or 3 mg/kg body weight of dexamethasone. (h) Administer antibiotics if the sputum culture is positive. The choice of antibiotic is dependent on culture and sensitivity.

(3) Replace lost volume. (a) Place an intravenous cannula, preferably gauge 14, in a peripheral vein. (b) Place a PAP or CVP catheter using a flow-directed catheter. (c) Start infusions of Ringer's solution containing 44 mmol/l of sodium bicarbonate in both catheters.* (d) Give blood as soon as it is available, keeping the haematocrit at 30% or above.

(4) Monitor the vital functions. (a) Maintain and measure pulmonary artery pressure through the CVP catheter. (b) Measure urine output every hour. Maintain a urine output of 50–75 ml/h. If the urine output falls below 30 ml/h and there is no response to an increased infusion of Ringer's bicarbonate solution, infuse 12.5 g of mannitol over a period of 5 minutes. If mannitol fails to produce diuresis, give 50 mg of frusemide (furosemide) intravenously. If diuresis still does not occur, double the dose every 2 hours up to 400 mg. If there is no effect, acute renal failure has developed. Treatment of established renal failure should be instituted. (c) Monitor blood pressure by cuff or, if warranted, by arterial catheter. (d) Measure pH, $PaCO_2$ and PaO_2 by either femoral or radial artery cannula. (e) Determine lactic acid level and serum glucose every 2 hours until resuscitation is complete.

(5) Position the patient either with head and feet both at 30 degrees or supine.

(6) Keep the patient normothermic using a rectal thermistor-controlled water blanket.

(7) Administer antibiotics intravenously when there are definite indications. When this therapy has to be 'blind' the writer then gives Cefamandole or cefoxitin, 2 g every 4 hours. Alternative drugs are described in Chapter 3.

(8) To patients with previous heart disease, those over the age of 50 or those with increased PAP or PAWP after resuscitation, give 0.5 mg of digoxin immediately and 250 μg every 6 hours until digitalization occurs – usually after 1.5 mg is given.

(9) If the blood pressure is below 50 mmHg, give cardiotonics such as dopamine, dobutamine hydrochloride, and isoprenaline (isoproterenol, USP).

---

* Editor's note: The composition of Ringer's bicarbonate is as follows: sodium 19, potassium 4.1, calcium 2.24, bicarbonate 44 mmol/l. Two readily available and inexpensive colloids could be used as alternatives to Ringer's solution; they are polygeline and dextran 70

(10) Vasodilators, such as phentolamine, should be given at a constant infusion rate of 0.5 mg per minute if (a) the patient is unresponsive to general therapy; (b) there are clinical signs of sympathetic over-activity; (c) the measured peripheral resistance has increased.

(11) After resuscitation has been instituted, infuse hyperalimentation fluids every 8 hours through a PAP catheter. The formula should contain the following: (a) 1000 ml of 20% glucose, (b) 44 mmol of potassium chloride, (c) 250 mg of thiamine hydrochloride, (d) 50 mg of riboflavin, (e) 1.0 g of ascorbic acid, (f) 1.25 g of nicotinamide, (g) 50 mg of pyridoxine hydrochloride, (h) 500 mg of sodium pantothenate.

(3) Specific therapy

Treatment for hypovolaemic shock

(1) Replace lost volume with a balanced salt solution as long as the haematocrit remains above 30%. Give packed cells if the haematocrit falls below 30%. (2) Give additional bicarbonate if the pH drops below 7.36. (3) Maintain a urine output of 50–75 ml per hour.

Treatment for septic shock

(1) Give 3 mg/kg body weight of dexamethasone or 30 mg/kg body weight of methylprednisolone in a single bolus as soon as septic shock is diagnosed, and repeat after 4 hours if there is no beneficial response. Do not repeat again, unless the septic shock is episodic[13].* (2) Intravenously infuse gentamicin, 5.0 mg/kg body weight daily, and clindamycin, 35 mg/kg body weight daily. Monitor gentamicin levels with serial serum determinations, and sensitivities to antibiotics with Kirby–Bauer and bactericidal assays. (3) Obtain six blood cultures and sensitivity tests. Remember to obtain anaerobic cultures. (4) Treat the hypovolaemic phase of septic shock as hypovolaemic shock, using only balanced salt solution. (5) Maintain blood pressure without increasing PAP or PAWP. If either pressure increases abnormally, cardiotonics must be given to maintain cardiac output, 500 μg digoxin given immediately and followed by 250 μg every 6 hours, and/or 5 mg glucagon at a rate of 3–5 mg per hour. The cardiotonic chosen may be 1.0% solution of isoprenaline (isoproterenol) given to maintain systolic

* Editor's note: The author and his colleagues are quite convinced of the value of steroids in septic shock in man. Others remain sceptical of the use of these drugs in man, although in the animal model their efficacy is not doubted. [Thompson, W. L. (1978). In *Recent Advances in Clinical Pharmacology,* Turner, P. and Shand, D. G. (eds.). p. 137. (Edinburgh: Churchill Livingstone)]

pressure above 80 mmHg or dopamine at a rate of 5–10 μg/min/kg body weight for no longer than 8 hours or dobutamine at a rate of 10 μg/min/kg body weight.

Treatment for distributive shock

(1) Place the patient in either a supine or jackknife position at 30 degrees head and feet. (2) Intravenously or intramuscularly administer 10–20 mg methoxamine hydrochloride. (3) If there is no improvement, give Ringer's solution with 44 mg of potassium chloride via a large bore venous catheter. (4) Give 8–10 litres of oxygen by mask.

Treatment for anaphylactic shock

Emergency treatment
(1) Immediately and quickly initiate endotracheal intubation of the patient, otherwise glottal oedema becomes so severe that a tracheostomy procedure may be necessary.* Therefore, emergency disposable endotracheal intubation set-up should be immediately available to the physician either in the private office or the emergency room. (2) To counteract histamine and serotonin release, administer adrenaline (epinephrine) 1:1000 at a dose of 0.5 ml. (3) If shock resulted from an injection into a limb, apply tourniquet proximally to the injection site. (4) Ventilate patient via Ambu bag with 8–10 l/minute of oxygen. (5) Transport patient to nearest hospital, maintaining constant ventilation.

Treatment in the ICU
(1) Insert Foley catheter, and either a pulmonary artery catheter, or a central venous pressure catheter. Monitor respiratory patency, volume, vital functions and therapeutic efficacy, as described in hypovolaemic shock. (2) Infuse Ringer's bicarbonate solution. The amount of volume replacement should be based on pulmonary artery pressure and wedge pressure measurements. (3) Administer the following drugs: diphenhydramine, intramuscularly, in dosages of 50–100 mg, to prevent further histamine release; aminophylline, intravenously, at a dose of 6 mg/kg body weight. Repeat aminophylline, if necessary, at a dose of 1 mg/kg body weight hourly. If the patient shows any evidence of recent or present cardiac

---

* Editor's note: When prompt intubation is not possible then transtracheal ventilation should be used. A 14 gauge cannula is inserted into the trachea and oxygen at a pressure of 50 lb/sq. in. is injected at normal respiratory frequency (Spoerel et al. (1971), Br. J. Anaesth., **43**, 932)

failure, administer either dopamine in dosages of 1.0–10 μg per minute, or isoprenaline (isoproterenol), 2.0 mg per litre, in 5% glucose in water, at a rate of 0.5–0.1 ml per minute, to support cardiac function. Corticoids such as hydrocortisone succinate, in dosages of 100 mg every 1–2 hours to relieve bronchospasm, laryngeal oedema and hypotension.

If the patient in anaphylactic shock survives the first twenty-four hours, then the prognosis is good. The reported mortality rate in these patients is 24% indicating the gravity of this type of shock.

Treatment for cardiogenic shock

(1) Institute volume resuscitation by infusing saline or colloid via peripheral venous catheters at 10 minute intervals using the following criteria:

PAWP $\langle$ 12 mmHg – 200 ml
PAWP $\rangle$ 12 $\langle$ 16 mmHg – 100 ml
PAWP $\rangle$ 16 mmHg – 50 ml

Thereafter, continue to monitor PAWP and adjust infusion rate to maintain PAWP at 20 mmHg. Serum lactate, arterial pressure and urine output should return to normal levels. (2) If there is no improvement after volume replacement, administer the following pharmacological agent: nitroprusside in dosages of 20 μg/min – vasodilation decreases workload on the heart. Cardiac output should measure 3.0–4.0 l/min or cardiac index should measure 3.0. Monitor lactate levels as well as toe temperature–ambient temperature gradient ($\rangle$ 2 °C – survival; $\langle$ 2 °C – death)[14]. (3) If there is no improvement after drug therapy, institute mechanical support via an intra-aortic balloon pump to reduce afterload and increase coronary blood flow. The treatment of the shock which may follow acute myocardial infarction is detailed in Chapter 13.

References

1. Schumer, W. and Kukral, J. C. (1968). Metabolism of shock. *Metabolism*, **63**, 630
2. Schumer, W. (1976). The shock syndrome. *Compr. Ther.*, **2**, 18
3. Fuhrman, F. A. and Crismon, J. M. (1951). Muscle electrolytes in rats following ischemia produced by tourniquet. *Am. J. Physiol.*, **167**, 289
4. Holden, W. D., DePalma, R. G., Drucker, W. R. and McKalen, A. (1965). Ultrastructural changes in haemorrhagic shock. Electron microscopic study of liver, kidney and striated muscle cells in rats. *Ann. Surg.*, **162**, 517
5. Page, I. H. (1961). Some neurohumoral and endocrine aspects of shock. In

Seeley, S. F. and Weisiger, J. R. (eds.). Proceedings of a conference on recent progress and present problems in the field of shock. *Fed. Proc.*, **20,** 75

6. Youmans, P. L., Green, H. D. and Denison, A. B., Jr. (1955). Nature of the vasodilator and vasoconstrictor receptors in skeletal muscle of the dog. *Circ. Res.*, **3,** 171

7. Moore, F. D. (1959). *Metabolic Care of the Surgical Patient.* p. 172. (Philadelphia: W. B. Saunders)

8. Shires, G. T., Canizaro, P. C. and Carrion, C. J. (1979). Clinical manifestations of shock. In Schwartz, S. I., Shires, G. T., Spencer F. C. and Storer, E. H. (eds.). *Principles of Surgery*, pp. 135–184. (New York: McGraw-Hill)

9. Wright, A. and Kanegasaki, S. (1971). Molecular aspects of lipopolysaccharides. *Physiol. Rev.*, **51,** 748

10. Müller-Eberhard, H. J. (1976). The serum complement system. In Miescher, P. A. and Müller-Eberhard, H. J. (eds.). *Textbook of Immunopathology*, pp. 45–73 (New York: Grune Stratton)

11. Schumer, W. (1979). Septic shock. *J. Am. Med. Assoc.*, **242,** 1906

12. Schuler, J. J., Erve, P. R. and Schumer, W. (1976). Glucocorticoid effect on hepatic carbohydrate metabolism in endotoxin-shocked monkey. *Ann. Surg.*, **183,** 345

13. Schumer, W. (1976). Steroids in the treatment of clinical septic shock. *Ann. Surg.*, **184,** 333

14. Henning, R., Valdes, S., Wiener, F., Thompson, M. and Weil, M. H. (1978). Toe temperature as a prognostic indicator of circulatory shock. *Am. J. Cardiol.*, (Abstract) **41,** 440

6
Blood transfusion

BARBARA BAIN

Transfusion of blood and blood products can have deleterious effects in any patient. Some ICU patients require rapid or massive blood transfusion which increases the likelihood of adverse reactions. When a large part of the blood is approaching the end of its shelf life then the reduced capacity to deliver O_2 may also be a problem. Because of the complex clinical state, transfusion reactions are more difficult to recognize in the critically ill patient. Furthermore, adverse reactions to blood transfusion may be more serious in the ICU patient with circulatory or respiratory failure. The nature and management of the coagulation defect following massive transfusion were described in Chapter 4. This chapter describes the other complications of massive transfusion and other adverse effects of transfusion relevant to intensive therapy. Those complications which do not have an increased incidence or unusual features are omitted.

(I) COMPLICATIONS OF RAPID OR MASSIVE BLOOD TRANSFUSION

The definition of massive blood transfusion is arbitrary but a useful definition is the transfusion of more than 5 litres of blood, or more than 1.0-1.5 times the estimated blood volume during 24 hours.

129

(1) Incompatible blood transfusion and the use of uncrossmatched blood

The likelihood of an incompatible transfusion is increased when trauma-tized or bleeding patients require large volumes of blood during short periods. When multiple casualties are being dealt with the problems are similar but greater. The use of either uncrossmatched blood or of O blood in recipients of other groups increases the risk but this must be assessed in relation to the clinical situation[1]. The risk of either procedure is minimal in a young male trauma victim who has not previously been transfused, but more considerable in a middle-aged multiparous or previously transfused female.

(a) Group O blood in recipients of other groups

Giving group O blood to recipients of other blood groups, or of unknown blood group, may be indicated when dealing with mass casualties. Group O blood has sometimes been regarded as 'Universal Donor', but not all group O blood is suitable for transfusion into recipients of other groups. Some donors (including those who have recently had tetanus vaccinations) have a high titre of lytic anti-A or anti-B antibodies capable of causing haemolysis in the recipient. Blood which is to be transfused into recipients other than group O should be screened to exclude these donors, sometimes designated 'dangerous universal donors'. In transfusing young, previously healthy males group O Rh positive blood may be used with reasonable safety, although some recipients will subsequently develop anti-D. The develop-ment of anti-D is much more serious in a premenopausal woman or girl, so that group O Rh negative blood should be used if women of other blood groups are to be given group O blood. The likelihood of donor antibodies reacting with recipient red cells is reduced, but not eliminated, if packed cells or plasma reduced blood are used. However, packed red cells are not very satisfactory for emergency use since their high viscosity hinders rapid infusion. If group O blood has been transfused into a patient of another group then the withholding of type-specific blood (i.e. blood of the same ABO group as the patient) for 2 weeks will prevent any risk of lysis of donor cells by passively acquired antibodies.

(b) Transfusion of type-specific uncrossmatched blood

Vigorous efforts should be made to avoid using uncrossmatched blood. This can be done by using plasma protein solution, polygeline or dextran 70 for initial therapy and by employing rapid crossmatching techniques. The introduction of low ionic strength (LISS) techniques has considerably shortened the time needed for a full crossmatch. If there is insufficient time for a full crossmatch then an urgent crossmatch should be done by means of an immediate-spin–saline technique. This test only takes 5–10 minutes and will eliminate ABO incompatibility. If the patient has had a previous antibody screening then its safety approaches that of a standard crossmatch. If blood is to be used uncrossmatched, then a choice has to be made between group O blood and type-specific blood. The use of uncrossmatched group O blood has a good safety record when young males are being transfused. However, in civilian practice most directors of transfusion services advise the use of type-specific blood; this is both for logistic reasons and to avoid reactions of donor antibodies with recipient cells. An ABO and Rh group can be determined in 2–3 minutes if a potent and complete anti-D is used. If uncrossmatched blood is to be used, then there is serious risk of ABO incompatibility. Both the donor and recipient group must be known with certainty; patient identification must be meticulous; descriptions, such as 'unidentified adult male' must only be used with a registration number. It is of interest that when dealing with mass casualties of warfare, the number of adverse reactions increased considerably when type-specific rather than group O blood was used. The increased incidence of reactions was due to 'administrative' rather than technical errors. During a very rapid transfusion when virtual exchange occurs, a crossmatch against the initial serum sample becomes less relevant and often not feasible. In this situation a rapid crossmatch using the immediate-spin technique is appropriate. It is preferable to obtain a fresh serum sample but a crossmatch against an initial sample will at least exclude ABO incompatibility. The risks of the use of uncrossmatched blood are much higher in parous women or in patients who have previously been transfused but not recently had their sera screened for atypical antibodies.

(c) Detection of incompatible transfusion in critically ill patients

The signs of incompatible transfusion in the critically ill patient can be masked by coma or muscle relaxants. In these patients the urine should be tested for haemoglobin and the body temperature monitored. In some cases, haemorrhage may be the first warning of an incompatible transfusion.

(2) Microaggregates

After several days storage ACD blood develops microaggregates. At first these are composed of platelets, then leukocytes plus platelets. Microaggregates develop somewhat more rapidly in CPD blood and much more rapidly in heparinized blood. There is no agreement as to the harm caused by microaggregates when transfused into a patient, but the possibility is greatest in the critically ill patient. Standard filters used in blood transfusion have a pore size of 170–200 μm, so that smaller microaggregates will not be removed by the filter, but may be trapped in the pulmonary capillaries. Various microaggregate filters are available which will filter out particles down to a size of 10–40 μm. The number of microaggregates in stored blood can be determined by counting single particles of 20 μm or larger in size by means of a particle counter. Alternatively, they can be detected indirectly by measuring the screen filtration pressure. Blood is passed through a nickel screen with 20×20 μm holes and a build up in pressure indicates the presence of microaggregates, which block the pores.

The relationship of microaggregates to adult respiratory distress syndrome (ARDS) remains controversial. Animal experiments have given conflicting results. Experiments in dogs show convincing evidence of pulmonary damage by stored blood and this damage is prevented by using microfilters[2]. However, experiments in primates have shown that any damage is very minor[3-5]. In man, an association has been observed[7] between massive blood transfusion and ARDS, but this does not necessarily indicate that microaggregates are causative. Rosario[8] found no relationship between the number of units transfused and the occurrence of ARDS. The relationship to other factors, such as the type of injury[6] or the presence of bacterial infection[8] may be closer. The pathophysiology is further described in Chapter 8.

Conclusive evidence of the benefit from microfilters in man is not available. Reull[9] in a controlled study found less hypoxaemia when microfilters were used but, as pointed out by Collins[6], the injuries in the two groups were not really comparable. Virgilio (quoted by Collins[6]) in a prospective controlled trial of patients having elective aortic surgery found little relationship between volume of transfusion and hypoxaemia, and no differences between standard filters and microfilters. On the other hand Barrett et al.[10] found that when surgical patients were transfused 20% or more of their blood volume, their tests showed an increase in venous admixture. This was not seen when microfilters were used.

It must be conceded that microaggregates are potentially harmful. Organ damage is particularly likely to occur in patients who have other adverse factors (shock, thoracic injury, DIC, infection). On the other hand, all microfilters slow the rate of flow and become occluded with debris after 1–5 units of blood; they add to the cost of transfusion. Hypovolaemia and hypotension present a graver threat to the traumatized patient than transfusion of blood containing microaggregates, so that the use of microfilters should never be allowed to interfere with the adequacy of resuscitation. On the other hand, current knowledge suggests it is wise to use a microfilter when transfusion of more than half the blood volume or 5 units is certain or probable, particularly if there is a thoracic injury or pre-existing pulmonary disease.

Flow through microfilters can be improved by prewarming the blood which decreases the viscosity[11]. It is essential that the blood warmer cannot overheat the blood. Microfilters may lower the platelet count of fresh blood[12]. They do not invariably remove platelets from concentrates stored at room temperature[12], but this may not apply to platelets stored at 4 °C. It is preferable to remove microfilters from the circuit when either fresh blood or platelets are transfused.

(3) Citrate toxicity

The likelihood of citrate toxicity and the need for calcium injections in massively transfused patients remains controversial. Some clarification has been achieved since the calcium-sensitive electrode made it possible to measure ionized calcium precisely. The toxicity of citrate is due predominantly, if not entirely, to its calcium binding. ACD and CPD blood both contain an excess of citrate in order to ensure complete anticoagulation and CPD blood contains approximately 20% less citrate than does ACD blood. In the normal subject approximately 47% of the serum calcium is ionized, about 39% is bound to albumin, and a further 14% is complexed to various anions[13]. If blood is transfused at a too rapid rate for citrate to be metabolized, then the excess citrate will bind some of the recipient's ionized calcium, causing functional hypocalcaemia. In health, although citrate is rapidly metabolized, the maximum rate can be exceeded during plateletphoresis with a standard ACD solution. By the end of the procedure the donors have citrate levels of 26.7 mg/dl, a prolongation of the QT interval and not infrequently have symptoms of hypocalcaemia. The ionized serum calcium levels have been noted to fall by about one third[14]. The decrease in ionized calcium causes tetany, myocardial depression and, if severe enough, a coagulation defect. In the ICU patient the metabolism of citrate may be slow due to liver damage, hypotension or hypothermia[15]. The toxicity of citrate is increased by haemorrhage and acidosis and the depressant effects on the myocardium are increased if hyperkalaemia coexists[16]. Hyperphosphataemia (which may result from rapid blood transfusion) will aggravate the calcium binding effect of citrate[16] and lactate also has some calcium binding effect[17].

Massive transfusions have been given, without supplementary calcium, without apparent ill-effects[18,19]. However, more detailed studies have shown that the rapid transfusion of even one unit of CPD or ACD blood may cause a 27% fall in the ionized calcium and depression of myocardial function[20]. Wilson et al.[21] observed shock in massively transfused patients which was refractory to all measures until calcium chloride was given. Hubbard[22] observed severe hypotension and ECG signs of hypocalcaemia followed by cardiac arrest in a patient being transfused with ACD blood at a rate of 65 ml/min; recovery followed cardiac massage and calcium chloride.

It has been stated that coagulation defects due to a low ionized calcium are not seen, as cardiac arrest occurs first. However, occasionally patients are seen in whom a coagulation defect appears to be due to hypocalcaemia and is improved by calcium infusion[23,24]. Such patients may have a whole blood clotting time prolonged out of proportion to other tests as no calcium is added in this test. The likelihood of citrate toxicity can be reduced by using the minimum amount of citrate necessary to anticoagulate the blood and by avoiding premature formation of microaggregates. Blood stored in plastic bags requires less citrate than blood stored in glass bottles[25]. The use of ACD-A or CPD blood reduces the citrate load[25].

Supplementary calcium should be given if blood is transfused at a rate faster than 100 ml/minute. This is particularly important if the patient is hypotensive or has impaired liver function. The appropriate dose is 500 mg of $CaCl_2$ or 3 g of calcium gluconate (30 ml of 10%) per unit of blood. Weight for weight, calcium gluconate contains one quarter the amount of calcium chloride and is only two thirds ionized[20]. Calcium may be given simultaneously with the blood if two intravenous lines are open; otherwise it should be given after each unit. The papers by Howland et al.[18,19] are sometimes quoted as evidence that the administration of calcium may increase mortality. However, Mollison[26] pointed out that this was a retrospective study and the groups were not comparable. A high total serum calcium during the 24 hours after massive transfusion is not a cause for concern, since most of it is bound to citrate and the free calcium remains normal[20]. However, cardiac arrest may occur if recommended doses of calcium chloride or gluconate are greatly exceeded[27].

(4) Acid–base and electrolyte imbalance

Many critically ill patients have a metabolic acidosis when transfusion is started. Whether transfusion aggravates the acidosis depends on the state of the circulation. If hypotension is corrected then there is only a transient worsening because the lactic and other acids are metabolized. During rapid transfusion for haemorrhage, Collins[17] found that when hypotension was corrected, or in some instances of persistent shock, the arterial pH returned towards normal even though the transfused blood had a low pH. In contrast, when haemorrhage was uncontrolled and hypotension persisted, then the acidosis persisted. CPD blood gives less of an acid load than ACD blood. Sodium bicarbonate should not be given empirically, but only when a documented acidosis needs partial correction.

Stored blood has a high plasma potassium due to the leakage of potassium from red cells. Hyperkalaemia in the recipient is usually only a problem in patients with renal failure or severe burns, who should not receive rapid transfusions of old stored blood.

Massive transfusions are often followed by hypokalaemia and a metabolic alkalosis within 24 hours[21]. If hypokalaemia is left uncorrected the metabolic alkalosis will be aggravated. Metabolism of citrate is largely responsible for the metabolic alkalosis but it may be partly due to sodium bicarbonate being given empirically.

(5) Alterations in oxygen affinity

Anticoagulant solutions for the storage of blood were developed to ensure adequate viability of red cells after transfusion. Modern resuscitation methods enable patients to survive exsanguinating haemorrhage and virtually complete blood replacement, thus the O_2 delivering capacity of transfused red cells has also assumed importance. The HbO_2 dissociation curve ensures that at normal PaO_2 small changes in PO_2 have only a slight effect on O_2 saturation, whereas at the normal PvO_2 small reductions in PO_2 lead to a rapid reduction of HbO_2 saturation with ready delivery of O_2 to the tissues. It is known that acidosis and hyperthermia cause a right shift of the O_2 dissociaton curve which facilitates the delivery of oxygen to the tissues; alkalosis and hypothermia have the reverse effect. The P_{50} is a measure of the position of the HbO_2 dissociation curve, being the pressure at which half the haemoglobin is in the form of HbO_2. A left shifted curve is indicated by a low P_{50}. Recently, it has been found that blood stored in ACD shows a rapid fall of 2,3-diphosphoglycerate (2:3 DPG) with a consequent left shift of the HbO_2 dissociation curve. Following transfusion of the stored blood 2:3 DPG is returned to half the normal level within 24 hours and is fully restored by the 4th day[28]. Blood stored for three weeks in ACD has a P_{50} of 1.9 kPa (14.5 mmHg) and CPD blood of the same age has a P_{50} of 2.46 kPa (18.5 mmHg) compared with a normal P_{50} of 3.53 kPa (26.5 mmHg)[28]. The acid conditions of storage inhibit synthesis of 2:3 DPG. Massive transfusion of 2:3 DPG depleted blood leads to a fall of P_{50} to approximately 2.53 kPa (19 mmHg). In extensively transfused patients the effect of post-transfusion alkalosis is often greater than the effect of low 2:3 DPG, but the effects are additive.

The significance of a left shifted curve has not yet been fully determined[29]. It is most likely to be of significance when compensating mechanisms are exhausted and when adequate O_2 delivery is critical at the time of transfusion or during the next few hours. Experiments suggest that at normal haematocrit levels animals can compensate for a left shifted HbO_2

dissociation curve caused by exchange transfusion of stored blood, by an increased cardiac output. But under conditions of reduced haematocrit, with or without haemorrhagic shock, a left shifted curve increased mortality[17]. In an isolated perfused organ a right shifted curve has an adverse effect during severe hypoxic hypoxia. A left shifted curve has an adverse effect during moderate hypoxic hypoxia, moderate and severe stagnant hypoxia and during moderate anaemic hypoxia[29]. In man, a left shifted curve diminishes exercise tolerance; cardiac output is increased and $P\bar{v}O_2$ is reduced[17]. The basal cardiac output and the response of the heart to volume loading is decreased in patients transfused with blood low in 2:3 DPG for emergency resection of aortic aneurysms[29]. Massive transfusion with stored blood requires a 50% increase in coronary blood flow, but this is only half that required to compensate for an acute reduction of haemoglobin at $10\,g/dl$[30]. Patients with coronary artery disease are particularly at risk. To compensate, the cardiac output must increase and the $P\bar{v}O_2$ fall; the coronary sinus PO_2 may already be close to the minimum functional level.

Undesirable left shift of the O_2 dissociation curve can be minimized by not giving blood with low 2:3 DPG levels; by preventing hypothermia or alkalosis; and by correcting severe acidosis and hypophosphataemia, both of which impair synthesis of 2:3 DPG. Hypophosphataemia may occur in the acutely ill patient or as a consequence of hyperalimentation without phosphate supplementation[31]. Hypophosphataemia should also be avoided because of the reduction of ATP which occurs with adverse effects on red cell flexibility and survival[17].

(6) Hypothermia

Blood must be warmed in all patients who are being rapidly or massively transfused. If 10 litres of blood at 4 °C are transfused over 2 hours and are warmed by the body to 37 °C then the metabolic rate is doubled[17]. If cold blood is transfused rapidly through a central venous line then ventricular fibrillation can occur. One of the potential advantages of intraoperative autotransfusion is that the blood is warm. To be effective a blood warmer must be able to warm blood to at least 32 °C at flow rates of 150 ml/min. The design of blood warmers has been reviewed by Russell[32].

(II) ADDITIONAL COMPLICATIONS

There are several other complications of blood transfusion which are of particular importance in the postoperative traumatized or critically ill patient.

(1) Adverse effects on blood viscosity

Following trauma and acute illness the plasma viscosity increases due to a marked elevation of the acute phase reactants (fibrinogen, α_2-macroglobulin). It is possible that the suppression of erythropoiesis which occurs in this situation compensates for the increased plasma viscosity, since reduction of whole blood viscosity follows a reduction in the haematocrit. Certainly critically ill patients should not be transfused so that the haemoglobin is higher than normal, as the increased viscosity is likely to be disadvantageous. It is controversial whether a modest degree of anaemia (Hb 10 g/dl; PCV 0.30) is advantageous in operative and postoperative patients leading to improved flow through the microcirculation; or is disadvantageous, since O_2 delivery to tissues can only be maintained by increased cardiac output or hypervolaemia[30,33,34].

A decision as to whether blood transfusion is desirable in these circumstances must await further evidence. Anaemia of this degree does not impair wound healing in experimental animals[35], so that the postoperative state does not in itself provide a reason to raise the PCV above 0.30.

(2) Immunologically-mediated reactions (other than red cell incompatibility)

Reactions to blood transfusion which appear to be immunologically-mediated include reactions to donor plasma proteins, white cells and platelets. These reactions are not especially common in critically ill patients, but an awareness of them is necessary, since diagnosis may be difficult when they occur in an already complex clinical situation. Immediate hypersensitivity reactions may be due to antibodies against IgA or other plasma proteins. Antibodies against HLA antigens or other granulocyte or lymphocyte antigens may occur in patients who have been previously transfused or have been immunized by pregnancy; the commonest clinical manifestation is a febrile reaction but white cell antibodies are also suspected as being the cause of acute pulmonary oedema unrelated to circulatory overload[36].

(III) PLASMA PROTEIN SOLUTION

Plasma protein fraction (PPF) or stable plasma protein solution (SPPS) is available for volume replacement or restoration of serum proteins. Its proteins are 85–90% albumin, the remainder being globulins. It is free of risk of transmission of hepatitis so that it should replace dried plasma. SPPS may cause adverse reactions with flushing, headache, hypotension, back pain and abdominal pain[37]. The reactions are probably due to kinins and occur with some but not all batches of SPPS. Kinin content decreases with storage. Reactions have been most commonly seen in patients or donors undergoing plasmaphoresis and during cardiopulmonary bypass; the latter may be related to the bypassing of the lung, which is the main site of inactivation of kinins. If an adverse reaction to SPPS is suspected, the infusion should be stopped and another colloid or a crystalloid should be substituted.

(IV) ALBUMIN SOLUTION

In some countries albumin is available as a 5% solution for resuscitation and replacement of serum proteins. The choice of SPPS or albumin solution rather than a crystalloid in resuscitating injured patients remains controversial. The use of very large amounts of albumin to keep serum albumin levels normal in patients with oligaemic shock is of no benefit and may be deleterious[38]. Adverse reactions to albumin are infrequent; occasional patients suffer chills, fever and urticaria with variable alterations in blood pressure and pulse rate.

(V) FRESH-FROZEN PLASMA

Fresh-frozen plasma (FFP) is indicated for the replacement of coagulation factors; complement components and antithrombin III will also be supplied. Despite testing for hepatitis surface antigen, FFP carries some risk of transmission of hepatitis, the risk from one donation of plasma being the same as that from a single donation of whole blood. (SPPS and albumin solution are free of hepatitis risk but do not contain coagulation factors). Adverse reactions to FFP are uncommon and are usually mild; occasional patients suffer fever, urticaria or hypotension. SPPS and albumin can be given without regard to ABO group, but FFP should be either from an AB donor or of ABO group appropriate to the recipient.

(VI) CRYOPRECIPITATE

Cryoprecipitate contains most of the factor VIII of blood and about a third of the fibrinogen of whole blood – 200–250 mg per donation. It is indicated, as a supplement to FFP, when these factors are consumed during disseminated intravascular coagulation (Chapter 4). Cryoprecipitate also contains high concentrations of fibrinonectin or opsonic glycoprotein[39] It has been suggested that fibrinonectin may mediate the clearance of bacteria, fibrin, microaggregates and other debris. When cryoprecipitate was given to correct the opsonic defect in the injured patient with bacterial infection, cardiorespiratory function was improved and infection lessened[39]. Adverse reactions to cryoprecipitate are rare but there is a risk of transmitting hepatitis.

(VII) FIBRINOGEN

Fibrinogen is rarely necessary. It is indicated when serious haemorrhage is associated with severe hypofibrinogenaemia. Adverse reactions are pathological clotting and the transmission of hepatitis. Because fibrinogen is made from large plasma pools it carries a relatively high risk of transmission of hepatitis. Cryoprecipitate is an alternative source of fibrinogen, the yield from 8 to 10 donations of blood being approximately equivalent to a 2 gram bottle of fibrinogen.

References

1. Barnes, A. (1980). Transfusion of universal donor and uncrossmatched blood. *Bibl. Haematol.* **46**, 132
2. Dhurandher, H. N., Brown, C., Barrett, J. and Litwin, M. S. (1979). Pulmonary structural changes following microembolism and blood transfusion. *Arch. Pathol. Lab. Med.*, **103**, 335
3. Tobey, R. E., Kopriva, C. J., Horner, L. D., Solis, R. T., Dickson, L. G. and Herman, C. M. (1974). Pulmonary gas exchange following hemorrhagic shock and massive blood transfusion in the baboon. *Ann. Surg.*, **179**, 316
4. McDanal, J. T. and McNamara, J. J. (1976). Pulmonary and systemic effects of stored or fresh blood in traumatized shocked baboons. *Surg. Forum*, **27**, 178
5. McNamara, J. J. (1977). *International Forum.* Does a relationship exist between massive blood transfusion and the adult respiratory distress syndrome? *Vox Sang.*, **32**, 311
6. Collins, J. A., James, P. M., Bredenberg, C. E., Anderson, R. W., Heisterkamp, C. A. and Simmons, R. L. (1978). The relationship between transfusion and hypoxaemia in combat casualties. *Ann. Surg.*, **188**, 518
7. Fulton, R. L. (1977). *International Forum* Does a relationship exist between massive blood transfusion and the adult respiratory distress syndrome? *Vox Sang.*, **32**, 311
8. Rosario, M. D., Rumsey, E. W., Arakaki, G., Tanoue, R. E., McDanal, J. and McNamara, J. J. (1978). Blood microaggregates and ultrafilters. *J. Trauma*, **18**, 498
9. Reull, G. J. (Jnr.), Beall, A. C. and Greenberg, S. D. (1974). Protection of the pulmonary microvasculature by fine screen blood filtration. *Chest,* **66**, 409
10. Barrett, J., Jahir, A. H. and Litwin, M. S. (1978). Increased pulmonary

arteriovenous shunting in humans following blood transfusion. *Arch. Surg.*, **113**, 947

11. Linko, K. (1979). In-line blood warming and microfiltration devices. *Acta Anaesthesiol. Scand.*, **23**, 46

12. Snyder, E. L., Grum, P., Cooper-Smith, M. and James, R. (1979). Transfusion of platelets through microaggregate filters. *Anaesthesiology*, **51** (Suppl.), 205

13. Szymanski, I. O. (1978). Ionized calcium during plateletpheresis. *Transfusion*, **18**, 701

14. Olson, P. R., Cox, C. and McCullough, J. (1977). Laboratory and clinical effects of the infusion of ACD solution during plateletpheresis. *Vox Sang.*, **33**, 79

15. Ludbrook, J. and Wynn, V. (1958). Citrate intoxication. A clinical and experimental study. *Br. Med. J.*, **2**, 523

16. Bunker, J. P. (1966). Metabolic effects of blood transfusion. *Anesthesiology*, **27**, 446

17. Collins, J. A. (1974). Problems associated with massive transfusion of stored blood. *Surgery*, **75**, 274

18. Howland, W. S., Bellville, J. W., Zucker, M. B., Boyon, P. and Cliffton, E. E. (1957). Massive blood replacement. V. Failure to observe citrate intoxication. *Surg. Gynecol. Obstet.*, **105**, 529

19. Howland, W. S., Jacobs, R. G. and Goulet, A. H. (1960). An evaluation of calcium administration during rapid blood replacement. *Anesth. Analg.*, **39**, 557

20. Olinger, G. N., Hottenrott, C., Mulder, D. G., Maloney, J. V., Patterson, R. W., Sullivan, S. F. and Buckberg, G. D. (1976). Acute clinical hypocalcaemic myocardial depression during rapid blood transfusion and postoperative haemodialysis. *J. Thorac. Cardiovasc. Surg.*, **72**, 503

21. Wilson, R. F., Mammen, E. and Walt, A. J. (1971). Eight years of experience with massive blood transfusion. *J. Trauma*, **11**, 275

22. Hubbard, T. F., Neis, D. D. and Barmore, J. L. (1956). Severe citrate intoxication during cardiovascular surgery. *J. Am. Med. Assoc.*, **162**, 1534

23. Simmons, R. L., Collins, J. A., Heisterkamp, C. A., Mills, D. E., Andren, R. and Phillips, L. L. (1969). Coagulation disorders in combat casualties. *Ann. Surg.*, **169**, 455

24. Perkins, H. A. (1966). Postoperative coagulation defects. *Anesthesiology*, **27**, 456

25. Mishler, J. M., Darley, J. H., Haworth, C. and Mollison, P. L. (1979). Viability of red cells stored in diminished concentration of citrate. *Br. J. Haematol.*, **43**, 63

26. Mollison, P. L. (1979). *Blood Transfusion in Clinical Medicine.* 6th edn. p. 637 (Oxford: Blackwell Scientific Publications)

27. Wolf, P. L., McCarthy, L. J. and Hafleigh, B. (1970). Extreme hypercalcaemia following blood transfusion combined with intravenous calcium. *Vox Sang.*, **19**, 544

28. McConn, R. (1975). The oxyhaemoglobin dissociation curve. *Surg. Clin. N. Am.*, **55**, 627

29. International Forum (1978). What is the clinical importance of alterations of

the haemoglobin oxygen affinity in preserved blood – especially as produced by variations of red cell 2,3 DPG content. *Vox Sang.*, **34**, 111

30. Lundsgaard-Hansen, P. (1979). Hemodilution – new clothes for an anemic emperor. *Vox Sang.*, **36**, 321
31. Watkins, G. M., Rabelo, A., Plzak, L. F. and Sheldon, G. F. (1974). The left shifted oxyhaemoglobin curve in sepsis: a preventable defect. *Ann. Surg.*, **180**, 213
32. Russell, W. J. (1974). A review of blood warmers for massive transfusion. *Anaesth. Intens. Care*, **2**, 109
33. Rose, D., Forest, R. and Coutsoftides, M. D. (1979). Acute normovolemic hemodilution. *Anesthesiology*, **51**, (Suppl.), 91
34. Messmer, K. (1975). Hemodilution. *Surg. Clin. N. Am.*, **55**, 659
35. Heughan, C., Grislis, G. and Hunt, T. K. (1974). The effect of anemia on wound healing. *Ann. Surg.*, **179**, 163
36. Byrne, J. P. and Dixon, J. A. (1971). Pulmonary edema following transfusion reaction. *Arch. Surg.*, **102**, 91
37. Isbister, J. P. and Biggs, J. C. (1976). Reactions to rapid infusion of stable plasma protein solution during large volume plasma exchange. *Anaesth. Intens. Care*, **4**, 105
38. Johnson, S. D., Lucas, C. E., Gerrick, S. J., Ledgerwood, A. M. and Higgings, R. F. (1979). Altered coagulation after albumin supplements for treatment of oligemic shock. *Arch. Surg.*, **114**, 379
39. Saba, T. M. and Jaffe, E. (1980). Plasma fibrinonectin (opsonic glycoprotein); Its synthesis by vascular endothelial cells and role in cardiopulmonary integrity after trauma as related to reticuloendothial function. *Am. J. Med.*, **68**, 577

7
Intermittent positive pressure ventilation

PAUL LAWLER

Intermittent postive pressure ventilation (IPPV) was invented at least 200 years ago, but it was not until the 1950s that prolonged IPPV was used to treat poliomyelitis[1], the acute respiratory failure of chronic lung disease[2], and tetanus[3]. The commonest use of IPPV remains during anaesthesia, but the treatment is also applied to very varied diseases in the general intensive care unit (ICU). IPPV is now considered whenever the respiratory status of the patient is in jeopardy, is likely to become so, or when respiratory failure effects other body systems. This chapter reviews the general principles and new developments. The author trained in both general medicine and anaesthesia. He spent several years researching in intensive care and is now establishing a multi-disciplinary unit.

(I) CHOICE OF A VENTILATOR

Personal prejudice often plays a large part in the choice of a ventilator. However, questions which should be posed when choosing a ventilator are given in Table 7.1. Opinion varies on the advantages of equipping an ICU with a single type of ventilator. While familiarity with one type of ventilator is important, the teaching element of intensive therapy and the experience of those 'on the ground', the nursing and junior medical staff, must be considered. Unfortunately, cost often plays a decisive part in the choice. Nevertheless, the purchase of relatively cheap all-purpose ventilators, such as the Brompton Manley[4], may allow the purchase of one or two newer machines of the 'servo' type, which can be necessary for the management of complex cases. 'Servo' ventilators continuously monitor both inspired and expired flow and tidal volume, and ensure that the patient receives the prescribed ventilation. Because of their advanced design, these ventilators may provide on-line measurement of respiratory mechanics. Nevertheless, a simple ventilator capable of an inspiratory 'hold' enables the compliance to be assessed, and a 'top hat' flow pattern will enable the airway resistance to be calculated[5].

Table 7.1 The choice of a ventilator

Is it safe and reliable?

Can the controls be understood by those most likely to use them?

Does the ventilator require high pressure gas sources for operation?

Which patients are likely to require IPPV? How old are they? Will they have normal lungs?

Can the ventilator be decontaminated? Does it require bacterial filters?

Will it continue to deliver the same minute and tidal volume despite moment-to-moment changes in the patient's condition? Can the gas flow pattern be altered?

Are there alarms for disconnection, power failure and high airway pressure?

Are there any weaning facilities?

How much does it cost to buy and run?

In this unit, primarily for cost considerations, the Blease Brompton Manley ventilator (costing under £1000) has been chosen as the workhorse. In addition a 'servo-type' ventilator, the Siemens Servo ventilator, was purchased because of the facility to extract electrical analogue signals and to add on 'black boxes' capable of monitoring lung mechanics, CO_2 output

143

and oxygen consumption. This ventilator can also cycle at rates up to 60/min and is thus capable of providing high frequency positive pressure ventilation (HFPPV). A simple Bird ventilator was also obtained.

(II) PHYSIOLOGY

(1) Mechanics

IPPV is usually undertaken with the patient in the supine or semi-erect position; weaning from mechanical ventilation is usually undertaken in the semi-erect or erect position. It is therefore necessary to know how posture affects pulmonary physiology. In the erect position the normal lungs can be compared to a loosely coiled spring (e.g. a 'slinky'*) supported at the apex. At functional residual capacity (FRC), gravity ensures that the airways at the apex of the lung are held open by the weight of the lung, while at the base, the weight of the lung tends to reduce airway size. Inspiration from FRC tends to direct gas to the basal airways because the apical airways, like the spring, are already under considerable tension and further expansion is limited. This analogy is also true in the supine position, although the lung is then under less tension. The anterior (superior) airways are then stretched, but gas will be more evenly distributed between the anterior and posterior regions of the lung, because of the reduced pressure gradient.

Gravity and pulmonary artery pressure (PAP) determine the maximum height to which blood can be pumped within the lung. Thus, there is a gravity dependent gradation of blood flow from apex to base, although local changes in pulmonary vascular resistance (PVR) can alter flow to individual areas. Stretching of the lung during inspiration reduces PVR proportionally, so that flow to the bases increases and the blood flow is directed towards the gas flow. The lung is held open by the opposing forces of the chest wall (rib cage and the diaphragm), which tends to spring open. A consequence is that the pressure in the pleural space will be subatmospheric. Gravity will cause a pressure gradient in the pleural space, the apical pressure being less than the basal. In the supine position the gradient will be from anterior to posterior. Allowing time for normal inspiration air enters the lung because the lung stretches as the pleural pressure falls progressively below atmospheric; expiration is the reverse of this process. A change in the elastic properties of the lung or chest wall will alter the pleural pressure, the FRC and the relationship between lung volume and pleural pressure. These events assume that gas flow occurs without a pressure gradient, which is untrue. Consequently, there will be a larger change in pleural pressure to achieve the tidal volume in a finite time. Allowing time for an

---

* Editor's note: for the uninitiated this is a walking spring toy.

infinitely long inspiration, the pleural pressure required for the tidal volume will depend solely on the elastic properties of the lung. The 'time constant' of the lung (compliance × airway resistance) defines the rate at which volume changes actually take place. Of the volume change, 95% is accomplished within three time constants, at which time pleural pressure lies extremely close to that which might be predicted from the elastic properties of the lung.

During IPPV, the pressure gradient from mouth to pleura – the transpulmonary pressure – is reversed. The same transpulmonary pressure produces the same volume change, but during inflation of the lungs the pleural pressure rises rather than falls. Alveolar pressure and mouth pressure rise. In the upright position there is once more an apex to base gradation of pleural pressure and again apical ventilation will be relatively less than basal. However, the flow pattern produced by the ventilator may, theoretically at least, alter the gas distribution described above. Because of the spring effect, apical airways are wider than basal. Therefore at high flow the apical airways may be preferentially ventilated because of their low resistance. Theoretically, a combination of high frequency and high inspiratory flow rates would lead to preferential apical ventilation; in practice, flow pattern seems to be of less importance.

IPPV and spontaneous respiration are broadly similar in terms of gas distribution when the lung is considered in the upright position. The adoption of the supine posture uncovers differences which are at least partly explained by the fact that the diaphragm is no longer 'suspended' from the edges of the rib cage. Thus in the supine position FRC is reduced, the cause of which is only partially explained by the above. During spontaneous breathing, in the supine position, the action of the diaphragm ensures that the posterior parts of the lung (now the 'base') are best ventilated. Thus diaphragmatic excursion is greatest posteriorly. Ventilation and perfusion are again matched. During IPPV, at least with paralysis, the position, shape and movement of the diaphragm differs[6]. The shape and position are now governed by the pressure gradient between the abdomen and chest. This gradient is greatest posteriorly, because of the weight of the abdominal viscera. The superior (i.e. anterior) part of the diaphragm tends to move caudad, while the inferior (i.e. posterior) part tends to move cephalad. The distribution of gas during IPPV remains dependent on compliance and gravity, so that in the supine position IPPV tends to ventilate the superior (i.e. anterior) parts of the lung and this causes a ventilation–perfusion imbalance.

(2) Circulation

The distribution of pulmonary blood flow is determined by the PAP, pulmonary venous pressure, alveolar pressure (PA) and the PVR. The latter depends on lung volume and gravity. At the apex PAP is insufficient to keep the pulmonary capillaries open against the PA which, during spontaneous respiration, is close to atmospheric. In the mid-zone of the lung PAP exceeds PA and flow depends on this pressure difference. At the base, venous pressure exceeds PA and flow then depends upon the pressure difference between artery and vein. From the above, it can be seen that the pulmonary blood flow and distribution depend on PA. The increase in PA which occurs during IPPV increases the volume of the 'apical' compartment, thus increasing dead space (V_D) and altering ventilation–perfusion ratios. A reduction in PAP will have a similar effect, while an increase in pulmonary venous pressure will decrease flow at the base and may divert blood towards the apex.

For many years it has been known that IPPV reduces cardiac output and does so by reducing venous return[7]. It is only recently that the mechanisms of some respiratory effects have become clear[8-10]. For example, during normal respiration, arterial pressure decreases during inspiration and increases during expiration. It is therefore surprising that positive pressure breathing which increases mean intrathoracic pressure, can also increase systemic arterial pressure. Let us first consider the left side of the heart. During spontaneous inspiration, the pleural pressure falls and the left side of the heart must then increase intraventricular pressure by the same amount in order to maintain arterial pressure, that is, the left ventricle sustains an increased afterload during inspiration. On the right side of the heart, the fall in pleural pressure increases the extrathoracic to intrathoracic venous pressure gradient. However, the inflow is not increased by the expected amount because extrathoracic veins are compressed by atmospheric pressure. Nevertheless, this small increase in venous return increases right ventricular preload, distends the right ventricle and increases right ventricular output. The extra distension of the right ventricle causes a shift in the ventricular septum to the left and hence reduces left ventricular compliance. This increase in stiffness of the left ventricle leads to an immediate reduction in end-diastolic volume and diminishes stroke work. Thus, small reductions in pleural pressure have immediate effect by increasing right heart output and decreasing left heart output. This information may explain the occurrence of left ventricular failure in asthma[11] and why a negative (subatmospheric) end-expiratory pressure fails to increase cardiac output markedly during IPPV[12]. When a negative end-expiratory pressure is used during IPPV, the reduction in mean intrathoracic pressure increases left ventricular afterload. On the right side the reduction in mean intrathoracic pressure, although increasing the extrathoracic to intrathoracic pressure drop, does not increase venous return proportionately.

During inflation of the lungs by a positive pressure, the pleural pressure rises acutely with the following effects. On the left side of the heart afterload is decreased and the left ventricle empties more fully, so increasing arterial pressure by an amount similar to the increase in intrathoracic pressure. On the right side of the heart venous return is reduced, the right ventricle fills less and puts out less. The ventricular septum is deviated to the right, effectively altering left ventricular compliance and thus left ventricular output.

(III) MANAGEMENT

(1) General nursing care

Patients requiring IPPV are often sedated or paralysed and may be unconscious. They present an extremely heavy nursing load. The eyes, mouth and skin need obsessional care. The eyes of unconscious or paralysed patients can remain open and the corneas are easily damaged by equipment or during turning. Because the corneal reflex is obtunded and the eyes remain open, the corneas can become dry. The use of 'artificial tears' (methyl cellulose eye drops) may suffice; it is preferable to tape the eyelids together as an added precaution. Mouth care may be difficult in patients in whom an oral endotracheal tube has been inserted; such a tube must not be allowed to drag on the corner of the mouth. Although acute parotitis is now rare, inadequate mouth care and inappropriate fluid restriction enhance its likelihood. The teeth must be kept brushed, and the pharynx clear of secretions, which may be of gastric origin.

Skin care is of critical importance[13]. Patients requiring IPPV are often immobile and can be hypotensive, hypothermic and hypoxaemic. They may also be incontinent. They are thus prime candidates for developing pressure sores. As the name suggests, pressure sores develop where the weight per unit area is greatest. The combination of a large weight applied over a small area is most likely where bony prominences lie close to the skin. In the supine position, the heels and sacrum are most likely sites for the development of pressure sores, while in the lateral position the site most at risk lies beneath the greater trochanter. The point of contact between upper and lower limbs in the knee area is a further site at risk. Prevention of pressure sores is considerably easier than cure, and attention to detail is the most important aspect of care. The sheets must be uncreased, clean and dry. Regular turning and the use of lambskin to distribute weight should eliminate pressure sores. Water-beds and high air loss beds are not always appropriate for the critically ill patient who may require external cardiac massage although a fluidized bead bed may be used[14]. Wet skin, whether caused by incontinence or spilled intravenous fluids, is particularly vulnerable. Although urinary catheterization is necessary to monitor fluid balance, it also prevents wet beds. If wet, the skin must be gently dried, and talcum powder used for lubrication and not as a substitute for gentle drying.

One final aspect of general nursing care not to be forgotten is that patients requiring IPPV, although heavily sedated, or apparently unconscious, must be assumed conscious and treated as such. Unfortunately this is more often forgotten by the medical staff!

(2) The gastrointestinal tract

After starting IPPV many patients develop gastrointestinal stasis which may persist for up to 48 hours. Whether this is caused by IPPV or by drugs is not clear. A nasogastric tube is a wise precaution to prevent regurgitation of gastric contents and to warn of gastric dilatation. Continuous aspiration of the nasogastric aspirate may give an early indication of upper gastrointestinal bleeding, which is a serious complication in the critically ill[15,16]. Antacids (e.g. Mist. Mag. Trisil. 20 ml 4 hourly) are of prophylactic value against stress bleeding in these patients provided that the gastric pH is maintained above 5.0[17,18]. Cimetidine is less effective than antacid therapy[19]. Once bowel sounds return, nasogastric feeding should be commenced, and a bowel action may be expected. Simple enemata may be required to prevent faecal impaction and overflow incontinence (Chapter 12).

(3) The urinary tract

Aseptic bladder catheterization should be performed in patients requiring IPPV, unless specifically contraindicated. Fluid management is complex and the monitoring of urine output may be mandatory, particularly in the hypotensive patient. It is important that a closed system of drainage is used in order to prevent infection.

(4) Sedation during IPPV

The presence of an endotracheal tube, the intermittent inflation of the lungs and bronchial suction are unpleasant if not painful, even for those patients with insight[20-22]. The absolute dependence upon a machine for life can be terrifying and cause considerable psychological problems[23]. In addition, patients requiring IPPV have often been subject to painful surgery, or are likely to undergo painful or distressing procedures, perhaps without adequate explanation. It is humane for patients to be heavily sedated, at least during the early period after starting IPPV. Since many procedures are painful, the ideal sedative is a potent analgesic, an opiate given i.v. Over short periods, accumulation and addiction are relatively unimportant and respiratory depression irrelevant. 'Background' sedation in the form of intermittent intramuscular injection of opiates or benzodiazepines, for example, lorazepam, can be helpful, the latter having a potent amnesic effect[24]. Benzodiazepines are, however, notoriously cumulative, and some are painful when given i.m. During the early phase of treatment circulatory failure may make absorption from i.m. sites unpredictable, and the intravenous route is essential for all medication. Although providing adequate sedation, opiates may not suppress spontaneous respiratory efforts. In certain circumstances, for example, crushed chest or head injury, ventilator compliance is necessary and coughing must be suppressed. It is therefore necessary to add a muscle relaxant (e.g. pancuronium bromide) to the drug regime. However, it is still necessary to determine the reasons for 'fighting'. When muscle relaxants are given it is mandatory that conscious patients also receive adequate sedation. Muscle relaxants have no sedative action, a point which must not be forgotten by the nursing staff[25]. Recently, continuous intravenous sedation has been used in the management of these patients, either thiopentone[26], etomidate[27] or Althesin. Continuous intramuscular sedation[28] is not advised in these circumstances. Nitrous oxide, either as Entonox or as a 1:80 mixture with oxygen/air is gaining popularity[29], although anxiety remains about bone marrow depression following prolonged useage. The site of depression by nitrous oxide appears to be in a B_{12} pathway[30,31].

(5) Physiotherapy

Chest physiotherapy is of paramount importance during IPPV, although regular passive movements of arms and legs must not be omitted. Physiotherapy is best undertaken by a physiotherapist specifically allotted to the ICU. In my view one daily session of chest physiotherapy should be carried out by the physiotherapist in conjunction with an intensive care doctor. In addition to postural drainage and 'vibratory expression', patients with endotracheal tubes should be 'bagged' regularly by the nurses or physiotherapist. Any radiological evidence of absorption collapse requires bagging, although potential hazards (pneumothorax, low cardiac output, raised intracranial pressure) are relative contraindications. Endotracheal suction should be carried out during each sequence of 'bagging' or 'vibration', and at regular intervals. Since the normal lung defences in these patients are compromised, a rigidly 'clean' technique should be used. A sterile disposable suction catheter should be used at the start of each sequence and discarded at the end. Suction into a mucus trap at the start of physiotherapy is required for bacteriological monitoring. However, the flora of the trachea and main bronchus can differ from that in the smaller airways and these can be obtained by using a long fine-bore tube[33]. The external diameter of the suction catheter should not exceed half the internal diameter of the endotracheal tube, otherwise suction can cause a sub-atmospheric airway pressure leading to atelectasis or rarely pulmonary oedema. Trauma to the tracheal and bronchial mucosa is inevitable during suction particularly if the suction catheter has sharp edges. The advantages of catheters with both end and side holes and a 'beaded' tip are not proven. The trauma produced by these catheters is comparable to that produced by conventional catheters, suggesting that damage results from factors other than tip design[34,35]

(6) Humidification

In health, inspired gas is fully saturated with water vapour by the time it reaches the subglottis. An endotracheal or tracheostomy tube bypasses the upper respiratory tract and thus the tracheal and bronchial mucosae are subjected to the drying effect of cold, completely dry air. During anaesthesia at least, it has been shown that following endotracheal intubation, humidification of gases is completed by the time the inspired gas reaches the carina[36]. During this short journey the exposed mucosa must supply 44 mg of water vapour to fully saturate 1 l of dry gas at a temperature of 37 °C. With a minute volume of 10 litres this amounts to 670 ml of water per 24 hours. Higher minute volume, which may be needed in some patients, will need correspondingly larger volumes.

Numerous methods of humidification are available. Condenser humidifiers (the 'Swedish nose') are simple but relatively inefficient when exposed to a completely dry gas. Their dead space and resistance may be excessive for children and when they become fouled with secretion their resistance may even be too high for adults. Nebulizers can be designed to produce water droplets varying in size. A droplet size of less than 5 μm is necessary to ensure that water droplets reach the alveoli. 'Sidestream' humidification, in which a small volume of humidified gas is added to the main gas stream, is inadequate for anything other than giving nebulized drugs. Hot water humidifiers, usually designed as 'blow over' humidifiers, are simple and remarkably efficient. When heated to 50 °C to produce an airway temperature of 37 °C, the water content of the gas may be as high as 40 mg/l. A recently introduced humidifier (Fisher Paekel) incorporates a heating element in the inspiratory hose and has a bath temperature of 37 °C. Coaxial tubing which insulates the inspiratory hose is also available. This combination allows full humidification to be accomplished without condensation of water in the inspiratory hosing which occurs in 'overheated' hot water humidifiers. A pasteurization temperature is not required as the paper element and dome are sterile and disposable.

(7) Infection

Intubation bypasses the defence mechanisms of the upper respiratory tract. The ICU patient, often immune-incompetent (Chapter 2), is then at an increased risk of developing pulmonary infections. An ICU harbours potential reservoirs of infections, some of which are difficult to eliminate. The sources of infection have been frequently described and only a brief recapitulation is required. The chief sources are the environment – the ventilator, suction machines, air, bed linen, hand basins, and the patient's own bacterial flora, especially in the colon and nose. Transmission is by the gas inflating the lungs and by his fingers, lotions or tube feeds. In those patients with ileus the stomach becomes a reservoir and the gram-negative bacteria reach the pharynx and trachea by direct spread[37].

Decontamination of complex ventilators may be difficult or impossible. The 'new generation' ventilators have separate autoclavable circuits and work on a 'bag in bottle' system thus ensuring that cross-infection cannot occur. While older ventilators can be adapted to the 'bag in bottle' system, the use of bacteriological filters is often more practical than either the 'bag in bottle' system or ethylene oxide sterilization[38]. Bacteriological isolation of the ventilator from the patient circuit can be obtained by means of autoclavable or disposable filters. These ensure that the sterility (or otherwise) of the internal 'plumbing' of the ventilator can be ignored. The inspiratory filter, situated between ventilator and humidifier, remains dry during use, but the expiratory filter, between patient and ventilator, will become wet. The condensation in some expiratory filters will increase their resistance to gas flow unless the filter is heated. Siliconized filters (e.g. the Williams filter) are not affected by moisture[39]. This filter has a sufficiently low resistance (less than $0.01 \text{ kPa l s}^{-1}$ ($0.1 \text{ cmH}_2\text{O l s}^{-1}$) at 0.75 l s^{-1} (45 l min^{-1})), to be acceptable during spontaneous respiration. However, each filter has an internal volume of 700 ml thus adding 1400 ml of compressible volume to the circuit (personal observations).

Ideally, filters, inspiratory hoses and the humidifier should be changed daily and autoclaved between use. In the case of hot water humidifiers, sterilization may be achieved by boiling for 20 minutes and the humidifier changed between patients. The humidifier should be topped up once daily with aqueous chlorhexidine[40] (0.02%) and thereafter with sterile water. Hydrogen peroxide will sterilize the humidifier, but will not maintain sterility. In some units, humidifiers and tubing are changed daily, while filters are only changed between patients. While this system protects the patient from the ventilator and vice versa, the filter itself can remain a source of infection. Finally, even when filters are in use, all possible decontamination procedures should be carried out between patients.

(IV) AIRWAY

IPPV requires free access to the trachea via a cuffed oral or nasotracheal tube, or via a cuffed tracheostomy tube. When an emergency airway is needed, it is usual to employ a cuffed oral endotracheal tube because of the ease and speed with which this can be inserted. However, when intubation is elective this often requires local or general anaesthesia with or without a muscle relaxant. In some conditions the latter may be contra-indicated. Many patients require endotracheal intubation for surgery followed by intensive care. In these 'elective' cases it is better to use a plastic endotracheal tube for the initial intubation. Red rubber endotracheal tubes are not appropriate for prolonged intubation because they cause laryngeal and tracheal trauma. Nasotracheal intubation has advantages over the oro-tracheal route and is more widely used for prolonged intubation. It is more comfortable, allows better fixation and facilitates oral toilet. However, nasotracheal intubation requires greater skill and is contra-indicated in patients with anterior skull fractures or bleeding disorders. Anatomical reasons may make nasotracheal intubation impossible. Although erosion of the nasal cartilage by nasotracheal tube is rare, both this complication and that of angular stomatitis from oral intubation can be prevented by careful choice of tube size and meticulous fixation. Unfortunately, nasotracheal intubation requires a tube which is longer and narrower than the oral type. This does not matter during IPPV but spontaneous respiration and endo-tracheal suction may be hindered by choice of the nasotracheal route.

Modern plastic endotracheal tubes cause considerably less pharyngeal, laryngeal and tracheal damage than their predecessors. Plastic endotracheal tubes become soft and pliable at 37 °C and thus tend to take up the general shape and curves of the airway. For this reason the incidence of trauma has been reduced but not eliminated. Movement of the tube with respiration and the use of large diameter tubes can damage the anterior and posterior commissures of the larynx and the vocal cords, and lead to granuloma formation and subglottic stenosis. Endotracheal tube 'cuff' complications are more important, especially the long term complication of tracheal stenosis. Both stenosis and malacea result from prolonged ischaemia of the tracheal mucosa and supporting structures. Some form of tracheal narrowing can be demonstrated in over 50% of patients following long term intubation[41]. Various techniques were tried to overcome the problem, including the use of double cuffs. However, there was little progress until Geffin designed a high volume, large diameter, higher compliance cuff[42]. When inflated, the classical small volume, low compliance cuff lies in contact with a small area of the trachea. Assuming for a moment that the trachea is circular in outline, it should be possible to inflate the cuff until its diameter marginally exceeds that of the trachea and produces a seal. At this point the pressure applied to the tracheal mucosa will be minimal and will not seriously affect capillary blood flow. Unfortunately, the trachea is not circular and the cuff is only able to take up one shape, that is, circular in cross section. Thus a larger volume of gas must be inserted into the cuff to produce a seal, inevitably increasing the pressure on the mucosa. Furthermore, because the cuff has a low compliance and low volume, it is extremely difficult to detect a change in the pressure-volume relationship of the cuff at the point of seal. Large volume, large diameter, high compliance cuffs ('floppy') have two advantages. Firstly, the cuff is applied over a large surface area and this is more likely to create a seal. Secondly, the pressure–volume relationship of the cuff is such as to be practically irrelevant when the cuff is distended to its seal point. This is because only an extremely low pressure is required to distend the cuff to a diameter greater than that of the trachea. The pressure in the inflated cuff is related to tracheal wall distension and not to cuff distension. It is thus possible to ensure that cuff and tracheal wall pressures remain at a low level, just above the seal point during the inflation of the lungs. Other methods of reducing tracheal wall pressure have been attempted, e.g. the Kamen Wilkinson foam cuff[43] although this may not be as safe as expected[44]. The deflated size of the 'floppy' cuff of some endotracheal tubes can make intubation more difficult but the large cuff ensures that the tube lies centrally in the trachea so that 'tip' ulceration is reduced. Unfortunately, the seal produced by the 'floppy' cuff may not be as satisfactory as once thought. When inflated to the correct level folds may remain in the cuff material. While the cuff may remain leak-proof for gas, fluids may seep past the cuff[45,46]. Furthermore, during spontaneous respiration the changes in diameter of the trachea may lead to unforeseen leaks around the cuff[47]. The increasing use of nitrous oxide for sedation during IPPV has produced a further 'cuff' problem. Nitrous oxide within the airway diffuses into the cuff. When the diffusion of nitrous oxide into the cuff exceeds the diffusion of oxygen or nitrogen from the cuff (assuming the cuff was filled with air), the cuff volume and pressure will increase leading to unforeseen damage to the mucosa[48,49].

The length of time for which an oral or nasotracheal tube may remain in place before causing significant laryngeal damage is controversial. There is little doubt that red rubber endotracheal tubes cause damage to both trachea and larynx within 48 hours. However, the modern plastic endotracheal tubes are relatively inert and smooth and can safely remain in the larynx for longer periods. It is the author's practice to advise tracheostomy after 10–14 days of continuous intubation although such tubes have been left in place for as long as 2 months with little damage[50].

In certain circumstances, e.g. expected long term IPPV with weaning problems, it is probably wise to carry out an early tracheostomy, assuming the clinical condition of the patient is relatively stable. Tracheostomy will allow better endotracheal suction, better mouth care and better communication and thus improve patient morale. Tracheostomy is seldom an emergency procedure and is commonly performed with general anaesthesia and muscle relaxation, and with an endotracheal tube already in place. The tracheal incision must spare the cricoid ring and the first thyroid cartilage, otherwise late subglottic stenosis is inevitable. Tracheostomy is always followed by some degree of tracheal narrowing at the level of the stoma and this reduction in tracheal diameter appears to be greater when the stoma is large. The use of the modified Björk flap appears to reduce stenosis at the stoma level[52] and also enables the tracheostomy tube to be reinserted with relative ease before a clearly defined track has developed. Recently there has been a return to the simple tracheal window, which theoretically may cause less damage than a Björk flap of similar diameter. Whichever stoma is chosen, it is important to minimize movement between tube and trachea and avoid too large a tube. Retrospective studies have shown that there is some narrowing of the trachea at the stoma in up to 85% of cases, although less than a quarter of these patients admitted any symptoms[53].

(1) The catheter mount

With all types of tracheal tubes the constant dragging and movement of the ventilator tubes and the catheter mount will cause some movement of the tracheal tube. This movement will exacerbate laryngeal or tracheal injury and is particularly important in the case of tracheostomy tubes, which must remain centrally placed within the tracheostome and trachea to reduce trauma to a minimum. Careful fixation of tracheal tubes and catheter mount is mandatory. Disconnection or dislodgement is often fatal unless quickly rectified.

(V) INDICATIONS FOR ARTIFICIAL VENTILATION

The use of IPPV has increased with experience and so have the indications. It is now common practice to intervene earlier during the course of a disease. Originally, the sole indication for IPPV was acute respiratory failure, whether due to parenchymal disease, paralysis, or flail chest. IPPV is now considered when there is a likelihood of respiratory failure complicating another disorder or its treatment. Lastly, IPPV is sometimes used to treat brain oedema in the absence of respiratory failure. The indications for mechanical ventilation are threefold: respiratory failure, prophylaxis and mechanical stabilization. Additionally, IPPV is essential for cardiopulmonary resuscitation, when none of these indications hold.

154

(1) Respiratory failure

A physiological definition of respiratory failure was devised by Campbell and is widely accepted[54]. Failure is defined as a PaO_2 of less than 8.0 kPa or a $PaCO_2$ greater than 6.5 kPa (50 mmHg), when the patient was breathing air. The inexperienced or ignorant might conclude that blood gas analysis would provide clear-cut criteria for IPPV, but the contents of this book should convince the reader otherwise! It should be recalled that the normal range for PaO_2 is wide and that the values in health vary considerably both with age and the F_1O_2. The arterial blood gases are often inadequate indicators for IPPV, particularly if interpreted without the clinical findings. For instance, in acute severe asthma, the exhausted patient can have a normal $PaCO_2$ but still require IPPV. Similarly, when hypoxaemic failure complicates abdominal surgery or bacterial infection or toxaemia, the patient may need IPPV even when the PaO_2 is only moderately decreased and readily restored to normal by oxygen therapy. Progressive changes in the blood gases are of much greater importance and IPPV may be required before the blood gases deviate to those of 'failure'.

Respiratory failure is subdivided into ventilatory failure and transfer[55] or hypoxaemic failure[56]. Although treatment is essentially the same, it is valuable to distinguish between these varieties because the prognosis can differ as described below. Ventilatory failure is characterized by a rising $PaCO_2$ and a falling PaO_2. The principal causes of ventilatory failure are (i) a reduction in the neural input to the respiratory muscles, either of central or peripheral origin, e.g. self-poisoning, polyneuritis; (ii) impairment of the mechanical properties of the chest wall, e.g. flail chest; (iii) increase in the physiological dead space, e.g. pulmonary embolism.

'Transfer failure' is characterized by a low PaO_2 and a normal or low $PaCO_2$. This pattern is commonly seen in the ICU and is due to one or more of the following conditions: pulmonary oedema, pulmonary infection, absorption collapse, contusion of the lung. The adult respiratory distress syndrome (Chapter 8) is another cause of 'transfer failure'. In these circumstances a rising $PaCO_2$ then indicates the additional development of ventilatory failure.

As indicated earlier, the blood gases should not be considered in isolation from the patient. The ability to continue to breathe is of equal importance. 'Fatigue' is as important an indication for respiratory assistance as is a low PaO_2 or a high $PaCO_2$. A clinical scoring system for 'fatigue' has been developed[57] because measurement of the work of breathing is difficult in the intensive care patient.[58-60] Recent developments in the analysis of electromyograms of the respiratory muscles have shown that it is possible to detect 'fatigue' at an early stage, at least in the neonate[61,62]. At present the usual method of assessing respiratory power is by measurements of the vital capacity and the 'inspiratory force'. The latter is obtained by forced inspiration from an occluded mouthpiece. Using these, and other criteria, the Boston group have suggested guidelines for assessing the need for IPPV[63,64]. Table 7.2 summarizes the measurements, but the Boston group stress that trends are as important as isolated values. Furthermore, chronic lung disease may make these guidelines inappropriate when a $PaCO_2$ of 7.5 kPa may not be an indication for IPPV. The specific examples of the indications for IPPV are described in other chapters or the references given in Table 7.3.

Table 7.2 Physiological indications for artificial ventilation

Oxygenation	PaO_2 less than 9 kPa on high flow oxygen $P(\text{A-a})O_2$ greater than 60 kPa (450 mmHg) while breathing 100% oxygen
Ventilation	$PaCO_2$ greater than 7.5 kPa (55 mmHg) V_D/V_T greater than 0.6
Mechanics	FEV_1 less than 10 ml kg^{-1} Vital capacity less than 15 ml kg^{-1} Inspiratory force less than 25 cmH$_2$O (normal greater than 75 cmH$_2$O)

Table 7.3 Some uses of artificial ventilation

Extensive or prolonged surgery
Chest injury   (Chapter 11)
Head injury   (Chapter 9)
Acute poisoning   (Chapter 14)
Tetanus   (Chapter 16)
Guillain–Barré syndrome   (Chapter 15)
Adult respiratory distress syndrome   (Chapter 8)
Botulism   (Chapter 17)
Pulmonary burns
Pulmonary blast injury
Spinal cord injuries   (Chapter 12)
Liver failure
Malignant hyperpyrexia
Post cardiac arrest   (Chapters 13 and 18)
Renal donor   (Chapter 10)
Asthma*

* Editor's note: Asthma is dealt with in *Essential Intensive Care*. 1978. p. 303. (Lancaster: MTP Press)

(2) Prophylaxis

Prophylactic IPPV means elective ventilation in patients who have a high risk of developing respiratory failure. These patients commonly require potent analgesics and drugs to induce sleep; there is no such thing as a potent but safe narcotic analgesic! Such prophylactic IPPV is routinely used following cardiac surgery. In the general ICU prophylactic IPPV is used following extensive abdominal surgery in the critically ill or elderly. The rationale is to ensure proper gas exchange and allow pain to be fully relieved. The IPPV is commonly stopped after 8–12 hours. The treatment of head injuries or cerebral oedema by mechanical ventilation is considered by some to be prophylactic. IPPV with hyperventilation reduces intracranial pressure and suppresses struggling or coughing. Oxygenation can be assured and treatment with massive doses of barbiturate and hypothermia can be used with greater safety. There.is, as yet, no evidence in the head-injured that any of these treatments influence the outcome (Chapter 9).

(3) Mechanical stabilization

IPPV is now widely used as a means of 'internal pneumatic stabilization' of the flail chest. Indeed, the paper by Avery, Mörch and Benson is one of the classics on intensive therapy[65]. With increasing experience the complications of the treatment are fewer and there is less hesitation in starting. Recently, the need for mechanical ventilation following these injuries has been questioned by Schaal who suggested that the improvement in mortality was due to factors other than IPPV[66]. Nevertheless, blunt chest injury with rib fractures is often associated with parenchymal lung damage, and IPPV may then be appropriate for reasons other than stabilization. These problems are analysed in Chapter 11.

(4) When not to ventilate

The decision not to ventilate a patient in overt respiratory failure can be easy or difficult. It is correct to ventilate the patient with acute respiratory failure due to poisoning, asthma or chest injury. Nor should there be any doubt about ventilating the elderly patient following curative abdominal surgery even when the patient has chronic lung disease. The decision should be clear cut in patients with incurable cancer or incurable neurological disease; IPPV is then unethical. To decide whether or not to ventilate a patient severely disabled by chronic bronchitis or emphysema can be difficult. When the dyspnoea prior to the acute illness is extreme, the results from IPPV do not justify an unpleasant and expensive treatment. But the

157

doctor must also consider the patient's quality of life and the views of his relatives. To reach a decision may take time and an infusion of doxapram hydrochloride can be used to buy time[67].

(VI) MONITORING OF PATIENTS DURING IPPV

The aim of monitoring is to assess the following: tissue oxygenation, ventilation, alterations in respiratory function with time or treatment, and equipment failure.

(1) Tissue oxygenation

A high PaO_2 does not equate with adequate tissue oxygenation. Oxygen flux is determined by the equation:

$$\dot{V}_{O_2} = C(a\text{-}\bar{v})O_2 \times \dot{Q}$$

where $\dot{V}_{O_2}$ is the oxygen consumption or delivery
$C(a\text{-}\bar{v})O_2$ is the arterio-venous oxygen content difference
$\dot{Q}$ is the cardiac output

It can be seen that any factor which reduces cardiac output can cause a fall in oxygen delivery unless there is a corresponding increase in the $C(a\text{-}\bar{v})O_2$. This is of particular importance when using positive end-expiratory pressure (PEEP) which may reduce the cardiac output; a rise in the PaO_2 may not then signify improved oxygen flux.

An adequate PaO_2 can nearly always be achieved by ventilation with 100% oxygen. However, the prolonged use of an F_IO_2 above 50% causes pulmonary oxygen toxicity. Therefore an F_IO_2 of less than 50% is chosen which will produce a PaO_2 slightly in excess of 10 kPa (80 mmHg). Repeated measurements of PaO_2 are required during IPPV. The frequency will depend upon the clinical findings, but the PaO_2 should be measured whenever there is a change in F_IO_2, manipulation of the endotracheal tube or alteration to the ventilator. Following a change in the patient's position, F_IO_2 or physiotherapy, the measurement of PaO_2 should be delayed for 20 minutes to allow gas exchange to reach a steady state. Obviously, this '20 minute' rule does not apply when unexpected changes occur in the clinical condition of the patient. Measurement of the PO_2 of the blood sample should be performed immediately, otherwise the sample should be placed on ice during the waiting period. Frequent measurement of the PaO_2 requires multiple arterial punctures. It is therefore common practice to

158

insert an indwelling arterial cannula when multiple stabs are required over a short time. Of the cannulae available for this, a 20 or 22 G parallel-sided Teflon cannula will cause the least permanent sequelae[68]. Under certain circumstances, e.g. weaning, intermittent monitoring of PaO_2 may be considered inadequate and it is now possible to measure the PaO_2 continuously, using either an intra-arterial electrode[69] or a mass spectrometer. Transcutaneous oxygen ($TcPO_2$) has been used to monitor oxygenation of neonates but in adult practice the relationship between the $TcPO_2$ and PaO_2 may not be sufficiently close for clinical purposes[70]. Furthermore, some transcutaneous PO_2 electrodes are subject to considerable error in the presence of nitrous oxide, which is an increasingly popular sedative during IPPV.

The measurement of mixed venous oxygen content ($C\bar{v}O_2$) requires insertion of a pulmonary artery catheter. Nevertheless, when considered in conjunction with the PaO_2 this measurement provides the best guide to tissue oxygenation. Respiratory manipulations which raise both the PaO_2 and the $C\bar{v}O_2$ are a sign of improved tissue oxygenation. Continuous monitoring of mixed venous saturation has been undertaken in some centres using a fibre-optic catheter[71]; alternatively, $P\bar{v}O_2$ has been monitored continuously using an oxygen electrode. Measurement of the oxygen content of blood from the right atrium instead of the pulmonary artery gives only a rough guide to $C\bar{v}O_2$ because of 'streaming' of blood in the right atrium. Repeated measurement of arterial pH and base deficit may give some indication of failure of tissue oxygenation. An increasing metabolic acidosis is frequently a sign of lactic acidosis and tissue hypoperfusion or hypoxia.

Monitoring of the cardiac output is required to assess oxygen flux. Often the cardiac output has to be gauged clinically from measurements of blood pressure, pulse rate and volume, central venous pressure (CVP), urine output, and peripheral to core temperature gradient. These simple measurements are very valuable. Alternatively the cardiac output can be measured directly by the thermodilution method. Hypotension induced by IPPV or by the addition of PEEP is usually due to a fall in cardiac output. Its correction may require an i.v. infusion to increase the venous return and raise venous pressure.

Interpretation of the CVP is difficult during IPPV. A proportion of the raised airway pressure will be transmitted to the intrathoracic great vessels. The precise rise in CVP will depend upon the time constant of the lung, that is the compliance × airway resistance. Stiff lungs will therefore transmit little of the raised airway pressure to the great vessels. The measurement can be made either during IPPV or during a short period of disconnection from the ventilator. The latter technique gives a constant baseline at zero airway pressure, and the former measurement relates to function of the cardiovascular system during IPPV (see Section II). Changes in CVP measured in this way must be interpreted in the light of the mode of mechanical

159

ventilation (flow pattern, PEEP) and changes in lung mechanics.

A recurring problem during IPPV is the combination of a high CVP and hypotension. Is there pump failure? One approach is to rapidly infuse 200 ml of crystalloid and reassess[72]. When the blood pressure rises and signs indicate an improved cardiac output, then additional infusions are probably appropriate. Alternatively, the pulmonary capillary wedge pressure (PAWP) is measured. If normal or low then intravenous infusions are given; when high an inotrope alone is used by continuous intravenous infusion.

Decreased oxygen flux can be the result of hypoxaemia due to pulmonary oedema. When the pathophysiology is in doubt, measurement of the PAWP will help to distinguish the oedema of left ventricular failure (PAWP 15 mmHg, 2.0 kPa) from that of alveolar capillary leak, when the PAWP is normal. It should be recalled that a moderate increase in PAWP will cause pulmonary oedema when the serum albumin is low, and the cause of pulmonary oedema (leak or heart failure) can only be accurately diagnosed by measurement of both PAWP and the oncotic pressure, although the latter can be calculated from the serum albumin concentration. Recently an attempt has been made to diagnose alveolar capillary leak by measurement of rate of loss from the lungs of an inhaled isotope[73,74].

(2) Ventilation

Alveolar ventilation determines the P_ACO_2 and this is closely related to the $PaCO_2$; ventilation can thus be assessed by measurement of $PaCO_2$. Although end-expired PCO_2 and $PaCO_2$ are closely related in health, this may not be the case for patients requiring IPPV and peak expired CO_2 may be even further removed from $PaCO_2$. Monitoring of end-expired CO_2 during IPPV must be viewed with caution until the relationship between this measurement and the $PaCO_2$ has been established. Should this be established then minute to minute changes in the expired CO_2 may be useful in monitoring ventilation and could be used to 'close the loop' in true servo ventilation. Transcutaneous PCO_2 (TcPCO_2) unlike that for TcPO_2 bears a close relationship to $PaCO_2$, both in neonates and adults. Measurement of TcPCO_2 has proved to be of considerable use in monitoring IPPV and during weaning[75,76], although the time lag may be too long for the latter use. Developments in this field should be of considerable value in routine monitoring in the ICU.

(3) Alteration in respiratory function with time and treatment

Monitoring tissue oxygenation and ventilation as described above ensures that gas exchange will maintain life but gives little insight into changes in respiratory function which may be occurring with time. The two components of respiratory function, gas exchange and lung mechanics, need additional assessment and quantification.

Gas exchange

Changes in $PaCO_2$ with alterations to the mode or minute volume may or may not signify improvement. To quantify alveolar ventilation it is necessary to calculate the dead space/tidal volume ratio. This measurement is simple, requiring only a Douglas bag, a respirometer, a blood gas machine and a stop watch. The blood gas machine can be used to measure both the $PaCO_2$ and the CO_2 in the gaseous phase (mixed expired CO_2), although the latter is more usually measured with a capnograph. The results are inserted in the Bohr equation giving the dead space/tidal volume ratio.

$$\frac{V_D}{V_T} = \frac{PaCO_2 - P_{\bar{E}}CO_2}{PaCO_2}$$

where V_D is the physiological dead space volume

V_T is the tidal volume

and $P_{\bar{E}}CO_2$ is mixed expired carbon dioxide tension

If the tidal volume is known then the alveolar volume V_A can be calculated by subtraction. During IPPV, V_D/V_A can be 0.8. It is unlikely that weaning will succeed when V_D/V_T exceeds 0.6[77].

Oxygen transfer is difficult to compare on a day-to-day basis because changes are made in the inspired oxygen concentration. In the normal lung the relationship between F_IO_2 and PaO_2 is non-linear and greater deviations may be expected in disease. Three simple indices of oxygen transfer are used, of which the $P(A-a)O_2$ is the best known. Measurement of this gradient after 20 minutes of ventilation with 100% oxygen enables day-to-day comparisons to be made[63]. Unfortunately, it has become evident that oxygen itself may alter venous admixture ('Hyperoxic shunt') so that the value of this measurement is suspect. Benumof[81] used an alternative index labelled the 'respiratory index'. This is calculated by dividing $P(A-a)O_2$ by the PaO_2. 'Virtual shunt' is a third index of oxygenation[82]. However, these indices are simply a means of comparing venous admixture and their calculation assumes many variables. Since the Swan–Ganz catheter became more widely used, venous admixture at a known F_IO_2 can be measured directly, using the equation given in Table 7.4.

Table 7.4 Calculation of venous admixture as a fraction of the cardiac output

$$\frac{\dot{Q}_S}{\dot{Q}_T} = \frac{(CcO_2 - CaO_2)}{(CcO_2 - C\bar{v}O_2)}$$

where	$\dot{Q}_S$	is the shunt flow
	$\dot{Q}_T$	is the total cardiac output
	CcO_2	is the pulmonary end capillary oxygen content (calculated from the ideal alveolar PO_2)
	CaO_2	is the measured arterial oxygen content
and	$C\bar{v}O_2$	is the measured mixed venous (pulmonary artery) oxygen content

Lung mechanics

The continuous monitoring of airway pressure warns of disconnection or obstruction. However, airway pressure monitoring may yield useful indices of changes in lung mechanics. 'Effective compliance' is the simplest measurement of lung mechanics and is the ratio of tidal volume (measured at the airway) and peak airway pressure[83]. Obviously this measurement is a hybrid, and relates to both airway resistance and to compliance. The flow pattern of many ventilators can be adjusted to produce an inspiratory 'hold' during which total static compliance may be calculated from the plateau pressure and tidal volume. Measurement of compliance in this way is the simplest method available for determining the 'best PEEP', which is that level of PEEP at which oxygen flux is maximal[84]. When 'top hat' flows are used, the difference between the peak and plateau pressure can be used to calculate airway resistance. When the ventilation settings are constant, then a change in this gradient indicates a change in airway resistance. Unfortunately, compliance and airway resistance measured in this way include a factor related to external respiratory equipment. Nevertheless, reasonable conclusions can be drawn. Some modern ventilators (e.g. the Siemens Servo 900B) include an electronic 'black box', which is programmed to calculate airway resistance and compliance. This ventilator produces analogue signals which may be further processed to produce breath-to-breath measurements of respiratory work[85]. The latter measurement is of value in determining the likelihood of a successful wean[86].

(4) Equipment failure

Equipment used for mechanical ventilation may fail or disconnect. Simple 'pressure' alarms are useful in detecting disconnection or failure. Continuous observation by trained staff is always better than alarms; the latter can fail. Continuous monitoring of F_IO_2 is mandatory when high concentrations of nitrous oxide are used and should preferably be used routinely. Oxygen analysers using fuel cells are probably safest because the battery operated polarographic oxygen electrode can become sensitive to nitrous oxide when its battery has partly discharged[87].

(5) Additional monitoring

The routine daily monitoring during IPPV includes a full blood count, platelet count, serum and urinary electrolytes, and serum albumin. Clinical examination of the chest is not very helpful because of the noises transmitted from the ventilator, humidifier and hoses; signs of pneumothorax are the important exception. A daily chest X-ray is necessary. In order to compare the X-rays and to obtain most information, each X-ray should be taken with the lungs inflated to a known airway pressure with the patient in the same posture and with the same radiographic settings. If the chest X-ray can only be taken supine, a lateral decubitus view may be necessary to detect a pleural effusion.

(VII) OPTIMIZING GAS EXCHANGE

Oxygen toxicity limits the maximum continuous F_IO_2 to 50%. However, despite adequate bronchial toilet and humidification, the PaO_2 may still remain at an unsatisfactorily low level. Occasionally reducing minute ventilation (to increase the $PaCO_2$) improves the cardiac output, reduces venous admixture and thus increases PaO_2. The prone position also improves oxygenation[88]. The application of graded levels of PEEP may improve PaO_2 and oxygen delivery. 'Best PEEP' should be sought. A PEEP of 5–15 cmH$_2$O is often required, but levels as high as 60 cmH$_2$O ('super PEEP') have been used on occasion[89]. The effect of PEEP upon $PaCO_2$ is variable but the changes appear slight[90]. PEEP can be used in conjunction with an inspiratory 'hold' and an expiratory 'retard'. Both these manoeuvres have similar effects upon gas distribution. The increase in mean intrathoracic pressure can be detrimental to cardiac output and oxygen flux and an attempt to assess these should be made.

Variations in inspiratory flow pattern are theoretically important in reducing maldistribution of ventilation and maintaining cardiac output. However, in most ICU patients the pulmonary pathology is not uniformly distributed, so that the best pattern of ventilation for one area of lung is not so for another. Furthermore, the bacterial filters, humidifiers and long

163

corrugated hoses modify the airflow pattern of the ventilator. Nevertheless, what evidence there is suggests that a decreasing flow pattern is best[91,92], and that the addition of an inspiratory 'hold' may marginally improve gas distribution[93]. An adequate inspiratory time (1–2 seconds, 3 time constants) is just as important as the choice of flow pattern.

The use of negative end-expiratory pressure (NEEP) as a method of reducing mean intrathoracic pressure and thus improving cardiac output and oxygen flux has been shown to be of minimal benefit. This is not surprising, because maximum venous flow into the chest is flow limited. NEEP is now seldom used.

Unlike oxygen transfer, carbon dioxide output is hardly affected by large increases in venous admixture. The high V_D/V_T ratio found in many patients in the ICU, suggests that large tidal volumes (10–15 ml/kg) should be a routine practice. The further imposition of sighs may not have a significant effect[94].

The technique of high frequency positive pressure ventilation (HFPPV) allows adequate oxygenation and excellent carbon dioxide removal although the 'minute volumes' are higher than would normally be used. Ventilation using this technique maintains mean airway and intrathoracic pressure at a much lower level than conventional IPPV. HFPPV may thus be advantageous when cardiac output is compromised, or when the bronchial tree is disrupted, e.g. bronchopleural fistula[95-98].

(VIII) POSITIVE END-EXPIRATORY PRESSURE (PEEP)

Sporadic references to the use of PEEP, with or without IPPV, have appeared over many years[99-101]. However, its use did not become commonplace until Ashbaugh reported a reduced mortality from adult respiratory distress syndrome following the use of PEEP[102]. At first PEEP was often used indiscriminately as an adjunct to IPPV when F_iO_2 values above 50% were required to correct hypoxaemia. Little regard was paid to the effect on oxygen flux. In the majority of the early patients treated, lung damage was so severe that the increase in mean airway pressure produced by PEEP to IPPV was only partially transmitted to the great vessels. Although PEEP was known to reduce cardiac output, oxygen flux presumably increased in these severely ill patients[103].

PEEP exerts its beneficial effect by raising the functional residual capacity and improving gas distribution. Previously closed airways are opened, or remain open throughout the respiratory cycle. Venous admixture is correspondingly reduced. The increase in lung volume from PEEP will depend on mean lung compliance . Lung compliance will also determine the increase in mean airway pressure which is transmitted as the pleural pressure to the great vessels, and thus the consequent fall in cardiac output. The improvement in PaO_2 is thus partly offset by a fall in cardiac output. The effect upon oxygen flux will thus need to be evaluated. 'Best PEEP' was the term introduced by Suter for the value of PEEP at which oxygen flux was maximal[84]. 'Optimum PEEP' has been used by other workers for the level of PEEP at which venous admixture is minimal; however, the two terms are essentially interchangeable. Suter showed that at 'best PEEP' the total compliance was at a maximum and measurement of the total compliance remains the simplest means by which 'best PEEP' can be calculated. In the measurement of 'best PEEP', total compliance is considered acceptable because it is reasonable to assume that changes in compliance with PEEP will originate in the lung. However, recent work has suggested that it is necessary to measure lung compliance separately in order to calculate 'best PEEP'. Measurement of lung compliance is probably necessary when PEEP is applied independently and at different levels to each lung. This may be necessary when the severity of disease in each lung is different and warrants synchronous independent lung ventilation; the technical problems of management are then considerable[105-107], unless the asynchronous technique is used[108].

The problems of CVP measurement during IPPV have already been described, and similar comments apply when PEEP has been added. The measurement of PAWP during PEEP is also complicated. The reduction in cardiac output and redistribution of blood flow which occurs following the application of PEEP may 'strand' a catheter already placed in a pulmonary artery whose blood flow is reduced to negligible levels. The 'wedge pressure' recorded is erroneous and is, in fact, the alveolar pressure[109-111]. To overcome this problem it is the author's practice to increase PEEP to a high level while the catheter is being advanced along the pulmonary artery. 'Stranding' of the catheter will not then occur if PEEP remains below this level. The reduction in cardiac output which occurs with PEEP may be overcome by increasing the central venous pressure by giving a fluid load. However, since IPPV is associated with salt and water retention[112], further loads may be harmful, particularly if there is alveolar capillary leak. Any transfusion should thus be kept to a minimum and inotropic agents are more appropriate than fluid loading to increase the cardiac output. The use of dopamine in particular may reverse the deleterious effect of PEEP on renal function[113,114]. PEEP may have deleterious effects upon other systems, for example, hepatic function, and can increase intracranial pressure. The latter effect can be partially overcome by changing posture. Barotrauma is discussed on page 170.

(IX) WEANING

It is not always clear when IPPV should be discontinued. Weaning

165

problems are most likely to occur in those patients who, for whatever reasons, have required prolonged IPPV or in those who have chronic lung disease. There are three main reasons why an attempt to wean can fail. (1) There is insufficient central respiratory drive for the prevailing conditions of gas exchange. A reduction in respiratory drive can be due to depressant drugs or disease of the central nervous system. (2) Insufficient gas exchange (usually oxygen) may occur during spontaneous respiration despite a normal or increased minute volume. (3) There may be a mechanical deficit. This may be due to loss of chest wall integrity, to muscle weakness or fatigue, or due to disco-ordinate action of the respiratory muscles. Whether disco-ordination is a manifestation of muscle fatigue or is of neural origin is not yet known. Of the causes listed, mechanical insufficiency is the most difficult to predict and is the commonest reason for a return to a ventilatory support.

(1) Prediction and assessment

Table 7.5 lists the criteria for weaning suggested by the Boston group[115]. The criteria closely resemble the physiological indications for IPPV. Measurement of the work of breathing during IPPV has also proved helpful in predicting a successful transition to spontaneous respiration[86], and on-line measurements of respiratory work can now be made[85]. Perhaps the most interesting and potentially most valuable aid in prediction of fatigue and failure to wean has come from the diaphragmatic electromyogram[116,117]. Diaphragmatic electromyograms may be obtained with difficulty using surface electrodes, and analysis may reveal a 'fatigue' pattern under conditions of severe inspiratory loading. The technique has been used to successfully predict the weaning patterns in both neonates and adults[62,117]. Diaphragmatic electromyograms are much more easily obtained by using an oesophageal balloon electrode, but unfortunately the discomfort may limit the use of this technique.

'Failure to wean' is most often recognized on clinical grounds, blood gas measurement being secondary. Gilston described a clinical scoring system based upon respiratory, cardiovascular and central nervous system signs; blood gas results did not distinguish successful from unsuccessful weaning[57,118]. The pattern of events following the discontinuation of IPPV is not well described. It is usual for respiratory frequency to increase, and tidal volume to fall to low values[119]. A respiratory acidosis due to an increase in $PaCO_2$ of about 1.0 kPa (8 mmHg) occurs in the first hour, even in those patients who are weaned successfully. In one series the $P(A-a)O_2$ when breathing 100% oxygen increased by a mean of 13 kPa (100 mmHg)[15]. The response of the cardiovascular system to weaning varies. Patients who wean successfully usually increase their heart rate by less than 10 and

Table 7.5 Criteria for weaning from IPPV

Measurement of V_D/V_T may be required in some circumstances. Weaning is unlikely to be successful if V_D/V_T exceeds 0.6.

Oxygenation	$P(\text{A-a})O_2$ less than 45 kPa (350 mmHg) while breathing 100% oxygen
Ventilation	vital capacity greater than 10 ml kg^{-1}
Mechanics	inspiratory force greater than 20 cmH$_2$O

---

their blood pressure by less than 15 mmHg[120]. The effect of weaning on cardiac output is controversial[121]. In theory a small increase in cardiac output should be expected following the reduction in intrathoracic pressure and a rise in the $P\text{aCO}_2$.

(2) Techniques for weaning

(a) 'Crash' wean

The respiratory system and circulation are assessed and the indications reviewed, with particular reference to respiratory depressants. The patient is placed in the sitting position, the weaning explained and IPPV is stopped. Humidified oxygen, at an F_1O_2 10% higher than that given during IPPV, is supplied via a T-piece. When success is in doubt, then the crash method is modified by giving doxapam by continuous intravenous infusion. Careful clinical observation is made during the first 20 minutes of weaning, at which time the arterial blood gases are measured. Severe hypoxaemia, hypercapnoea, hypertension, tachycardia, arrhythmias, peripheral vasoconstriction, deterioration in conscious level, or obvious fatigue indicate the need for a return to IPPV.

(b) Intermittent mandatory ventilation (IMV)

The 'sink or swim' technique of the crash wean often causes concern and can delay the final weaning. Kirby[122] described an alternative technique of 'continuous flow ventilation' in neonates, and Downs[123] applied this technique as IMV to adult practice. During IMV, weaning takes place in a gradual fashion by a stepwise reduction in the frequency of mechanical ventilation (IMV rate), the mechanical tidal volume remaining constant.

The patient is able to breathe spontaneously between each mechanical breath. Weaning is no longer an 'all or none' technique and can be stopped at any stage. Although a considerable literature describes the successful use of this technique[124,125], many of the claims are disputed[126]. There is little doubt, however, that IMV is safer than the conventional 'crash wean', particularly as IMV avoids the issue of whether the patient is ready to wean. Because the technique is used from the start of IPPV, it has been claimed that IMV must speed the weaning process. However, the claim that incoordinate breathing is reduced by IMV may have a physiological basis[127]. Ventilators with IMV facilities are now readily available and simple modifications can be made to existing ventilators[128].

(c) Intermittent assisted ventilation (IAV)

A criticism of IMV is the possibility of desynchronization of patient and ventilator, with the result that the patient's expiration coincides with inflation by the ventilator. An increase in the incidence of pulmonary barotrauma would then be expected. IAV[129] eliminates this possibility. Intermittent mechanical inflation of a preset volume is triggered by the patient's inspiration and is not time-dependent, as in IMV. The 'mechanical' frequency is set at some fraction of the patient's own respiratory rate. Unlike IMV, which guarantees at least the mechanical minute volume, IAV requires continuous and accurate monitoring of the expired minute volume. Apnoea cannot trigger an assisted inflation and a failure of the expiratory flow transducer could be disastrous.

(d) Triggered ventilators

This weaning technique has been largely superseded by IMV or IAV. The greatest drawback of triggered ventilators used for weaning is that the tidal volume delivered by the machine bears no relationship to the inspiratory effort necessary to trigger the ventilator.

(e) Mandatory minute volume (MMV)

This technique[130] ensures that the patient receives the prescribed minute volume, whatever the current ability to breathe spontaneously. Failure of spontaneous efforts results in mechanical ventilation to 'top up' the minute volume. As the patient's ability to breathe improves, the volume of gas supplied by the ventilator is automatically reduced, until weaning is complete. Clinical experience with this system is limited[131], but it is unsuited to those patients who have a high respiratory drive but poor gas transfer. Many ventilators can be modified for MMV by the simple system devised by Ravenscroft[132]. However, this system has a potential disadvantage, namely, that the mechanical tidal volume varies from breath to breath. There is also a greater likelihood of the patient–ventilator desynchronization characteristic of IMV.

IMV, IAV and MMV are quite popular despite the lack of sound evidence of their advantages over a conventional 'crash' wean. However, there can be no doubt that systems achieving a gradual change from mechanical to spontaneous respiration reduce the errors in predicting the course of weaning.

(3) Continuous positive airway pressure (CPAP) and PEEP

When lung volume falls from total lung capacity towards residual volume, the normal subject is able to generate increasingly negative pleural and mouth pressures. The ability to overcome an inspiratory load (obstruction) therefore increases. However, at a point some 200–400 ml above residual volume, the ability to generate mouth and pleural pressures declines abruptly[133]. In patients with acute respiratory failure, lung volume is decreased and is usually found to be close to residual volume. Any technique which increases lung volume might therefore be expected to improve the ability to generate negative pleural and mouth pressures, and thus overcome the respiratory load. In this way the increase in lung volume found during weaning with PEEP might improve the ability to overcome a load. This was demonstrated, although unexplained, by Feeley[134]. The increase in lung volume with PEEP results in improved compliance. This potentially reduces both inspiratory and total respiratory work, but this is at least partly offset when inspiration occurs from atmospheric pressure, and expiration is to positive (sPEEP). Pressurization of inspiration (as CPAP) reduces inspiratory work and this technique is preferable to spontaneous PEEP (sPEEP) during weaning. The lung volume induced by CPAP or sPEEP improves gas exchange. PaO_2 rises, $P(\text{A-a})O_2$ fails, and venous admixture decreases. A fall in cardiac output should not be expected if the CPAP or sPEEP level is equal to the PEEP level used during IPPV, because the mean intrathoracic pressure will be less. CPAP or sPEEP may be used in an attempt to avoid IPPV[135,136]. In these circumstances an improvement in PaO_2 alone cannot be equated with an increase in oxygen flux. The assessment of 'best CPAP' requires the insertion of an oesophageal balloon or a pulmonary artery catheter. Non-invasive measurement of aortic blood velocity by ultrasound is an alternative[137].

(4) Extubation

Extubation should quickly follow successful weaning, unless the patient's power to cough is inadequate or the laryngeal or pharyngeal reflexes are compromised. Extubation should be postponed in the unconscious. Following extubation the larynx may remain incompetent for many hours[138], despite the alertness of the patient, and care is necessary for at least 8 hours following extubation. When a cuffed tracheostomy tube is present, laryngeal competence can easily be checked using the Ribena* test. The tracheostomy cuff is deflated and the patient asked to drink a small volume of Ribena. If this coloured fluid is found on tracheal suction then the larynx is incompetent. The cuff should be reinflated or other precautions observed if decannulation is to be performed. It is a common practice to replace the deflated cuffed tracheostomy tube with silver or plastic 'speaking' tube for a period of 24 hours prior to complete decannulation.

(X) BAROTRAUMA

Barotrauma can cause a leakage of air resulting in pneumothorax, mediastinal emphysema or subcutaneous emphysema. Kumar reported an incidence of 10%[139]. However, this figure included patients in whom barotrauma may have been a consequence of a coincidental event such as central venous catheter placement or chest trauma, and the true incidence of barotrauma may be less than 1%[140,141]. Surprisingly, the incidence of barotrauma appears similar with or without PEEP and does not appear to be related to the duration of ventilation. During extremes of straining and obstruction the pleural pressure may momentarily reach $+220\,cmH_2O$ and $-120\,cmH_2O$ respectively, with mouth pressure only a few centimetres different[133]. Although these values contrast sharply with those during spontaneous respiration when the pleural pressure falls to 3.0–5.0 cm below atmosphere and the mouth pressure remains atmospheric, it is not altogether surprising that, at least in terms of barotrauma, IPPV appears so innocuous.

(XI) INDEPENDENT LUNG VENTILATION

Occasionally, lung pathology is non-uniform and IPPV leads to preferential ventilation of one lung. If blood flows mainly to the opposite lung, then a gross disturbance of oxygenation occurs. In these circumstances, independent ventilation of each lung by a separate ventilator is appropriate, thus allowing adequate ventilation to the 'bad' lung. The introduction of a

* Ribena: a proprietary, highly coloured, blackcurrant drink.

170

plastic disposable double lumen endotracheal tube (Bronchocath, Mallinckrodt) has partially allayed worries concerning pharyngeal, laryngeal and tracheal trauma. This oral tube is relatively easy to insert and position, but fixation has to be meticulous. Because of fears of mediastinal tamponade, initial experience with this technique was gained by using twin synchronized ventilators ('synchronous independent lung ventilation'). Technical problems appeared formidable[105-107]. However, asynchronous ventilation of each lung appears to be relatively innocuous and brings the technique of independent lung ventilation within the range of all ICUs[108]. Adequate suction clearance down the relatively narrow lumina of these long endotracheal tubes remains a serious problem. PEEP may be applied independently and unequally to each lung. 'Best PEEP' should be assessed by independent measurements of compliance.

(XII) LOW FREQUENCY POSITIVE PRESSURE VENTILATION

Low frequency positive pressure ventilation (2-3 breaths/min) has been tried as a method which may be of value in severe lung disease as a means of preventing barotrauma[142]. Extracorporeal removal of CO_2 is required. Clinical experience, like that with high frequency positive pressure ventilation, is limited.

References

1. Lassen, H. C. A. (1953). A preliminary report on the 1952 epidemic of polio-myelitis in Copenhagen, with special reference to the treatment of acute respiratory insufficiency. *Lancet*, **1**, 37
2. Bjorneboe, M., Ibsen, B., and Astrup, *et al.* (1955). Active ventilation in treatment of respiratory acidosis. *Lancet*, **2**, 901
3. Lassen, H. C. A., Henriksen, E., Neukirch, F. and Kristensen, H. S. (1956). Treatment of tetanus – severe bone-marrow depression after prolonged nitrous oxide anaesthesia. *Lancet*, **1**, 527
4. English, I. C. W. and Manley, R. E. W. (1970). The Brompton system of artificial ventilation – a scheme for the intensive care unit. *Anaesthesia*, **25**, 541
5. Don, H. F. and Robson, J. G. (1975). The mechanics of the respiratory system during anaesthesia. *Anesthesiology*, **26**, 168
6. Froese, A. B. and Bryan, A. C. (1974). Effects of anaesthesia and paralysis on diaphragmatic mechanics in man. *Anaesthesiology*, **41**, 242
7. Cournand, A., Hurley, L. M., Werko, L. and Richards, D. W. (1948). Physiological studies of the effects of intermittent positive pressure breathing on cardiac output in man. *Am. J. Physiol.*, **152**, 162
8. Buda, A. J., Pinsky, M. R. and Ingels, N. B. *et al.* (1979). Effect of intrathoracic pressure on left ventricular performance. *N. Engl. J. Med.*, **301**, 453
9. McGregor, M. (1979). Pulsus paradoxus. *N. Engl. J. Med.*, **301**, 480

10. Laver, M. B., Strauss, H. W. and Pohost, G. M. (1979). Right and left ventricular geometry; adjustments during acute respiratory failure. *Crit. Care Med.*, **1**, 509
11. Stalcup, S. A. and Mellins, R. B. (1977). Mechanical forces producing pulmonary edema in acute asthma. *N. Engl. J. Med.*, **297**, 592
12. Scott, D. B., Stephen, G. W. and Davie, I. T. (1972). Haemodynamic effects of a negative (subatmospheric) pressure expiratory phase during artificial ventilation. *Br. J. Anaesth.*, **44**, 171
13. Agate, J. N. (1978). Aging and the Skin (b) Pressure Sores. *Textbook of Geriatric Medicine and Gerontology.* 2nd Edn. Ch. 15, p. 640. (Edinburgh, London & New York: Churchill Livingstone)
14. Thomson, C. W., Ryan, D. W., Dunkin, L. J. and Smith, M. (1980). Fluidised-bead bed in the intensive therapy unit. *Lancet*, **1**, 568
15. Harris, S. K., Bone, R. C. and Ruth, W. E. (1977). Gastrointestinal hemorrhage in patients in a respiratory intensive care unit. *Chest*, **72**, 301
16. Editorial (1978). Gastrointestinal bleeding in acute respiratory failure. *Br. Med. J.*, **1**, 531
17. Hastings, P. R., Skillman, J. J., Bushnell, L. S. and Silen, W. (1978). Antacid titration in the prevention of acute gastrointestinal bleeding. *N. Engl. J. Med.*, **298**, 1041
18. MacDougall, B. R. D., Bailey, R. J. Williams, R. (1977). H$_2$-receptor antagonists and antacids in the prevention of acute gastrointestinal haemorrhage in fulminant hepatic failure. Two controlled trials. *Lancet*, **1**, 617
19. Priebe, H. J., Skillman, J. J. and Bushnell, L. S. *et al.* (1980). Antacid versus cimetidine in preventing acute gastrointestinal bleeding. *N. Engl. J. Med.*, **302**, 426
20. Robinson, J. S. (1976). The psychological effects of intensive care (a personal account). *Scott. Soc. Anaesth. J.*, **17**, 10
21. Henschel, E. O. (1977). The Guillain-Barre syndrome, a personal experience. *Anesthesiology*, **47**, 228
22. Paiement, B., Boulanger, M., Jones, C. W. and Roy, M. (1979). Intubation and other experiences in cardiac surgery: the consumer's view. *Can. Anaesth. Soc. J.*, **26**, 173
23. Gaudinski, M. A. (1977). Psychological considerations with patients on respirators. *Aviat. Space, Environ. Med.*, **48**, 71
24. Cormack, R. S. (1979). Awareness during surgery – a new approach. *Br. J. Anaesth.*, **51**, 1051
25. Miller Jones, C. M. R. (1980). Paralysis or sedation for controlled ventilation? *Lancet*, **1**, 312
26. Carlow, G. C., Kahn, R. C. and Goldiner, P. L. *et al.* (1978). Long-term infusion of sodium thiopental. Hemodynamic and respiratory effects. *Crit. Care Med.*, **6**, 311
27. Edbrooke, D. L., Newby, D. M. and ebron, B. S. *et al.* (1981). Etomidate infusion: a method of sedation for the intensive care unit. *Anaesthesia*, **36**, 65
28. Davenport, H. T. and Wright, B. M. (1979). Relief of postoperative pain. *Br. Med. J.*, **1**, 1561
29. Hewlett, A. M. (1979). Personal communication
30. Minty, B., Deacon, R., Lumb, M. *et al.* (1978). Effect of nitrous oxide on

B12-requiring enzymes. *Br. J. Anaesth.*, **50**, 65

31. Deacon, R., Lumb, M., Perry *et al.* (1978). Selective inactivation of vitamin B12 in rats by nitrous oxide. *Lancet*, **2**, 1024

32. Clement, A. J. and Hubsch, S. K. (1968). Chest physiotherapy by the 'bag squeezing' method: a guide to technique. *Physiotherapy*, **54**, 355

33. Matthew, E. B., Holmstrom, P. M. G. and Kasper, R. L. (1977). A simple method for diagnosing pneumonia in intubated or tracheostomized patients. *Crit. Care Med.*, **5**, 76

34. Sackner, M. A., Landa, J. F., Greeneltch, N. and Robinson, M. J. (1973). Pathogenesis and prevention of tracheobronchial damage with suction procedures. *Chest*, **64**, 284

35. Jung, R. C. and Gottlieb, L. S. (1976). Comparison of tracheobronchial suction catheters in humans. *Chest*, **69**, 179

36. Boys, J. E. and Howells, T. H. (1972). Humidification in anaesthesia. *Br. J. Anaesth.*, **44**, 879

37. Atherton, S. T. and White, D. J. (1978). Stomach as a source of bacteria colonising respiratory tract during artificial ventilation. *Lancet*, **2**, 968

38. Holdcroft, A., Lumley, J. and Gaya, H. *et al.* (1974). Respiratory filters in clinical practice. *Lancet*, **1**, 25

39. Mitchell, J. N. (1973). Evaluation of the new 'Williams' filter. *Br. Med. J.*, **2**, 653

40. Ayliffe G. A. J., Collins, B. J. and Green, S. (1975). Hygiene of babies' incubators. *Lancet*, **1**, 923

41. Lindholm, C. E. (1970). Prolonged endotracheal intubation. *Acta Anaesthesiol. Scan. Suppl*, **33**, 1

42. Geffin, B. and Pontoppidan, H. (1969). Reduction of tracheal damage by the prestretching of inflatable cuffs. *Anesthesiology*, **31**, 462

43. Kamen, J. M. and Wilkinson, C. J. (1971). A new low pressure cuff for endotracheal tubes. *Anesthesiology*, **34**, 482

44. MacKenzie, C. F., Klose, S. and Browne, D. R. G. (1976). A study of inflatable cuffs on endotracheal tubes. *Br. J. Anaesth.*, **48**, 105

45. Pavlin, E. G., van Mimwegan, D. and Hornbein, T. F. (1975). Failure of a high-compliance low-pressure cuff to prevent aspiration. *Anesthesiology*, **42**, 216

46. Mostert, J. W. (1977). Cuffs do not seal the trachea airtight. *Anesthesiology*, **42**, 309

47. Egnatinsky, J. (1975). Overinflating low-pressure cuffs to prevent aspiration. *Anesthesiology*, **42**, 114

48. Revenas, B. and Lindholm, C. E. (1976). Pressure and volume changes in tracheal cuffs during anaesthesia. *Acta Anaesthesiol. Scand.*, **20**, 321

49. Stanley, T. H. (1975). Nitrous oxide and pressures and volumes of high and low pressure endotracheal-tube cuffs in intubated patients. *Anesthesiology*, **42**, 637

50. Vogelhut, M. M. and Downs, J. B. (1979). Prolonged endotracheal intubation. *Chest*, **76**, 110

51. Goldberg, M. and Pearson, F. G. (1972). Pathogenesis of tracheal stenosis following tracheostomy with a cuffed tube – an experimental study in dogs. *Thorax*, **27**, 678

52. Dukes, H. M. (1970). Tracheostomy. *Thorax*, **25**, 573
53. Fridan, L., Hedenstierna, G. and Schildt, B. (1976). Stenosis following tracheostomy. *Anesthesia*, **31**, 479
54. Campbell, E. J. M. (1965). Respiratory failure. *Br. Med. J.*, **1**, 1451
55. Milledge, J. S. and Nunn, J. F. (1980). Anaesthesia and the patient with respiratory disease. In Gray, T. C., Nunn, J. F. and Utting, J. E. (eds.). *General Anaesthesia*. 4th edn., pp. 511–530. (London: Butterworth)
56. Sykes, M. K., McNicol, M. .W. and Campbell, E. J. M. (1976). *Respiratory Failure*. 2nd edn. (Oxford: Blackwell)
57. Gilson, A. (1976). A clinical scoring system for adult respiratory distress. Preliminary report of its use in heart disease. *Anaesthesia*, **31**, 448
58. Peters, R. M., Hilberman, M., Hogan, J. S. and Crawford, D. A. (1972). Objective indications for respirator therapy in post-trauma and postoperative patients. *Am. J. Surg.*, **124**, 262
59. Peters, R. M. (1974). Work of breathing and abnormal mechanics. *Surg. Clin. N. Am.*, **54**, 995
60. Henning, R. J., Shubin, H. and Weil, M. H. (1977). The measurement of the work of breathing for the clinical assessment of ventilator dependence. *Crit. Care Med.*, **5**, 264
61. Gross, D., Grassino, A., Ross, W. R. D. and Macklem, P. T. (1979). Electromyogram pattern of diaphragmatic fatigue. *J. Appl. Physiol: Respirat. Environ. Exercise Physiol.*, **46**, 1
62. Muller, N., Gulston, G. and Cade, D. *et al.* (1979) Diaphragmatic muscle fatigue in the newborn. *J. Appl. Physiol: Respirat. Environ. Exercise Physiol.*, **46**, 688
63. Pontoppidan, H., Geffin, B. and Lowestein, E. (1972). Acute respiratory failure in the adult. *N. Engl. J. Med.*, **287**, pp. 690–698, 743–752 and 799–806
64. Wilson, R. S. and Pontoppidan, H. (1974). Acute respiratory failure: diagnostic and therapeutic criteria. *Crit. Care Med.*, **2**, 293
65. Avery, E. E., Morch, E. T., Head, J. R. and Benson, D. W. (1959). Severe crushing injuries of the chest; a new method of treatment with continuous mechanical ventilation by mean of intermittent positive endotracheal insufflation. *Q. Bull. Northwest. Univ. Med. Sch.*, **39**, 301
66. Schaal, M. A., Fischer, R. P. and Perry, J. F. (1979). The unchanged mortality of flail chest injuries. *J. Trauma*, **19**, 492
67. Moser, K. M., Luchsinger, P. C. and Adamson, J. S. *et al.* (1973). Respiratory stimulation with intravenous doxapram in respiratory failure. *N. Engl. J. Med.*, **288**, 427
68. Bedford, R. F. (1977). Radial arterial function following percutaneous cannulation with 18 and 20 gauge catheters. *Anaesthesiology*, **47**, 37
69. Armstrong, R. F., Hutchinson, J. M., Lincoln, C., Ingram, D. and Soutter, L. (1976). Continuous measurement of the arterial oxygen tension during one lung anaesthesia. *Br. J. Anaesth.*, **48**, 1005
70. Al-Diaidy, W., Skeates, S. J., Hill, D. W. and Tinker, J. (1977). The use of transcutaneous oxygen electrodes in intensive therapy. *Intens. Care Med.*, **3**, 35
71. Krauss, X. H., Verdouw, P. D., Hugenholtz, P. G. and Nauta, J. (1975). On-

line monitoring of mixed venous oxygen saturation after cardiothoracic surgery. *Thorax,* **30,** 636

72. Sykes, M. K. (1963). Venous pressure as a clinical indication of adequacy of transfusion. *Ann. R. Coll. Surg.,* **35,** 185
73. Jones, J. G., Berry, M., Hulands, G. H. and Crawley, J. C. W. (1978). The time course and degree of change in alveolar–capillary membrane permeability induced by aspiration of hydrochloric acid and hypotonic saline. *Am. Rev. Respir. Dis.,* **11,** 1007
74. Jones, J. G., Minty, B. D., Lawler, P. *et al.* (1980). Increased alveolar epithelial permeability in cigarette smokers. *Lancet,* **1,** 66
75. Severinghaus, J. W. (1977). Transcutaneous (non-invasive) measurement of arterial PCO_2. In *Abstracts of Scientific Papers. American Society of Anaesthesiologists Annual Meeting*, p. 1
76. Eletr, S., Jimison, H., Ream, A. K. *et al.* (1978). Cutaneous monitoring of systemic PCO_2 on patients in the respiratory intensive care unit being weaned from the ventilators. *Acta Anaesthesiol. Scand., Suppl.* **68,** 123
77. Downs, J. B., Perkins, H. M. and Sutton, W. W. (1974). Successful weaning after five years of mechanical ventilation. *Anesthesiology,* **40,** 602
78. Wagner, P. D., Larauuso, R. B., Viyl, R. R. and West, J. B. (1974). Continuous distribution of ventilation perfusion ratios in normal subjects breathing air and 100% oxygen. *J. Clin. Invest.,* **54,** 54
79. Kerr, J. H. (1975). Pulmonary oxygen transfer during IPPV in man. *Br. J. Anaesth.,* **47,** 695
80. Suter, P. M., Fairley, H. B. and Schlobohm, R. M. (1975). Shunt, lung volume and perfusion following short periods of ventilation with oxygen. *Anesthesiology,* **43,** 617
81. Benumof, J. L., Rauscher, A. and Herren, A. (1977). Comparison of respiratory index $(P(AaDO_2)/PaO_2)$ with transpulmonary shunt. *Abstracts of Scientific Papers. American Society of Anesthesiologists Annual Meeting*, pp. 185–186
82. Benatar, S. R., Hewlett, A. M. and Nunn, J. F. (1973). The use of iso-shunt lines for the control of oxygen therapy. *Br. J. Anaesth.,* **47,** 711
83. Bendixen, H. H., Egbert, L. D. and Hedley-Whyte, J. (1965). *Respiratory Care.* p. 145. (St Louis: The C. V. Mosby Company)
84. Suter, P. M., Fairley, H. B. and Isemberg, M. D. (1975). Optimum and expiratory airway pressure in patients with acute pulmonary failure. *N. Engl. J. Med.,* **292,** 284
85. Kenny, G. N. C., Davis, P. D. and Campbell, D. (1979). Monitoring respiratory function with a microcomputer. *Br. J. Anaesth.,* **51,** 996
86. Proctor, H. J. and Woolson, R. (1973). Prediction of respiratory muscle fatigue by measurements of the work of breathing. *Surg. Gynaecol. Obstet.,* **136,** 367
87. Piernan, S., Roizen, M. F. and Severinghaus, J. W. (1979). Oxygen analyser dangerous – senses nitrous oxide as battery fails. *Anesthesiology,* **50,** 146
88. Douglas, W., Rehder, K., Froukje, M. B., Sessler, A. D. and Marsh, M. M. (1977). Improved oxygenation in patient with acute respiratory failure: the prone position. *Am. Rev. Respir. Dis.,* **115,** 559
89. Kirby, R. R., Downs, J. B., Civetta, M. *et al.* (1975). High level positive end

expiratory pressure (PEEP) in acute respiratory insufficiency. *Chest*, **67**,156

90. Tenaillon, A., Labrousse, J., Coriat, P. and Lissac, J. (1979). PEEP and PaCO$_2$. *Anesthesiology*, **50**, 554

91. Johansson, H. (1975). Effects of different gas flow patterns on central circulation during respirator treatment. *Acta Anaesthesiol. Scand.*, **19**, 96

92. Baker, A. B. Colliss, J. E. and Cowie, R. W. (1977). Effects of varying inspiratory flow waveform and time in intermittent positive pressure ventilation. II. Various physiological variables. *Br. J. Anaesth.*, **49**, 1221

93. Dammann, J. F., McAslan, T. C. and Maffeo, C. J. (1978). Optimal flow pattern for mechanical ventilation of the lungs. II. The effect of a sine versus square wave flow pattern with and without an end-inspiratory pause on patients. *Crit. Care Med.*, **6**, 293

94. Katz, J. A., Ozanne, G. M., Zinn, S. E. and Fairley, H. B. (1981). Time course and mechanics of lung-volume increase with PEEP in acute pulmonary failure. *Anesthesiology*, **54**, 9

95. Heijman, K., Heijman, L. and Jonzon, A. *et al.* (1972). High frequency positive pressure ventilation during anaesthesia and routine surgery in man. *Acta Anaesthesiol. Scand.*, **16**, 176

96. Bjerager, K., Sjostrand, U. and Wattwil, M. (1977). Long-term treatment of two patients with respiratory insufficiency with IPPV/PEEP and HFPPV/PEEP *Acta Anaesthesiol. Scand. (Suppl.)*, **64**, 55

97. Carlon, G. C., Ray, C. and Kahn, R. C. *et al.* (1979). High frequency positive pressure ventilation for prolonged respiratory support. *Anesthesiology*, **51**, 189

98. Kirby, R. R. (1980). High-frequency positive pressure ventilation (HFPPV): what role in ventilatory insufficiency? *Anesthesiology*, **52**, 109

99. Auer, J. and Gates, F. L. (1917). Experiments on the causation and amelioration of adrenalin pulmonary oedema. *J. Exp. Med.*, **26**, 201

100. Poulton, E. P. (1936). Left-sided heart failure with pulmonary oedema. Its treatment with the 'pulmonary plus pressure machine'. *Lancet*, **2**, 981

101. Barach, A. L., Martin, J. and Eckman, B. S. (1938). Positive pressure respiration and its application to the treatment of acute pulmonary edema. *Ann. Intern. Med.*, **12**, 754

102. Ashbaugh, G., Boyd Bigelow, M. D., Petty, T. L. and Levine, B. E. (1967). Acute respiratory distress in adults. *Lancet*, **2**, 317

103. Kumar, A., Falke, K. J. and Geffin, B. *et al.* (1970). Continuous positive pressure ventilation in acute respiratory failure. *N. Engl. J. Med.*, **283**, 1430

104. Katz, J. A., Zinn, S. E. and Ozanne, G. M. *et al.* (1979). Components of PEEP-induced lung-thorax volume increase. *Anesthesiology*, **51**, 5361

105. Powner, D. J., Eross, B. and Grenvik, A. (1977). Differential lung ventilation with PEEP in the treatment of unilateral pneumonia. *Crit. Care Med.*, **5**, 170

106. Carlon, G. C., Kahn, R. and Howland, W. S. *et al.* (1978). Acute life-threatening ventilation–perfusion inequality: an indication of independent lung ventilation. *Crit. Care Med.*, **6**, 380

107. Cavanilles, J. M., Carrigosa, F., Prieto, C. and Oncins, J. R. (1979). A selective ventilation distribution circuit (SVDC). *Intens. Care Med.*, **5**, 95

108. Hillman, K. M. and Barber, J. B. (1980). Asynchronous independent lung ventilation (AILV). *Crit. Care Med.*, **8**, 390

109. Roy, R., Powers, S. R., Feustal, P. J. and Dutton, R. E. (1977). Pulmonary wedge catheterisation during positive end-expiratory pressure ventilation in the dog. *Anesthesiology*, **46**, 385

110. Kane, P. B., Askanazi, J. and Neville, J. F. *et al.* (1978). Artifacts in the measurement of pulmonary artery wedge pressure. *Crit. Care Med.*, **6**, 36

111. Kronberg, G. M., Quan, S. F., Schloborm, R. M. *et al.* (1979). Anatomic locations of the tips of pulmonary artery catheters in supine patients. *Anesthesiology*, **51**, 467

112. Sladen, A., Laver, M. B. and Pontoppidan, H. (1968). Pulmonary complications and water retention in prolonged mechanical ventilation. *N. Engl. J. Med.*, **279**, 448

113. Marquez, J. M., Douglas, M. E., Downes, J. B. *et al.* (1979). Renal function and cardiovascular response during positive airway pressure. *Anesthesiology*, **50**, 393

114. Hemmer, M. and Suter, P. (1979). Treatment of cardiac and renal effects of PEEP with dopamine in patients with acute respiratory failure. *Anesthesiology*, **50**, 399

155. Feeley, T. W. and Hedley Whyte, J. (1975). Weaning from controlled ventilation and supplemental oxygen. *N. Engl. J. Med.*, **292**, 903

116. Schweitzer, T. W., Fitzgerald, J. W., Bowden, J. A. and Lynne-Davies, P. (1981). Spectral analysis of human inspiratory diaphragmatic electromyograms. *J. Appl. Physiol: Respirat. Environ. Exercise Physiol.*, **46**, 152

117. Andersen, J. B., Kann, T., Rasmussen, J. P. *et al.* (1978). Respiratory thoraco-abdominal cordination and muscle fatigue in acute respiratory failure. *Am. Rev. Respir. Dis.*, **117**, 89

118. Gilston, A. (1976). Facial signs of respiratory distress after cardiac surgery. A plea for the clinical approach to mechanical ventilation. *Anaesthesia*, **31**, 385

119. Gilbert, R., Aychincloss, J. H., Peppi, D. *et al.* (1974). The first few hours off a respirator. *Chest*, **65**, 152

120. Skillman, J. J., Malhotra, I. V., Pallotta, J. A. and Bushnell, L. S. (1971). Determinants of weaning from controlled ventilation. *Surg. Forum*, **22**,198

121. Beach, T., Millen, E. and Grenvik, A. (1973). Hemodynamic response to discontinuance of mechanical ventilation. *Crit. Care Med.*, **1**, 85

122. Kirby, R., Robinson, E., Schultz, J. and De Lomes, R. A. (1972). Continuous flow ventilation as an alternative to assisted or controlled ventilation in infants. *Anesth. Analg.: Curr Res.*, **51**, 871

123. Downs, J. B., Klein, E. F., Desautels, D. *et al.* (1973). Intermittent mandatory ventilation: a new approach to weaning patients from mechanical ventilators. *Chest*, **64**, 331

124. Downs, J. B., Perkins, H. M. and Modell, J. H. (1974). Intermittent mandatory ventilation. An evaluation. *Arch. Surg.*, **109**, 519

125. Civetta, J. M., Barnes, T. A. and Smith, L. O. (1975). 'Optimal PEEP' and intermittent mandatory ventilation in the treatment of acute pulmonary failure. *Respir. Care*, **20**, 551

126. Petty, T. L. (1975). IMV vs IMC. Editorial. *Chest*, **67**, 630

127. Lawler, P., Jones, J. G., Loh, L. and Lonn, M. (1979). Inability to maintain ventilation against large inspiratory threshold loads: muscle fatigue or progressive failure of co-ordination. *Br. J. Anaesth.*, **51**, 994

128. Lawler, P. G. P. and Nunn, J. F. (1977). Intermittent mandatory ventilation. *Anaesthesia*, **32**, 138

129. Harboe, S. (1977). Weaning from mechanical ventilation by means of intermittent assisted ventilation. IAV. *Acta Anaesthesiol. Scand.*, **21**, 252

130. Hewlett, A. M., Platt, A. S. and Terry, V. G. (1977). Mandatory minute volume – and new concept in weaning from mechanical ventilation. *Anaesthesia*, **32**, 163

131. Higgs, B. D. and Bevan, J. C. (1979). Use of mandatory minute volume ventilation in the operative management of a patient with myasthenia. *Br. J. Anaesth.*, **51**, 1181

132. Ravenscroft, P. J. (1978). Simple mandatory minute volume. *Anaesthesia*, **33**, 246

133. Campbell, E. J. M., Agastoni, E. and Newsom Davis, J. (1970). *The Respiratory Muscles – Mechanics and Neural Control.* pp. 63–66. (London: Lloyd-Luke (Medical Books) Ltd)

134. Feeley, T. W., Saumarex, R., Klick, J. M. *et al.* (1975). Positive end-expiratory pressure in weaning patients from controlled ventilation. A prospective randomised trial. *Lancet*, **2**, 725

135. Carg, G. P. and Hill, G. E. (1975). The use of spontaneous continuous positive airway pressure (CPAP) for reduction of intrapulmonary shunting in adults with acute respiratory failure. *Can. Anaesth. Soc. J.*, **22**, 284

136. Greenbaum, D. M., Millen, J. E., Eross, B. *et al.* (1976). Continuous positive airway pressure without tracheal intubation in spontaneously breathing patients. *Chest*, **69**, 615

137. Light, L. H. (1977). Aortic blood velocity measurement by transcutaneous aortvelography and clinical applications. In Bon, M. (ed.). *Echocardiology*, pp. 233–243. (The Hague: Martinus Nijhoff)

138. Burgess, G. E., Cooper, J. R., Marino, R. J. *et al.* (1979). Laryngeal competence after tracheal extubation. *Anesthesiology*, **51**, 73

139. Kumar, A., Pontoppidan, H., Falke, K. *et al.* (1973). Pulmonary barotrauma during mechanical ventilation. *Crit. Care Med.*, **1**, 181

140. Cullen, D. J. and Caldera, D. L. (1979). The incidence of ventilator-induced pulmonary barotrauma in critically ill patients. *Anesthesiology*, **50**, 185

141. Kirby, R. R. (1979). Ventilatory support and pulmonary barotrauma. *Anesthesiology*, **50**, 181

142. Gattinoni, L., Presenti, A., Rossi, G. P. *et al.* (1980). Treatment of acute respiratory failure with low-frequency positive pressure ventilation and extracorporeal removal of CO_2. *Lancet*, **2**, 292

8
Respiratory distress syndrome of shock and trauma

JAMES W. HOLCROFT AND F. WILLIAM BLAISDELL

(I) DEFINITION

The respiratory distress syndrome (RDS) of shock and trauma defines itself. It goes by many other names, including shock lung, post-traumatic pulmonary insufficiency, wet lung, daNang lung, adult hyaline membrane disease and haemorrhagic lung syndrome. We prefer the term RDS of shock and trauma because we believe that the syndrome occurs only after severe shock and trauma and because this term by itself does not denote a specific aetiology. The RDS of shock and trauma should be distinguished from other causes of ventilatory failure that can follow shock and trauma. These other entities include pulmonary contusion, aspiration, atelectasis, pulmonary oedema secondary to congestive heart failure, pneumonia and embolism by large thrombi or fat. The differential diagnosis of these conditions will be considered in Section VI.

(II) AETIOLOGY

We believe that the RDS of shock and trauma is due to embolization of the lungs by platelet microaggregates from traumatized tissue (Figure 8.1). The severity of the respiratory distress that develops is related to the severity of both the shock and the tissue trauma. Both shock and trauma activate the coagulation system, generate intravascular coagulation, and lead to extension of thrombi in the microvasculature (Chapter 4). These thrombi are then washed into the pulmonary microvasculature where they are filtered out. Here, under certain circumstances, the natural protective mechanisms may be blocked by shock or low perfusion. The microemboli then activate a number of secondary factors, leading to extravasation of fluid and protein into the interstitium. The end result is pulmonary dysfunction[1].

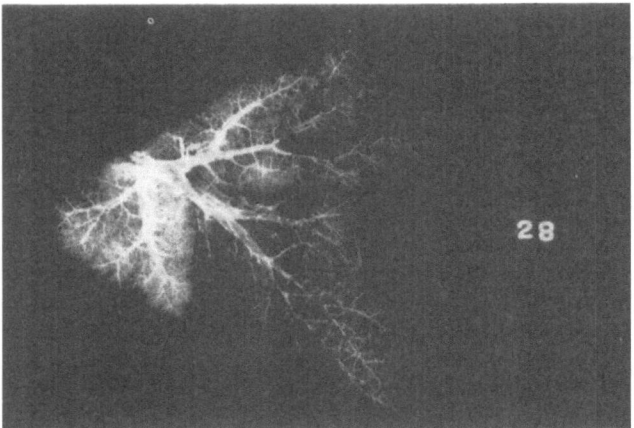

Figure 8.1 Microradiograph of a dog shock model (Lim, R. C., *Surg. Forum*, **17**, 13, 1966. Reproduced with permission). 24 hours following shock, multiple filling defects (thromboemboli) can be seen in the small pulmonary arterioles (H&E; × 10)

Other hypothetical causes of the RDS of shock and trauma include infection, lung hypoperfusion and ischaemia, oxygen toxicity, ventilator use, neurological abnormalities, fluid overload and humoral agents.

Infection frequently develops in patients who have suffered shock and trauma. Infection or bacterial toxaemia can also cause respiratory failure. Which comes first? We believe that shock, trauma and intravascular coagulation, of themselves, cause respiratory insufficiency. At the same time, shock, trauma and intravascular coagulation predispose the patient to infection by saturating the reticuloendothelial system with microthrombi and, perhaps, by damaging other immune defences (Chapter 2). The resulting infection worsens the respiratory insufficiency already present.

Others believe that the bacterial infection or toxaemia is the initiating event and that patients develop little or no respiratory failure until the infection is fully developed[2]. We disagree with this concept. In some patients, the respiratory failure is fully developed within 48 hours, well before infection has had a chance to establish itself. In other patients, the respiratory failure may worsen 4 or more days after the injury or may initially manifest itself 4 or more days after the injury. In these patients infection is usually the cause of the respiratory failure, but even then, we believe that it works through the mechanism of intravascular coagulation and pulmonary microembolism[3]. Gram-negative bacteraemia is one of the most potent stimuli known for producing intravascular coagulation.

Lung hypoperfusion and ischaemia cannot explain the respiratory failure, as demonstrated by patients who have been on cardiopulmonary bypass. Typically, these patients do not develop ventilatory insufficiency despite the fact that their lungs are not perfused at all during bypass. Transplantation experiments have also demonstrated that the lung is resistant to ischaemic damage. Moreover, in experimental models, occlusion or the circulation to one lung during and following shock and trauma, prevents rather than aggravates, the lung changes.

Oxygen toxicity could contribute to the respiratory failure[4] but we do not believe that it is a primary cause. Most patients who develop the respiratory failure of shock and trauma have multiple arterial blood gas determinations and most hospitals have effective devices for mechanical ventilation. It is unusual nowadays for patients to have either unrecognized excessively high PaO_2 or excessively high inspired concentrations of oxygen.

Ventilators have been implicated as causing the RDS of shock and trauma, but if anything, it would appear that early or even the prophylactic use of IPPV *lessens* the severity of the RDS of shock and trauma rather than causes it[5]. Thus, patients on IPPV for long periods of time with neurological disorders, such as the Guillain–Barré syndrome, maintain normal pulmonary parenchymal function (Chapter 15).

Neurological abnormalities have also been implicated in the production of the RDS of shock and trauma. Occasionally a patient with an isolated head injury will develop pulmonary oedema and respiratory failure but these patients are unusual. Once again, however, brain tissue is the most potent thromboplastin in the body, and damaged or devitalized brain is capable of activating intravascular coagulation and pulmonary microembolism.

Fluid overload has been suggested as a cause of the respiratory failure of shock and trauma and can indeed contribute to the severity of the ventilatory insufficiency. The introduction of the Swan–Ganz catheter has put into perspective the role of volume replacement in these patients. In the typical patient the pulmonary artery wedge pressure will be low rather than high, even though they can have received large amounts of fluid during resuscitation. That is, the typical patient has not been overloaded. Another point of evidence against the hypothesis that fluid overload causes the RDS of shock and trauma concerns the type of pulmonary oedema produced by fluid overloading, when compared with the pulmonary oedema actually seen in the syndrome. The pulmonary oedema that results from pure fluid overload is easily mobilized. As an example, patients who present with acute myocardial infarction and acute pulmonary oedema usually clear their pulmonary oedema within 24 hours. In contrast, the pulmonary oedema associated with the RDS of shock and trauma is difficult to mobilize and usually takes days to clear.

It has been postulated that many humoral agents can cause the RDS of shock and trauma. We believe that metabolites of arachidonic acid may well play a role in the aetiology and could be a mechanism by which platelet microaggregates damage the pulmonary microvasculature. The arachidonic acid metabolite most likely to be involved is thromboxane A_2. Embolization of an isolated lung causes the lung to release arachidonic acid metabolites. Some of these metabolites are capable of producing both pulmonary vaso-constriction and platelet aggregation, thus aggravating the vascular lesion and producing a vicious cycle.

Other humoral factors capable of damaging the lung have been suggested: serotonin, histamine and kinins. These factors may interact with arachidonic acid metabolites or may function independently. Complement has also been implicated and some believe that microaggregates of white blood cells, interacting with the complement system, produce increased vascular permeability and thus the RDS[6]. Once again, however, the complement system is activated by intravascular coagulation through factor XII.

(III) PATHOPHYSIOLOGY

Immediately after the insult of shock and trauma the lungs are morpho-logically normal except for the appearances of microaggregates in the pulmonary vasculature and congestion (Figure 8.2). Pathological changes develop after the injury[7]. The pathology is non-specific, and reflects an inflammatory response in the lung. The lungs all show interstitial oedema with progression to alveolar flooding. The microvasculature becomes congested and red cells extravasate into the interstitium. Subsequently, hyaline membranes and diffuse bronchopneumonia may appear. Interstitial fibrosis is rare and occurs in only about five per cent of all cases of the RDS of shock and trauma; this appears as a late manifestation and presumably

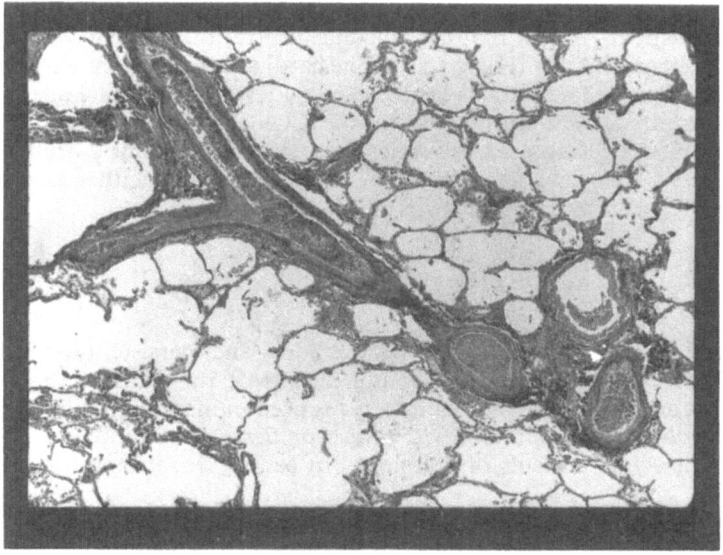

Figure 8.2 Lung biopsy following open chest resuscitation in a patient following major trauma with hypovolaemic shock. Amorphous material staining positively for platelets and fibrin are shown in the pulmonary arterioles (H&E; × 50)

results from persistent inflammation and infection.

The fundamental pathophysiological abnormality is a breakdown of the integrity of the pulmonary microvasculature with extravasation of plasma and blood into the interstitial space, with the later development of alveolar flooding. This oedema manifests itself functionally with decreased lung compliance and with ventilation–perfusion maldistribution leading to hypoxaemia. The pulmonary oedema inactivates surfactant and alveoli become atelectatic with a loss of functional residual capacity.

(IV) SYMPTOMS AND SIGNS

24 hours after the initial injury, illness or infection, convalescence is interrupted by progressive respiratory failure. The patient becomes dyspnoeic and tachypnoeic, with hyperventilation, grunting expiration, and intercostal and/or suprasternal retraction on inspiration. The patient may become cyanotic and the cyanosis may not improve with administration of oxygen. Since bronchial oedema is rarely present, auscultation often reveals no rales or rhonchi. Chest X-rays show a diffuse bilateral alveolar infil-

183

tration which is similar to that seen in the acute pulmonary oedema of cardiogenic shock, except that the alveolar infiltration of the RDS is distributed more peripherally (Figure 8.3). The cardiac silhouette on chest X-ray is usually normal. The PaO_2 is low but the patient will ventilate adequately as demonstrated by a normal or low $PaCO_2$ associated with a slightly elevated pH, reflecting mild to moderate respiratory alkalosis. Pulmonary vascular resistance may be increased. Cardiac output is either normal or elevated except in patients with circulatory collapse.

(V) COMPLICATIONS

Secondary bacterial colonization of the lung and persistent pulmonary infection are the most common complications of the RDS of shock and trauma. Gram-negative bacterial infections predominate, particularly those due to *Klebsiella*, *Pseudomonas*, *Proteus* or *Serratia*. Pulmonary fibrosis develops rarely as a result of secondary infection, barotrauma or oxygen toxicity.

Pneumothorax, in particular tension pneumothorax associated with the use of IPPV and PEEP, may develop and cause cardiopulmonary collapse in a matter of minutes. Any patient on a ventilator with PEEP who suddenly develops cardiopulmonary collapse must be assumed to have a tension pneumothorax until proven otherwise. The tension pneumothorax is usually associated with the development of both hyper-resonance and diminished breath sounds on the involved side, deviation of the trachea toward the uninvolved side, and distended neck veins. In patients on a volume ventilator many of these signs are absent or they are not picked up in the emergency situation. Often, time does not permit a chest X-ray. Under these circumstances a large bore needle should be inserted into both pleural cavities as a manoeuvre to rule out a tension pneumothorax. Pneumothoraces which develop late in the course of the RDS of shock and trauma are ominous, since they are usually associated with high ventilator pressures and severe lung damage.

Other complications of the RDS of shock and trauma are those associated with the need for prolonged IPPV (Chapter 7). These complications include erosion of the nasal alae, oral cavity, or vocal cords when nasal or oral endotracheal tubes are used. If tracheostomies are used, infection can develop around the stoma with contamination of both airways or intravenous lines. Other complications are associated with ischaemia of the tracheal mucosa leading to tracheo-oesophageal fistula, erosion of the innominate artery or, much later, tracheal stenosis.

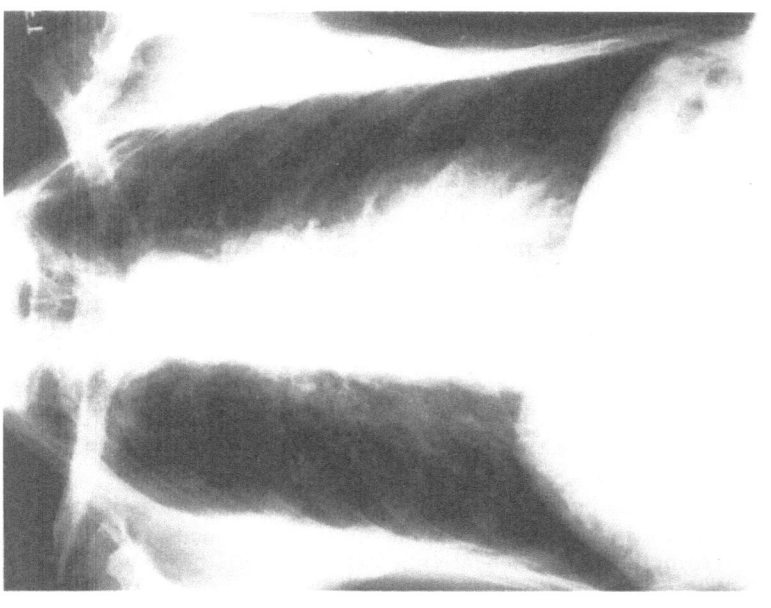

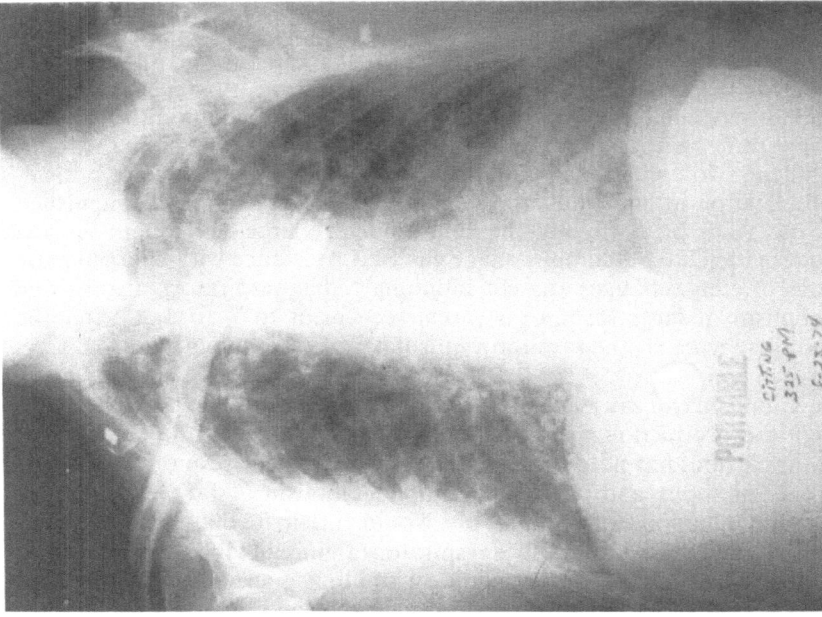

Fig 8.3 Chest X-ray during the acute phase of respiratory distress (a) and following recovery several weeks later (b)

(VI) DIAGNOSIS

Early diagnosis requires a high index of suspicion aroused by the onset of dyspnoea following a known aetiological disorder. Frequent clinical examinations, chest X-rays and serial arterial blood gases should enable an early diagnosis to be made. The most sensitive sign is a decreasing PaO_2 despite a high inspired O_2 concentration. The characteristic symptoms, X-ray findings and blood gas patterns then confirm the diagnosis. When there is doubt whether or not the patient's distress is due to heart failure, a catheter should be placed in the pulmonary artery. If the pulmonary arterial wedge pressure (PAWP) is high – greater than 15 mmHg – the probable aetiology is heart failure. If the PAWP is less than 12 mmHg the aetiology is probably the RDS of shock and trauma.

The RDS can be distinguished from pulmonary contusion because pulmonary contusion shows chest X-ray abnormalities promptly after the injury whereas the chest X-ray in the patient with the RDS of shock and trauma is initially normal.

Similarly the RDS can be distinguished from aspiration because the initial chest X-ray in aspiration will be abnormal. In addition, suctioning of gastric contents from the endotracheal tube will confirm the diagnosis of aspiration.

Atelectasis can mimic the RDS and indeed atelectasis is an integral part of the pathology associated with the syndrome. Atelectasis usually clears easily with treatment, whereas the RDS is more refractory.

Pneumonia can also mimic the RDS and, as in atelectasis, a pneumonia may well complicate the development of the syndrome. A lobar pneumonia can be distinguished on the basis of the chest film but pneumonitis will have much the same radiographic picture as the syndrome. Again, since the treatment of the two conditions is similar, the distinction is usually not critical.

Embolization of large clots to the pulmonary artery can be distinguished from the RDS primarily by the time course. Large pulmonary emboli produce acute changes in pulmonary vascular resistance with characteristic findings of e.c.g. changes and cor pulmonale. The respiratory distress due to embolism of large thrombi is rarely seen prior to 7–10 days after the initial injury whereas the respiratory insufficiency of the syndrome appears earlier.

Fat embolism can cause respiratory failure but the mechanism of action is through the production of intravascular coagulation and microembolism. Therefore it does not need to be distinguished from the respiratory distress syndrome of shock and trauma. If simple embolism of fat were indeed a major cause of respiratory failure, one would anticipate that intramedullary rodding of the femur would cause respiratory failure in all patients in whom it is used. The fact that intramedullary rodding is usually well tolerated suggests that most patients who are not in shock can tolerate a fair amount of fat, at least transiently, in the pulmonary circulation without the development of respiratory insufficiency.

(VII) TREATMENT

(1) Treatment of the underlying cause

Hypovolaemic shock must be treated aggressively to restore perfusion and to lessen the stimulus for intravascular coagulation. Adequate restoration of vascular volume can be assumed only when blood pressure, urine output, and skin perfusion have returned to normal. If the RDS of shock and trauma develops it is frequently necessary to pass a pulmonary artery catheter to measure PAWP. Pulmonary hypertension and increased pulmonary vascular resistance develop in severe cases. Although right atrial pressures may suggest that the patient's vascular volume has been adequately replenished, measurements of wedge pressure and cardiac output usually show that the patient still has hypovolaemia. Measurements of cardiac output as a function of filling pressures allow one to construct Frank–Starling curves and determine if the patient requires inotropic support (Chapter 5). Should inotropic support be indicated, isoprenaline (isoprotenerol USP) in doses which increase the heart rate to 120–140, depending on the patient's age, or dopamine in a maximum dose of 5 μg kg^{-1} min^{-1} can be used. Dopamine in higher doses can lead to alpha-adrenergic effects and lead to decreased perfusion of the splanchnic organs and of the kidneys. The PAWP can be used by itself as an indicator of whether inotropic support is needed or whether more fluid should be administered. Wedge pressures greater than 15 mmHg associated with inadequate perfusion indicate a need for inotropic support. Wedge pressures less than 12 mmHg associated with inadequate perfusion indicate the need for infusing more fluid.

Bacterial infection should be treated with appropriate surgical drainage and antibiotics. Frequent culturing of tracheal aspirates helps to detect pulmonary infection early and guide antibiotic therapy. It should be kept in mind, however, that any patient with an endotracheal tube in place will eventually grow organisms in material obtained by endotracheal suctioning. One should not treat solely on the basis of organisms in such material. The criteria that we use in deciding whether or not to treat positive sputum cultures are: (1) character of the sputum – is it purulent or thin and watery? (2) evidence of worsening pulmonary function as demonstrated by either deteriorating arterial blood gases or by the need to alter settings on the ventilator so as to maintain adequate blood gases; (3) a worsening chest X-ray; (4) signs of bacteraemia or bacterial toxaemia indicated by fever, leukocytosis, increasing requirements for fluid to maintain intravascular volume, or, if the patient is on total parenteral nutrition, decreasing glucose tolerance. If the patient has evidence of pneumonia on the basis of only one or two of the above criteria we do not start antibiotics. Antibiotics which are used injudiciously or too frequently, cause superinfection with organisms that are difficult to treat. Further information on the recognition and management of bacterial infection is given in Chapter 3.

Patients who are at risk of developing the RDS of shock and trauma may benefit from prophylactic IPPV used early after their initial episode of shock and trauma. Patients who suffer particularly severe injuries should not be extubated in the immediate postoperative period but should be maintained on IPPV for 24 hours, until it is clear that their pulmonary function is adequate. We prefer to use low levels of PEEP (4–5 cmH$_2$O) in all such patients to maintain functional residual capacity and, in almost all of our patients with the syndrome, we will use at least some PEEP in management.

Maintenance of adequate nutrition is also important in preventing or ameliorating the respiratory distress syndrome of shock and trauma. In patients who are nutritionally depleted, total parenteral nutrition or other forms of nutritional replenishment, should be instituted early (Chapter 1). Nutritional support should also be initiated early in patients who have sustained major injuries and in whom likelihood of establishing oral nutrition is unlikely within 7 days of the accident. Maintenance of adequate nutrition should help the host immune responses and the muscles of respiration.

(2) Treatment of the respiratory failure

Most patients with the RDS of shock and trauma require intubation and IPPV with a volume-controlled ventilator. The ventilator should be capable of delivering peak inspiratory pressures of up to 80 cm of water and accurately specified oxygen concentrations. Our indications for tracheal intubation and positive pressure ventilation are shown in Table 8.1. IPPV may require the use of large tidal volumes up to 20 ml kg^{-1} and of large minute volume ventilation – up to 20 l min^{-1}.

We use positive end-expiratory pressure (PEEP) in almost all these patients. The level of PEEP is initially determined by the use of the optimum compliance technique of Suter et al.[9]. Static compliance measured between PEEP levels is varied. The level of PEEP selected is that which gives the best lung compliance[9]. In critically ill patients with very poor pulmonary function, we adopt a more elaborate procedure of measuring cardiac output and arterial O$_2$ content as a function of different levels of PEEP. We select the level of PEEP that maximizes oxygen transport (the product of cardiac output and arterial O$_2$ content). Mixed venous O$_2$ saturations can also be used in the same way. The level of PEEP that maximizes the mixed venous O$_2$ saturation is usually the level of PEEP that

Table 8.1 Indications for tracheal intubation and mechanical ventilation

---

Indications for tracheal intubation
  1. Prevention of aspiration in coma
  2. Relief of upper airway obstruction
  3. Suctioning trachea in patients who cannot clear secretions
  4. Need for IPPV

Indications for mechanical ventilation
  1. Laboured respirations not relieved by conventional measures
  2. Respiratory rate greater than 35 breaths per minute
  3. $PaCO_2$ greater than 6.4 kPa (48 mmHg)
  4. Vital capacity less than 10 ml kg^{-1}
  5. Maximum inspiratory force less than 30 cmH_2O

---

maximizes oxygen transport. We will go to high levels of PEEP if we find that it is necessary to do so in order to maintain the inspired oxygen concentration at 50% or less. If the patient's oxygenating capacity is so impaired that we find it necessary to increase the inspired oxygen concentration to more than 60% we will progressively increase the levels of PEEP until it is possible to reduce the inspired oxygen concentration to 0.5. Occasionally this means using PEEP values as high as 20 cmH_2O. The use of PEEP generally depresses cardiac output and should be used very cautiously in hypovolaemic patients. Correction of hypovolaemia will allow the safe and effective use of PEEP. If we have to use high levels of PEEP we usually do so in conjunction with the use of a pulmonary arterial catheter so as to assess the effects of end-expiratory pressure on cardiac output. High levels of PEEP are not used if the patient's pulmonary function is good enough so that inspired oxygen concentrations can be maintained at levels of 0.4 or less.

Intermittent mandatory ventilation (IMV) (Chapter 7) is helpful in weaning patients from the ventilator[10]. With IMV the patient can breathe spontaneously as often and as deeply as he wants but the ventilator will give him a specified number of breaths per minute. Initially the patient can be given 12 mandatory breaths per minute so that the patient's ventilation is controlled. The number of mandatory breaths can be gradually diminished over a period of several days until the patient is finally at the point where he is breathing completely on his own, independently of the ventilator. The advantages of IMV are that it forces the patient to use his muscles of ventilation and it allows the patient to maintain his own $PaCO_2$. The disadvantage of IMV is that some patients fight the ventilator.

Our criteria for extubation have become quite simple during the past several years[11]. Before extubation the patient must fulfil the following criteria: (1) The patient must be alert enough to maintain an airway.

(2) The patient must be able to maintain normal arterial blood gases without IPPV. (3) The patient must be able to generate a maximum inspiratory force of 20 cmH$_2$O. (4) The patient must have a FVC of 10 ml kg^{-1} or better.

We rarely use the alveolar–arterial O$_2$ gradient, venous admixture, physiological dead space, or functional residual capacity in deciding whether or not the patient can be extubated. These measurements are made for research purposes and for quantitating the degree of respiratory insufficiency; they are unnecessary in deciding whether or not the patient can be extubated.

(VIII) PROGNOSIS

Of patients with the RDS, only 10–20% survive without intensive therapy. When intensive therapy is started early then the survival rate is 80–90% in the absence of bacterial infection or toxaemia. Patients who respond promptly to treatment will have little or no residual pulmonary dysfunction or disability[8]. Those requiring prolonged treatment, however, may develop restrictive lung disease.

References

1. Blaisdell, F. W. and Lewis, F. R., Jr. (1977). *Respiratory Distress Syndrome of Shock and Trauma: Post-traumatic Respiratory Failure.* (Philadelphia: W. B. Saunders)
2. Fulton, R. L. and Jones, C. E. (1975). The cause of post-traumatic pulmonary insufficiency in man. *Surg. Gynecol. Obstet.* **140**, 179
3. Holcroft, J. W., Blaisdell, F. W., Trunkey, D. D. *et al.* (1977). Intravascular coagulation and pulmonary edema in the septic baboon. *J. Surg. Res.*, **22**, 209
4. Barber, R. E., Lee, J. and Hamilton, W. K. (1970). Oxygen toxicity in man – a prospective study in patients with irreversible brain damage. *N. Engl. J. Med.*, **283**, 1478
5. Schmidt, G. B. *et al.* (1976). Continuous positive airway pressure in the prophylaxis of the adult respiratory distress syndrome. *Surg. Gynecol. Obstet.*, **143**, 613
6. Craddock, P. R. *et al.* (1977). Complement and leukocyte-mediated pulmonary dysfunction in hemodialysis. *N. Engl. J. Med.*, **296**, 769
7. Hill, J. D. *et al.* (1976). Pulmonary pathology in acute respiratory insufficiency: lung biopsy as a diagnostic tool. *J. Thor. Cardiovasc. Surg.* **71**, 64
8. Lakshminarayon, S., Stanford, R. E. and Petty, T. L. (1976). Prognosis after recovery from adult respiratory distress syndrome. *Am. Rev. Resp. Dis.*, **113**, 7
9. Suter, P. M., Fairley, H. B. and Isenberg, M. D. (1975) Optimum end-

expiratory airway pressure in patients with acute pulmonary failure. *N. Engl. J. Med.*, **292**, 284

10. Downs, J. B. *et al.* (1973). Intermittent mandatory ventilation. *Chest*, **64**, 331
11. Pontoppidan, H. *et al.* (1977). Respiratory intensive care. *Anesthesiology*, **47**, 96

9
Head injuries

BRYAN JENNETT

Head injured patients require intensive care only if they are in coma; but less severely affected patients may be in ICU because of multiple injuries. Head injuries sufficient to cause coma result in a set of pathological processes intracranially, and a set of management needs clinically, which differ only in minor details from those resulting from other forms of acute brain damage associated with coma. These include intracranial haemorrhage, cerebral ischaemia (including that resulting from cardiac arrest), meningoencephalitis and the like. Much of what follows about head injury will therefore apply to the management of comatose patients with these other conditions.

Trauma is no respecter of geography, and some head injured patients, particularly the severe ones from high speed road accidents, occur far from regional neurosurgical services. Initial treatment must therefore be in general hospitals, and because many of these now have ICUs an argument has been advanced for retaining patients there, even when there is a major head injury. The counter argument is that optimal treatment calls for the skills of a neurosurgical team, including specially trained nurses and anaesthetists; and, in particular, specialized investigation or monitoring, even when there is no need for intracranial surgery. Further discussion of this controversial issue is best deferred until the end of this chapter, after most of the factors, on which the arguments rest, have been described.

The overall aim of intensive care for the head injured patient is to prevent secondary brain damage – nothing can be done to repair damage sustained at impact. There is, however, good evidence that secondary events, intra-cranial and extracranial, contribute significantly to mortality and morbidity in patients who reach hospital alive. More than half the deaths ascribed to head injury occur before the victim can be admitted to hospital, but investigation of such cases indicates that almost all had suffered overwhelming injuries to the head or elsewhere, or both; only an occasional case might have been saved by more skilled care at the scene of the accident[1].

Because these secondary events dominate the *raison d'etre* of intensive care for the brain damage, it will be best to begin with an account of the pathophysiological processes involved. Methods of assessing and monitoring the head injured patient are then reviewed, followed by a brief account of the value of radiological and laboratory investigations. In the light of this the practical diagnosis of head injured patients in ICU is discussed, and then the therapeutic measures – with due emphasis on the ordering of priorities in the patient with multiple injuries. Outcome and prognosis are then described, as a basis for assessing the efficacy of treatment. The chapter ends with comments on the scale of the problem, and the implication of this for where (and by whom) these patients are best treated. The contents are based on published evidence, on two decades of personal experience, and on the results of an international study of severe head injuries conducted by the writer over the last 12 years.

(I) PATHOLOGICAL CONSEQUENCES OF HEAD INJURY

Our knowledge of these processes depends largely on painstaking examination of the brains of fatal cases by neuropathologists. This is not only time consuming but it is administratively quite difficult to arrange. By definition deaths due to accidents are of concern to coroners (or their equivalent), and the demand for an immediate autopsy report leads many pathologists to slice the unfixed brain. This can reveal only the most crude lesions – contusions and haemorrhage; only when the intact brain has been fixed for 2–3 weeks and then dissected, and submitted to microscopy, can the pathologists discover the extent of impact injury to white matter, and of secondary hypoxic/ischaemic damage. Only then is it possible to ascribe the contribution to the cause of death of primary and secondary events. Without skilled autopsy of this kind as an audit it is all too easy to regard most deaths after head injury as inevitable (which some certainly are), and so to underestimate the errors of omission in their care.

Most injuries in civilian life (in Europe) result from acceleration/deceleration forces, which act on the head as a whole, and cause *diffuse* brain damage. Severe damage to white matter throughout the brain can occur without skull fracture, and without significant contusions of the cerebral cortex; the brain may look almost normal on gross examination. Patients with only this particular lesion form a small but a characteristic group – they are in deep coma from the moment of impact with bilaterally extensor motor responses in their limbs; if they survive the first week or so they may live for months or even years in a vegetative state.

At the other extreme is the patient with primarily focal brain damage, due to penetrating injury of the skull – perhaps due to an instrument such as a screwdriver, hammer or a piece of metal or glass. Although there may be brain oozing out of the wound he may be fully conscious throughout, and there will not be any focal neurological signs unless particular areas of brain are involved. The danger of such an injury lies in the risk of infection (meningitis or brain abcess) unless prompt and adequate debridement is done. This is also the risk with basal fractures associated with CSF rhinorrhoea or otorrhoea – which may readily be overlooked in the unconscious, or the patient with multiple injuries.

Most head injured patients in an intensive care unit will have less clear-cut injuries than these – they will have suffered a mixture of focal and diffuse injuries, with both white matter shearing and cortical contusion. Damage will frequently be bilateral, and seldom confined either to the side of a skull fracture or to the contre-coup area of brain; brain stem signs may occur, but injury confined to this part of the brain is rare. Secondary processes comprise a complex mixture of vascular engorgement, haemorrhage and oedema – combining to cause brain swelling, focal or widespread; and of hypoxic/ischaemic damage related to intracranial hypertension and systemic hypotension, aggravated by reduced oxygen-carrying capacity of the blood, due to extracranial factors (blood loss and respiratory insufficiency).

Autopsy of patients who have died in a neurosurgical unit after head injury reveals that almost 90% have pathological evidence of raised ICP, and over 80% have ischaemic brain damage[2]; the latter is usually widespread, affecting many areas of cerebral cortex and basal ganglia[3]. About a third of such a series of fatalities talked before they died, evidence that the impact damage was not overwhelming[4]. In patients who talked and died a discrete intracranial haematoma was found in three-quarters; other complications were brain swelling, intracranial infection, hypoxic/ischaemic lesions and fat embolism. A review of a large series of autopsied head injuries in hospital indicated that avoidable factors in management had contributed significantly to death in 50%; such factors were more common in those who talked and died (65%) than in those continuously in coma (40%)[1]. These avoidable factors related to intracranial events in two thirds of cases, most commonly delayed evacuation of a haematoma; in the rest,

194

systemic hypotension or hypoxia were the most frequent factors which might have been prevented (or more promptly treated), but which led to fatal brain damage. It is reasonable to assume that patients who survive head injury with disability have secondary lesions similar to those found in fatal cases, albeit less severe. Investigation reveals a high incidence of avoidable factors in the management of such surviving patients.

(1) Intracranial haematoma

This is the complication which has the most obvious effect on outcome after head injury, in that it may cause death or permanent disability in a patient whose impact injury was not serious. Because its effects can often be prevented by prompt surgery, it is not surprising that delayed evacuation of a haematoma should be one of the commonest causes of avoidable mortality or morbidity. The purpose of much of the monitoring of head injured patients is directed towards the early detection of this complication.

The classical syndrome is of the patient who is temporarily unconscious after injury, then has a lucid interval, followed by headache and drowsiness progressing to coma, with dilatation of the pupil on the side of clot and hemiparesis on the other side. Bradycardia, periodic breathing and systemic hypertension eventually occur. Like many a classical syndrome, this is comparatively rare, and many of the features are those of the final stage of brain stem compression, when it is already often too late to intervene successfully. Yet clinicians still sometimes watch the patient in the early stages of cerebral compression, waiting for enough of these sinister signs to develop before initiating intervention.

Intracranial haematomas may be extradural or intradural – either subdural, intracerebral or both; some patients have both extradural and intradural clots. The 'classical' syndrome is commonly believed to be typical of the pure extradural haematoma but even that is untrue. When a large number of haematomas are analysed, with the benefit of the data now available from CT scanning as well as operative findings, and that from autopsy in fatal cases, it seems that there is no one clinical presentation which is typical of a particular kind of haematoma[5]. Many intradural haematomas have a lucid interval, but not all extradurals have an initially mild injury; haematomas may occur in patients in coma from the outset, and CT scan may show a large haematoma in a patient who has not yet deteriorated. A skull fracture occurs in 90% of adults with an extradural haematoma, and in 75% of those with an intradural clot. Haematomas are more common in patients who have sustained falls and assaults than in those injured in motor vehicle accidents. For this reason haematomas are also less common in patients with major extracranial injuries.

It must be concluded that a haematoma should be suspected in any patient in coma, but is more likely if there is a vault fracture and/or any focal neurological signs (hemiparesis or pupillary inequality). In the talking patient who has a vault fracture it must also be suspected. The only reliable way to exclude this diagnosis is by CT scanning.

(II) ASSESSMENT AND MONITORING

The purposes of assessment and monitoring are several. Initial severity of brain damage provides, with the patient's age, the best indication of the potential for recovery – this enables therapeutic triage to be undertaken, which is essential in deciding what treatment (and where) is appropriate. It also provides a base line from which subsequent monitoring may show change. This may lead to a revision of the original prognosis – if there is improvement or lack of it. If there is deterioration, complications may be suspected – some of which call for prompt action. An assessment of the severity of brain damage, whether primary or secondary, is essential also for the evaluation of alternative therapeutic methods. Unless these are compared in sufficiently similar groups of patients, conclusions about their efficacy may be invalid. Three main features have to be recorded – evidence of general and/or focal brain dysfunction, evidence of intracranial, structural or mechanical abnormalities, and signs of systemic dysfunction that may be the result or the cause of brain damage (or both). Assessment may be based on clinical observation or on laboratory methods, including radiology. With the exception of CT scanning it must be admitted that no laboratory investigation has so far been evolved that comes anywhere near to competing with clinical assessment, and even the CT scan is often normal in seriously brain damaged patients.

(1) Brain dysfunction

This is a sensitive and readily available index of brain damage. When the brain as a whole suffers an impact, as commonly occurs with the acceleration/deceleration forces of most civilian accidents, the immediate dysfunction is altered consciousness – there is a continuum between full alertness, confusion, coma and brain death; the level of responsiveness and the duration of impaired consciousness provide the most reliable guides to the extent of the brain damage; a deteriorating conscious level is also the most reliable sign of intracranial complications. This has two important practical implications for the intensive care unit. One is that any measures likely to obscure the assessment of consciousness (e.g. depressant or relaxant drugs) are best avoided, if at all possible, unless they are deemed essential for other reasons, e.g. chest injury. The other is that methods of assessing conscious level must be appropriate – easily carried out, reliably reported by a wide range of staff, and readily recorded. It was for this purpose that the Glasgow Coma Scale was evolved. It is now used widely in many places, and has become a standard measure for comparing the severity of head injured patients[6].

Responsiveness of three kinds is recorded: eye opening, motor response and verbal behaviour. By allocating an ordinal number to each point on these scales, an overall coma score can be derived (Table 9.1). An advantage of this method is that assessment is still possible even if one of the responses is unavailable, e.g. the patient cannot speak because of an ET tube.

A patient is said to be in coma if he does not open his eyes, obey commands or utter any understandable words. Other aspects of brain dysfunction which should be observed in the comatose patient are any asymmetry in the motor responses in the four limbs; inequality in pupil size and the reaction of the pupils to light; and eye movements, spontaneous and reflex. These may also be put on hierarchical scales (Table 9.2). These additional features may indicate the site of focal brain damage, as well as the functional state of the brain stem.

The state of responsiveness of recently head injured patients may alter quite markedly, especially within the first 24 hours. Partly this may be due to recovery with time or to intracranial complications making the patient less responsive. But extracranial factors also have an important influence,

Table 9.1   Glasgow Coma Scale

Eye opening		
spontaneous	E	4
to speech		3
to pain		2
nil		1
Best motor response		
obeys	M	6
localizes		5
withdraws		4
abnormal flexion		3
extensor response		2
nil		1
Verbal response		
orientated	V	5
confused conversation		4
inappropriate words		3
incomprehensible sounds		2
nil		1
Coma score $(E + M + V) = 3\text{--}15$		

Table 9.2 Eye movement scales

Spontaneous	1	normal
	2	conjugate roving
	3	dysconjugate roving
	4	lateral deviation
	5	absent
Oculocephalic	1	nil (normal)
	2	full
	3	minimal
	4	absent
Oculovestibular	1	nystagmus (normal)
	2	conjugate tonic
	3	dysconjugate tonic
	4	absent

particularly alcohol, which may combine with a moderately severe head injury to produce a patient who is in deep coma. Many injured patients have recently ingested alcohol (25% of severely head injured patients in one large international series); only a blood level can determine how significant its influence may be – if < 200 mg/100 ml then coma should not be ascribed to alcohol.

Other extracranial influences are hypotension, hypoxia, and low haemoglobin – all of which are common when patients first present with multiple injury including a head injury[7]. These factors combine to impair brain oxygenation, and a comatose patient may rapidly regain responsiveness, including the restoration of reacting pupils, as a result of initial resuscitation. For these reasons initial assessment of severity should not be made until this has been completed. During the first week a day by day assessment of coma should include the best and worst state of the patient during each day, as some fluctuations are likely to occur.

(2) Signs of abnormal structural and mechanical events

Until the advent of CT scanning and of ICP monitoring the clinician had little option but to make informed guesses about what was happening in the head. If there was a vault fracture associated with contralateral hemiparesis, he might have to assume an intracranial haematoma – and to proceed to blind burr holes or angiography to exclude this potentially remediable complication; he would feel even more constrained to this line of action if there had been evidence of clinical deterioration, and/or dilatation of the pupil opposite to the hemiparesis. If there were no focal signs, but the patient was deeply subconscious, with extensor limb responses, he might have to assume raised intracranial pressure, and consider it necessary to embark on decongestant therapy.

What recent investigative methods have revealed is that these simple clinical assumptions are often wrong; moreover some patients have a haematoma clearly evident on CT scan before any of the classical signs have developed[8]. These discoveries have altered the management of head injuries so fundamentally that it must now be accepted that there are two standards of care – with CT scanning and without. So the question to be answered about the head injured patient in the general intensive care unit is not only whether he needs an operation, but whether he requires moving to a neuro-surgical unit where investigational and monitoring facilities are available.

(3) Signs of systemic dysfunction

Head injured patients frequently have abnormalities of respiration and cardiovascular function, sometimes of body temperature. As already indicated these may threaten brain function, and even cause secondary structural brain damage. It is often difficult to be certain with respiratory abnormalities just what is the relative contribution of focal brain damage, of raised ICP, and of local pulmonary factors (aspiration, infarction or chest injury).

A variety of abnormal patterns is seen but these are not related to site of injury or outcome, and therefore monitoring them is of little value[9]. Hypo-ventilation (evidenced by high $PaCO_2$) is rare, but hyperventilation is common; a high frequency of breathing is often observed, but this is not a reliable guide to the degree of hypocapnia. Hypoxaemia (breathing air), or a wide alveolar–arterial oxygen difference (with high F_1O_2), is common, and is sometimes seen soon after injury – but may become progressively more marked. It is important to monitor PaO_2 and A-a difference, in order to detect increase in pulmonary venous admixture, which may call for action. There may be both local (pulmonary) as well as neurogenic influences on this phenomenon – and it is often impossible to separate these[10].

Bradycardia and hypertension are the classical cardiovascular responses to brain stem compression, secondary to raised intracranial pressure associated with brain shift, as occurs with an intracranial haematoma. However, these are late signs and often there is a rapid pulse. Hypotension on the other hand is rarely found in head injured patients, but when it is a systemic cause should be sought. Most often this will be blood loss (which occasionally is from the scalp). Relief of raised ICP, by evacuation of an intracranial haematoma, may result in a dangerous fall in systemic blood pressure, and that is why blood replacement should always be available before operation is started.

Hyperpyrexia is an occasional response to brain damage, and it may be

199

aggravated by the heat production associated with repeated epilepsy or sustained decerebrate rigidity. Transfer of such a patient wrapped in the statutory layers of ambulance blankets may cause an alarming rise in temperature.

(III) INVESTIGATIONS

(1) Plain skull X-rays[11]

Different opinions are sometimes expressed about the value of finding (or excluding) a skull fracture in a patient already in hospital after head injury, particularly if CT scanning is readily available. A linear fracture significantly increases the likelihood that an intracranial haematoma will occur, and this should increase vigilance for signs of this. Where scanning facilities are restricted it is patients with a fracture who should get priority – in order to exclude a haematoma. A depressed fracture under a scalp laceration indicates an open injury, as does a basal skull fracture or the finding of air in the basal cisterns (best shown in a brow-up lateral view). Absence of a skull fracture in a patient who has been decerebrate and in deep coma from the time of impact makes the diagnosis of overwhelming damage to diffuse white matter probable. In the absence of CT scanning, the site of a fracture may provide a useful clue to the site of a haematoma if surgical intervention becomes necessary.

For these various reasons it is wise always to secure an X-ray of the skull, although this should never be a reason for delaying resuscitation, or rapid admission to the intensive care unit. It is quite feasible to take portable views, and if multiple injuries make it difficult to put the patient prone, it is acceptable to limit the views (initially) to A-P and brow-up laterals; angulated axial views should be taken to exclude pineal shift, if lateral views show calcification. The cervical spine should also be X-rayed at this stage, because there is a need to know that it is safe to move the neck freely, e.g. during intubation or eliciting reflex eye movements.

(2) CT Scanning

This may show contusions, haematomas, hydrocephalus, ventricular shift, oedema and infarction. It is therefore a valuable tool and is free of risk, unless an anaesthetic is required because the patient is restless. However, about a third of head injuries in coma have a normal CT scan, and this investigation in no sense excludes severe, even irrecoverable, brain damage. On the other hand, some patients who are awake and alert are shown to have intracranial haematomas on the scan[8]; whilst some of these patients recover without the need for surgical evacuation of the clot, others deteriorate rapidly – sometimes days after the haematoma has been shown on the scan. The dynamic nature of the intracranial pathophysiology has already been stressed, and a corollary of this is that one scan soon after injury does not exclude (if it is normal or nearly so) the subsequent development of abnormalities. Not only may haematomas develop but contusions become more obvious and extensive after 24 hours. Whilst a single scan is obviously helpful, there is a potential danger in managing patients in circumstances where only one scan, usually soon after injury, is done, and where repeated examination is difficult.

Sometimes large ventricles are found, suggestive of a posterior fossa lesion – and further cuts can then be directed to that part of the brain. Small ventricles are often found in children, and sometimes these are associated with vascular congestion or oedema. However, marked and obvious oedema of the kind commonly seen in association with tumours is seldom seen on scans after recent head injury. Perhaps the greatest value of the CT scan is when it excludes an intracranial haematoma or focal swelling, and thereby reassures the clinician that there is no need to contemplate opening the skull. One of the most important effects this investigation has had on those who are using it daily in the management of head injured patients is to undermine their confidence in making clinical judgements about these patients. Those who have become used to having this investigation available become very reluctant to make diagnostic statements about patients before they see the scan, although there is need for considerable clinical judgement in deciding what relative significance to attach to the scan and the clinical picture when these seem to conflict.

(3) ICP Monitoring

The final common pathology of many of the intracranial processes which occur after head injury is raised pressure; there is evidence of this in about 90% of autopsies on fatalities in hospital. One reaction to this is to treat all patients as though they had raised pressure. The other is to measure the ICP – which makes it possible to recognize which patients need treatment, to monitor the effect of whatever measures are instituted, and to gain additional prognostic information. Clinically feasible methods for continuous ICP measurement have been available for 20 years, and in the last 5 years or so have become routine in most large neurosurgical clinics. They have even been used in a general intensive care unit remote from neurosurgical facilities[17]. In these circumstances it is timely to review what has been learnt from all these measurements (and those made on experimental animals), and what the practical lessons are for the intensive care unit clinician.

201

Three main methods are available, intraventricular, subdural and extradural. A catheter in the ventricle gives the most sensitive and accurate measurement, and it allows measurement of intracranial compliance, and also CSF drainage. Its disadvantages are that it may be difficult to initiate or to maintain connection with small ventricles, and the risk of infection. Probably the most widely used method is the subdural, using a hollow bolt which is secured into a burr hole and connected to a transducer by a fluid-filled catheter. Extradural methods, also dependent on a device screwed into a burr hole, have rigorous technical requirements for measurements to be valid.

The recording and display of continuous ICP recording presents problems – visual interpretation of long traces can be difficult. Data processing methods have been evolved to present histograms of the profile of pressure over successive periods. There is also the need to correlate these with what has been happening to the patient – do rises of pressure indicate primary intracranial events or simply a reaction to measuring or other procedures? Is it the overall level that matters, or the rises in response to stimuli, or the occurrence of spontaneous A, B and C waves? These matters remain controversial, as does the fundamental question of whether high pressure is the cause of brain damage, or evidence that there is already irremediable intracranial haemostasis.

The most recent views of the findings in large series are those of Miller[13] and of Jennett and Teasdale[5]. These reveal differences of opinion about the significance of different levels of pressure, but it seems that under 15 mmHg can be regarded as normal, 15–30 mmHg as raised but not justifying major intervention, whilst over 30 mmHg requires that something definite be done. The question is whether it is necessary to have ICP measurements before initiating treatment designed to lower ICP. Many of the routine aspects of the care of the patient in coma, which may favourably affect ICP, certainly do not call for ICP measurements before they are used. But if patients are to be given depressant and relaxant drugs, ICP may be the only way to monitor the intracranial situation, unless repeated CT scanning is available. It is difficult to justify the use of hyperventilation or barbiturate-induced cerebral depression if ICP monitoring is not available.

The value of ICP measurements in the diagnosis of intracranial haematoma is sometimes raised, particularly in the patient with multiple injuries who may have to be given depressant drugs. Measurements may be of some use, but compared with repeated CT scanning they come as a poor second best. In regard to prognosis, ICP measurements are even more confusing, because recovery is possible after bouts of high pressure, particularly in children, whilst the victims of the most severe diffuse white matter damage who never recover rarely have raised ICP.

In the context of the general ICU, without access to CT scanning and neurosurgical facilities, it is difficult to regard ICP measurements as playing a useful role – unless there are enough cases being treated for expertise to be developed, not only in securing measurements but in interpreting them[14].

(4) Ultrasound encephalography

It was at one time hoped that this cheap and portable method of detecting midline shift of intracranial structures might prove useful. However, only in the hands of a few committed enthusiasts has it proved reliable and it cannot be recommended.

(5) E.e.g.

Recording of the spontaneous electrical activity of the brain when there is already severe brain dysfunction (i.e. patient in coma) is of little value – general and focal abnormalities are found, but their significance is seldom clear. However, evoked cerebral responses to peripheral stimuli (somato-sensory, auditory and visual) have been shown to have a good correlation with damage in the brain stem and/or cerebral hemispheres, and to have some prognostic significance. The apparatus required is costly, however, and considerable time and expertise is required to obtain useful data.

(IV) MANAGEMENT

(1) Primary care and supportive therapy

In a book on intensive therapy it would be superfluous to reiterate what is written elsewhere about the details of care of the airway, avoidance of infection, replacement of fluid and maintenance of nutrition. Instead it is intended only to outline the principles of such care, emphasizing where the presence of a head injury may make it necessary to vary the routine treatment given in the ICU; also when it is necessary to be aware of a possible conflict between the management routine normally recommended and the needs of the brain damaged patient. Also the relative priority to be given to the head injury and to other injuries in cases of polytrauma is indicated.

Immediate resuscitation

Immediate resuscitation must proceed, regardless of any head injury; a temporary head-down position may be accepted, to avoid aspiration and to restore normotension – but this will increase ICP and may aggravate intra-

203

cranial bleeding. Circulatory overload must be avoided, as the injured brain with impaired autoregulation and a defective blood brain barrier may be vulnerable to this. Patients have become neurologically worse and even developed dilated pupils as a result of injudicious treatment of 'shock'.

Many unconscious patients can maintain an adequate airway with a combination of suction, positioning and a mechanical airway. If the patient will tolerate an endotracheal tube without sedation, then he needs one. But initial resuscitation should, wherever possible, avoid the giving of depressant or relaxant drugs until the state of brain dysfunction has been assessed. It must be remembered that many head injured patients admitted in coma will be waking up within a few hours, and it is important not to over-react and thereby delay (and even imperil) their recovery. The same goes for the giving of i.v. fluids – unless the patient is hypovolaemic, as a result of other injuries, there is no urgency for this. Indeed brain swelling is less likely to develop if fluid intake is on the low side of calculated requirements.

Diagnosis and treatment

Once initial resuscitation is complete the diagnosis of both intracranial and extracranial injuries must be established – clinical examination, X-ray of skull, cervical spine and chest in all cases, and of other parts as indicated. It must then be decided what priority different injuries require. *Immediate intervention* is necessary for gut or bladder perforation, or bleeding from spleen or kidneys, and for intracranial haematoma. A compound fracture of the limbs or of the skull may be *deferred for 12–24 hours*, provided anti-biotics are given. Internal fixation of limb fractures and facio-maxillary injuries can almost always be *deferred for a few days*, even for a week or two.

What has to be avoided, if possible, in the head injured patient is the hazard of surgery and general anaesthesia in the first 24–48 hours. Not only is the patient not accessible for monitoring for as long as he is under anaesthesia, but he may be subjected to fluctuations in blood pressure and even in PaO_2 and $PaCO_2$, to which the damaged brain is peculiarly vulnerable.

In the patient who *remains in coma* after the first 24 hours, the question of the continued care of the airway and of intubation arises. Children can often be managed without an ET tube for long periods, given skilled nursing. At all ages an ET tube can be maintained for much longer periods than previously, using modern materials and techniques. Tracheostomy should be deferred as long as possible in the head injured patient, because, apart from its local hazards, it makes it much more difficult to deal with and to assess the patient emerging from coma if he cannot speak.

Nutrition

The nutritional and fluid requirements of the head injured patient who remains in coma do not usually differ markedly from those of other patients – apart from the need to avoid overload. For this reason, nasogastric rather than i.v. administration is preferable. However, some head injured patients develop temporary diabetes insipidus; salt-hoarding or salt-losing syndromes have also been described, which may sometimes reflect damage in hypothalamic and pituitary structures. More often they result from inappropriate management of fluid and nutritional requirements, and a regular check on electrolytes and urine is therefore of particular importance in head injured patients.

Restlessness

Restlessness is often a matter of concern to those looking after head injured patients. The patient may be thrashing about, causing concern about his i.v. line, about his limb fractures, and he may also be noisy. It is tempting to give such a patient depressant drugs – if only for the sake of staff and other patients. Before doing so, it should be considered whether some specific discomfort is the cause of his behaviour such as a full bladder, a painful lesion (e.g. limb fracture) or thirst (in the patient with diabetes insipidus). It should also be questioned what harm is coming from this restlessness – patients like this tend not to develop hypostatic pneumonia, pressure sores or limb contractures, because they are doing their own physiotherapy! A patient who is restless like this is emerging from coma and his recovery may be delayed by drugs, although these may be necessary at night.

Whether continued decerebrate or decorticate rigidity is in fact harmful is uncertain. It has been shown that some patients develop temporary increases in ICP during extensor spasms, but not all patients do. It is doubtful whether depressant or relaxant drugs are justified simply because a patient is having such spasms.

(2) Treatment of raised ICP and respiratory dysfunction

Because these phenomena are common, and because autopsy frequently shows ischaemic brain damage, there has emerged over the last 10 years or so a tendency to treat most severe (i.e. comatose) head injuries routinely with measures which are supposed to be effective against these complications. Controlled respiration (often at hypocapnic levels), steroids (recently in massive doses), and hyperosmotic agents, have become standard practice; more recently high doses of barbiturates have been

205

advocated for the most severe cases. It is now clear that these various measures came to be adopted because they were expected, on theoretical grounds, to be useful – not because rigorously controlled trials had shown them to be effective.

Ways and means of assessing therapy for severe head injuries are currently emerging, partly due to evolution of standardized means of assessing the severity of brain damage soon after injury. These will be discussed later, but their relevance here is that they are already throwing doubt on the efficacy of methods currently used in the management of severe head injuries.

Steroids

The role of steroids even in high doses could not be demonstrated in two carefully conducted trials[15,16], and this accords with the relative infrequency of oedema in CT scans or autopsies after head injury. 'Brain oedema' was a common clinical diagnosis in the last 20 years; this was not based on evidence but was a short-hand term for a badly brain damaged patient with high pressure who had no mass lesion. It now seems likely that other features contribute more importantly to brain swelling, in particular cerebral congestion (i.e. cerebrovascular dilatation).

Osmotics

The value of osmotics as a means of reducing ICP is undoubted, in the context of one infusion of 500 ml of 20% mannitol. This may produce clinical improvement, and if there is a remediable cause for the raised ICP (such as a haematoma) this may prove life-saving – if it buys enough time for surgical intervention to be carried out. It is much more doubtful whether repeated doses, to produce a continuing state of altered serum osmolality, is beneficial, especially as the local effect on the brain is dependent on the blood brain barrier, which may be defective in some areas.

High dose barbiturates

The value of high dose barbiturates is currently under review, but the hazards of this treatment are so considerable (particularly arterial hypotension) that it is not justified at present outside of a formal trial[17]. It should be noted that two other elaborate therapies that have been abandoned in recent years are hypothermia, and massive bony decompression.

206

Controlled ventilation

This leaves controlled ventilation as the most commonly used (but still unproven) method of treatment for the comatose head injury. There seems to be considerable confusion about both the rationale for, and the effects of, this particular measure, and writings about it tend to be longer on dogma than on data. To be sure the situation is complex, and the best that can be done at present is to set out the arguments. There are two main reasons for taking over the patient's ventilation. One is that his own breathing is inadequate or in some other way unsatisfactory; the other is in order to regulate the state of the cerebral vasculature, by manipulation of the $PaCO_2$.

As already mentioned (p. 199) hypoventilation is uncommon in severely head injured patients; most patients are hyperventilating, and they may be normoxic and hypocapnic. This may be an appropriate response to hypoxaemia, which is due to venous admixture in the lungs, and one result is that there will be cerebrovascular constriction, tending to reduce ICP. If the patient is still hypoxaemic in spite of hyperventilation, he may be restored to normoxia by the simple device of enriching the inspired air. It is sometimes claimed that this 'natural' hyperventilation is disadvantageous to the patient because of the burden of the work of breathing. However, this can be shown to be a relatively trivial contribution to metabolic demand, far outweighed by that due to muscle spasticity in the limbs[10].

However, there are some patients, usually those with chest injury or major chest complications, who remain hypoxaemic even when breathing high oxygen mixtures and in them it may be necessary to institute controlled ventilation in order to improve cerebral oxygenation. It is well to remember that this depends also on an adequate haemoglobin, and if there are multiple injuries it is important to restore the haematocrit. Cerebral oxygenation depends on the cerebral perfusion pressure, the resultant of ICP and inflow pressure to the head.

Controlled ventilation may be advised in order to lower $PaCO_2$, as a means of reducing ICP – although most patients already have a low $PaCO_2$. Indeed some have such a low $PaCO_2$ (less than 25 mmHg, 3.3 kPa) that controlled ventilation may be considered useful in order to reverse the possible ill-effects of such extreme hypocapnia. Most now recommend adjusting the respirator to keep $PaCO_2$ between 30 and 35 mmHg, 4.0–4.7 kPa.

The disadvantages of controlled ventilation are that clinical monitoring of brain function is seriously impaired; the patient needs to be examined once a day before the next dose of drugs, to check on motor response and pupillary reaction. There are also the hazards of reliance on machines, certainly small in a well-organized service but never negligible; the adverse pulmonary effects of prolonged mechanical assistance; and the complications of prolonged intubation or of tracheostomy. There are, of course, circumstances in which controlled ventilation is undoubtedly necessary, for example, when there are associated chest or neck injuries. On the other hand there is no good evidence that centres which use it on a much larger proportion of their comatose patients achieve any better outcome than those who restrict its use to the few cases where it is clearly needed[18].

(V) OUTCOME

Until recently it has been difficult to evaluate the efficacy of alternative treatment regimes because of the variety of terms used to describe the state of surviviors. The Glasgow Outcome Scale is now widely used for this purpose, both for head injury and for non-traumatic coma. It is a simple scale, which does not itemize the nature of the disability but rather its social implications. Thus disability is deemed to be severe if it makes a person dependent on another person, for some activities, during each day. Disability after brain damage usually has both a mental and a physical component. In most cases the mental handicap is the more significant, and many patients who have made a good recovery physically are handicapped by personality changes and/or problems with memory and intellect. However, these mental abnormalities are easily overlooked, especially in a routine follow-up clinic; only when relatives and associates of the patient are questioned may it become clear that the patient is nothing like as good as he looks, or says he feels. Euphoria and lack of insight frequently leads the patient himself to under-estimate his disability.

The distribution of patients on this outcome scale depends on the severity and cause of the initial brain damage. In a series of 1000 head injured patients who were in coma for at least 6 hours[19], the outcome at 6 months was 49% dead, 2% vegetative, 10% severely and 17% moderately disabled, whilst 22% made a good recovery. The outcome for a series of patients with non-traumatic coma was much less good, 85% being dead[2]; more such patients are older than the head injured, and may suffer from progressive degenerative diseases.

The figures quoted apply to the state 6 months after injury. A few patients may improve further after this stage, but analysis shows that two thirds of patients are already in their ultimate outcome category within 3 months and 90% by 6 months. This is not to deny that improvement within one category does not occur. The nature of disability after head injury has been discussed in more detail elsewhere[21].

(1) Prognosis

It is now possible to predict the outcome of head injured patients at 6 months, on the Glasgow Scale, using clinical data available in the first few days after injury, together with the patient's age[19,22,23]. Only about half the patients can be confidently predicted (0.97 probability) in the first 24 hours, but the proportion is 75% by the end of the first week. Predictions are based on statistical calculations derived from analysis of 1000 patients in an international data bank, about whom there is data on early severity and 6 months outcome. Predictions about new patients do not require access to the original data bank, but can be made using a hand-held calculator and tables derived from the data bank.

The value of such predictions is considerable. They enable the clinician to make appropriate triage for treatment, particularly the continuation or not of intensive therapy. They also provide a means of evaluating treatment which obviates some of the ethical problems of controlled trials. And they enable doctors to give relatives a more realistic forecast of what the future holds – early counselling about the nature and duration of disability after severe head injury may do much to minimize the disruptive and distressing consequences of the patient's eventual return home.

(VI) EVALUATION OF THERAPY

When dealing with conditions associated with a high mortality, there are inevitably pressures to use any (or all) of the therapeutic manoeuvres which might be beneficial and it is difficult to conduct controlled trials. This problem has been commented on in respect of cancer and the point made that rather than randomized prospective trials it may be more appropriate (and more ethically acceptable) to use historical controls; also to compare 'best conventional treatment' with new methods, because a 'no treatment' group is unthinkable.

The first step in any such study is to agree on what criteria of severity should be used, to apply to groups of patients to be compared. The international data bank has identified those features which relate to outcome[19]. It is then a matter of judgement to decide how closely two series should conform in order to make a valid comparison. In fact this is largely a statistical issue, which we have discussed elsewhere, depending on how great a difference in outcome it is required to show, and what sample sizes are likely to be available[24].

One device is to insist only on a minimum degree of severity, and then to compare series of patients differently treated. When this was done for the international series of head injuries and non-traumatic coma, it did not seem that the more intensive treatment used in some centres had made a significant impact (Tables 9.3 and 9.4). More detailed analysis of the head injured cases, subdivided according to degrees of severity, also failed to show a better outcome among patients treated with steroids, with osmotics,

Table 9.3 Non-traumatic coma

	American patients 152	British patients 158
Special tests	206	68
Steroid drugs	61%	8%
Mechanical ventilation	45%	3%
Dead at 1 month	69%	77%

Based on Bates *et al.*[20]

Table 9.4 Traumatic coma

	American patients 167	British patients 495
Steroids	99%	31%
Tracheostomy	66%	14%
Mechanical ventilation	62%	12%
Bone flap removed (after craniotomy)	55%	15%
Dead at 1 month	45%	41%

with controlled ventilation, with tracheostomy or with bony decompression[18]. Claims from other centres [25-27] that more favourable outcomes resulted from more 'aggressive' treatment are of doubtful validity, either because the sample sizes were inadequate or because the initial severity was not sufficiently closely matched[24].

Another approach is to use predicitons as a basis for comparison. Thus in the head injury series the outcome of patients treated with steroids was predicted, on the basis of those not so treated; those who had had steroids did not have a better outcome than was predicted from those who did not[18].

Prediction could also be useful in setting up prospective trials, as it would enable new treatments to be used on patients whose outcome was in doubt, and therefore likely to be susceptible to influence. It seems likely that the benefits of some methods of management may have been obscured by the inclusion in series under test of too many patients who had a high probability either of death or of satisfactory recovery - regardless of the nature of treatment.

(VII) LOGISTICS

In Europe where neurosurgical facilities are regionalized, only a small fraction of head injuries reach neurosurgical units (5% in UK in 1974). Even in North America where many community hospitals may boast of having a neurosurgeon on their staff, only a fraction of head injuries reach a unit equipped and staffed to the standard of a European regional unit. General intensive care facilities are much more widely dispersed than neurosurgical units in Europe, and a natural question is whether this is where most comatose head injuries, especially those with multiple injuries, should be cared for. Before answering that question it is first necessary to know how frequent are head injuries, how many have multiple injuries and what is their geographical distribution. Also one must consider what are the implications of transporting comatose patients from one hospital to another, and how these match up to the advantages of having the patient moved to the specialized facilities of a neurosurgical unit.

Epidemiological studies indicate that the annual admission rate of comatose head injuries per 10^5 population is about ten in Britain, and double this in parts of USA[28]. There is no evidence of any increase in the incidence of severe head injuries in the last 10 years; indeed there has been a slight decrease. In the international series of severe head injuries, major extracranial injuries occurred in 21%; they were more than twice as common in victims of road accidents (30%) as in other patients with head injury (only 12% had a major extracranial injury).

From these figures it is evident that severe head injuries are not very common, and those with multiple injuries infrequent – at least at the level of the general hospital. It is therefore not feasible for anyone there to develop expertise in the investigation and management of severe head injuries, quite apart from the technical limitations. For these reasons it is best to consider how to ensure the transfer to the regional neurosurgical unit of as many of these patients as possible. The best time for transfer is once initial resuscitation has been completed and the extent of extracranial injuries determined. The patient who is still in coma at that stage, or who has focal signs, or is confused and has a skull fracture, requires to be in a neurosurgical unit, if his head injury is to be managed optimally. If transfer is delayed until deterioration begins it may be too late to get the patient to the neurosurgical unit; in any event, emergency transfer of the deteriorating patient increases the risk of untoward incidents en route, partly because there may not appear to be time to make proper arrangements for the patient's care in the ambulance. In a series of 150 patients transferred in coma after head injury to the neurosurgical unit in Glasgow from other hospitals, only 28% had an ET tube whilst 28% had not even a mechanical airway[29]. Although most were accompanied by a doctor or nurse, half were supine; only a quarter had had a nasogastric tube to empty the stomach.

Sometimes major extracranial injuries are overlooked or managed (e.g. pneumothorax, fractured femur, ruptured spleen).

It is known that a number of these patients were being transferred because they had already deteriorated, and it must be assumed that the rush to get them to the neurosurgical unit led to an inappropriate ordering of priorities.

There is need for each hospital to have staff on call 24 hours a day whose responsibility it is to supervise the arrangements for seriously ill patients being transferred to other hospitals. This would include not only those in coma, but victims of shock and burns, and those with other conditions requiring special care (e.g. major chest injuries, acute renal failure requiring dialysis). Such staff might be anaesthetists or intensive care nurses (or both). They would assess the need for airway care, nasogastric intubation, position of the patient, need for oxygen administration, and would instruct whoever was to escort the patient in exactly what to do in various eventualities.

Another matter of concern is the time taken for a patient to be moved to the neurosurgical unit – a matter of concern if the patient is already deteriorating with cerebral compression. This will obviously depend on the local geography, the distribution of hospitals, site of the regional neurosurgical unit and the nature of the road network. In Glasgow, although some cases come from 200 miles distant, and some are from islands where weather may hinder sea and air evacuation, 90% of all admitted head injuries go into primary hospitals that are within one hour of road time from the neurosurgical unit (two thirds within half an hour). However, it may take time to summon an ambulance, especially as inter-hospital transfers are not treated as a priority, unless an understanding is reached with the local service. Making arrangements for safe transportation could contribute further delay, e.g. finding an anaesthetist to pass an ET tube, or a nurse to act as escort. It is for this reason that it is suggested that each hospital should have a standardized means worked out for dealing with these transfers; but no set rules can be written down – there must be a person responsible for balancing the risks, in the individual case.

References

1. Jennett, B. and Carlin, J. (1978). Preventable mortality and morbidity after head injury. *Injury*, **10**, 31
2. Adams, J. H., Graham, D., Scott, G., Parker, L. and Doyle, D. (1980). Brain damage in fatal non-missile head injuries. *J. Clin. Pathol.*, **33**, 1132
3. Graham, D. I. and Adams, J. H. (1971). Ischaemic brain damage in fatal head injuries. *Lancet*, **1**, 265
4. Reilly, P. L., Graham, D. I., Adams, H. J. and Jennett, B. (1975). Patients

with head injury who talk and die. *Lancet*, **2**, 375

5. Jennett, B. and Teasdale, G. (1980). *Management of Head Injuries*. (Philadelphia: F. A. Davies)

6. Jennett, B. (1979). Defining brain damage after head injury. *J. R. Coll. Physicians*, **13**, 197

7. Miller, J. D., Sweet, R. C., Narayan, R. and Becker, D. P. (1978). Early insults to the injured brain. *J. Am. Med. Assoc.*, **240**, 439

8. Galbraith S. and Teasdale, G. (1981). Predicting the need for operation in the patient with an occult traumatic intracranial haematoma. *J. Neurosurg.*, **55**, 75

9. North, J. B. and Jennett, S. (1974). Abnormal breathing patterns associated with acute brain damage. *Arch. Neurol.*, **31**, 338

10. Jennett, S. (1980). Monographs in anaesthesiology – head injuries. In Fitch, W. and Barker, J. (eds.). *Pulmonary Function in the Head-injured Patient*. (Amsterdam: Elsevier-North Holland)

11. Jennett, B. (1980). Skull X-rays after recent head injury. *Clin. Radiol.*, **31**, 463

12. Healy, T. E. J., Pathakju, G. S. and Weston, P. A. M. (1980). Intracranial pressure measurements in patients suffering head injury, managed in a non-neurosurgical unit. *Injury*, **12**, 96

13. Miller, J. D. (1978). Intracranial pressure monitoring. *Br. J. Hosp. Med.*, May, 497

14. Jennett, B. (1980). Annotation to 'Intracranial pressure measurements in patients suffering head injury, managed in a non-neurosurgical unit. *Injury*, **12**, 99

15. Cooper, P. R., Moody, S., Clark, W. K., Kirkpatrick, J., Maravilla, K., Gould, A. L. and Drane, W. (1979). Dexamethasone and severe head injury. A prospective double-blind study. *J. Neurosurg.*, **51**, 307

16. Gudeman, S. K., Miller, J. D. and Becker, D. P. (1979). Failure of high-dose steroid therapy to influence intracranial pressure in patients with severe head injury. *J. Neurosurg.*, **51**, 301

17. Miller, J. D. (1979). Barbiturates and raised intracranial pressure. *Ann. Neurol.*, **6**, 189

18. Jennett, B., Teasdale, G., Fry, J., Braakman, R., Minderhoud, J., Heiden, J. and Kurze, T. (1980). Treatment for severe head injury. *J. Neurol. Neurosurg., Psychiat.*, **43**, 289

19. Jennett, B., Teasdale, G., Braakman, R., Minderhoud, J., Heiden, J. and Kurze, T. (1979). Prognosis of patients with severe head injury. *Neurosurgery*, **4**, 283

20. Bates, D., Caronna, J. J., Cartlidge, N. E. F., Knill-Jones, R. P., Levy, D. E., Shaw, D. A. and Plum, F. (1977). A prospective study of non-traumatic coma: Methods and results in 310 patients. *Ann. Neurol.*, **2**, 211

21. Jennett, B., Snoek, J., Bond, M. R. and Brooks, N. (1981). Disability after severe head injury. Observations on the use of the Glasgow Outcome Scale. *J. Neurol. Neurosurg., Psychiat.*, **44**, 285

22. Jennett, B., Teasdale, G., Braakman, R., Minderhoud, J. and Knill-Jones, R. P. (1976). Predicting outcome in individual patients after severe head injury. *Lancet*, **1**, 1031

23. Teasdale, G., Skene, A., Parker, L. and Jennett, B. (1979). Age and outcome

of severe head injury. *Acta Neurochirurg.*, **28,** 140

24. Teasdale, G., Parker, L., Murray, G. and Jennett, B. (1979). On comparing series of head injured patients. *Acta Neurochirurg.*, **28,** 205

25. Becker, D. P., Miller, J. D., Ward, J. D., Greenberg, R. P., Young, H. F. and Sakalas, R. (1977). The outcome from severe head injury with early diagnosis and intensive management. *J. Neurosurg.*, **47,** 491

26. Bruce, D. A., Schut, L. Bruno, L. A., Wood, J. H. and Sutton, L. N. (1978). Outcome following severe head injuries in children. *J. Neurosurg.*, **48,** 679

27. Marshall, L. F., Smith, R. W. and Shapiro, H. M. (1979). The outcome with aggressive treatment in severe head injuries. Parts I and II. *J. Neurosurg.*, **50,** 20

28. Jennett, B. and MacMillan, R. (1981). Epidemiology of head injury. *Br. Med. J.*, **282,** 101

29. Gentleman, G. and Jennett, B. (1981). Hazards of inter-hospital transfer of comatose head-injured patients. *Lancet,* **2,** 853

30. Bartlett, J. R. and Neil-Dwyer, G. (1979). The role of computerized tomography in the care of the injured. *Injury,* **11,** 144

10
The brain-dead kidney donor: from death to donation

ANDREW LUKSZA

(I) INTRODUCTION

Renal transplantation usually offers a better quality of life than maintenance dialysis to the patient with terminal renal failure. Early attempts at renal transplantation took place in the 1950s using both cadaveric and living donors. In a series of cadaveric kidney transplants, Hume demonstrated that the transplanted kidneys could function for short periods during which symptoms of uraemia resolved[1]. Long-term survival was rare due to insurmountable episodes of rejection. Attempts at immuno-suppression using total body irradiation produced disastrous results[2]. At around this time, long-term survival was reported following kidney transplantation between identical twins, since there was no antigenic difference between the donor and the recipient[3].

Problems of immunosuppression thwarted progress until 1960 when Schwartz and Damashek showed that the administration of 6-mercaptopurine in mammals resulted in prolongation of skin allografts[4]. From that time onwards, the combination of 6-mercaptopurine, or its analogue azathioprine, in combination with steroids has been used successfully for immunosuppression following transplantation. As a result, the number of cadaveric renal transplantations performed has risen to several thousand each year worldwide.

At first kidneys were removed only after the donor heart had stopped beating. Since cessation of heart beat follows an unpredictable period of hypotension, many of these kidneys were irreversibly damaged by prolonged warm ischaemia. The warm ischaemia time is defined as the period without a blood supply at normal temperature, and results in irreversible renal damage when it is longer than 1 hour.

In the 1970s educational, legal and administrative bodies in most parts of the world accepted that the diagnosis of brain death meant that the patient was dead whether or not other organs were maintained by artificial means[5,6]. This permitted the removal of kidneys from brain-dead, heart-beating donors. As a result, the quality of kidneys for transplantation improved. Despite these advances, there exists a serious shortage of donor kidneys. By the very nature of their diseases, potential kidney donors are frequently treated in an intensive care unit. It is the responsibility of clinicians working in such units to recognize brain death and to obtain kidneys from appropriate cases.

The purpose of this chapter is to describe which groups of patients constitute potential donors and to define the steps that need to be taken to realise this potential. The information comes from a general hospital working in collaboration with a transplant surgeon for 6 years and includes the results of a personal study into the care of the brain-dead kidney donor[7]. This work includes the application of flow diagrams to the problem of managing the brain-dead donor.

(II) THE SUPPLY OF DONOR KIDNEYS

Although renal transplantation has become a standardized surgical procedure, less than 700 kidneys are transplanted annually while an estimated 2000 are needed[8] in the United Kingdom alone. Some patients have to wait as long as 8 years for a transplant[9]. Moreover, 17% of transplanted kidneys never start to function and this figure is said to be rising[10]. An important factor in this high failure rate is a prolonged period of ischaemia, probably resulting from inappropriate donor care.

When one considers that each year in the United Kingdom an estimated 6000 people below the age of 65 years die from head injury or spontaneous subarachnoid haemorrhage[11], it is evident that the need could easily be fulfilled. Responsibility for the provision of suitable kidneys lies with the medical profession, and particularly with those clinicians working in intensive care and neurosurgical units. Despite favourable public attitudes towards transplantation[12], the supply of kidneys consistently fails to meet the need. Regrettably it is the medical profession which is at fault.

Such a widespread reluctance by doctors to contribute to the transplantation programme must be based on one of the following:

(1) There is a lack of knowledge and skills required for donor selection, diagnosis of brain death, maintenance of circulation and urine flow or administration. These aspects of care will be described later.

(2) Attitudes of hospital medical staff are inappropriate. These are less tangible but two views predominate. First, some doctors consider that their responsibility ends upon the death of a particular patient and, in their disappointment, are unable to conceive of possible benefit to others arising from their failure. Such an attitude can only be changed by the example of others. Secondly, some doctors consider that renal transplantation is inferior to maintenance dialysis in the treatment of chronic renal failure. How can such a view be justified?

(III) TRANSPLANTATION VERSUS DIALYSIS

When comparing treatments, one must evaluate efficacy, patient acceptance and cost. The results of various treatments[13] for chronic renal failure in terms of patient survival are listed in Table 10.1. The percentage patient survival for home dialysis and for living donor transplants is approximately 70% at 6 years, and the percentage patient survival for hospital dialysis and for cadaveric transplants is approximately 50% at 6 years. Unfortunately, only 10% of patients with end stage renal failure have a suitably matched relative who is willing to donate a kidney. So for the vast majority, treatment comprises maintenance dialysis or cadaveric renal transplantation. The superior results of home dialysis reflect selection of patients rather than

Table 10.1 Cumulative survival at 6 years following various treatments of chronic renal failure

Mode of treatment	Result
Home dialysis	70% patient survival
Hospital dialysis	50% patient survival
Transplantation (living donor)	70% patient survival 55% graft survival
Transplantation (cadaver)	50% patient survival 30% graft survival

a better treatment. Patients chosen for home dialysis tend to be medically less complicated, more intelligent and better motivated to comply with treatment. Direct comparison is therefore not justified.

Originally, the treatments were exclusive of one another, hence patients undergoing transplantation were frequently uraemic and inappropriately prepared for surgery. More recently, the treatments have become complementary. Dialysis is now used to prepare patients for operation, and an early return to dialysis is advocated for cases where graft rejection fails to respond promptly to immunosuppressive therapy. The gratifying difference between graft survival and patient survival reflects the success of this approach. In Australia, where this system was adopted much earlier, patient mortality following transplantation is less than 10% at 5 years in some centres[14].

In view of the serious shortage of donor kidneys, choice has been limited and some kidneys taken from inappropriately treated donors have been used for transplantation. This has undoubtedly contributed to the high primary failure rate and consequently to an increased mortality. If the supply of cadaveric kidneys and the care of potential donors improves, the high failure rate could be expected to fall.

Transplantation has two important advantages and one disadvantage when compared with maintenance haemodialysis. The individual with a successful transplant enjoys an improved quality of life, being freed from the constant burden of dialysis and its associated restrictive diet and fluid intake. The anaemia of chronic renal failure corrects itself. Neuropathy improves. Freedom to travel and employment prospects improve. The degree of rehabilitation, as gauged by ability to work, is as good as for home dialysis and much better than for hospital dialysis[15]. Social and psychological adjustment following transplantation is far superior to either form of haemodialysis[16]. These views are best exemplified in an account by Dr J.A. Henry, who himself underwent transplantation following many years of maintenance dialysis[17].

The second advantage is that a treatment programme based on transplantation will enable more uraemic subjects to be treated by existing resources. The costs of technological medicine are high and cannot be met in full by the State. The treatment of chronic renal failure already receives a disproportionately large share of National Health Service resources[18], and financial support is unlikely to increase in the present economic situation. This is an unfortunate but realistic view. In the United Kingdom, only 14.5 patients per million population commence maintenance dialysis each year[16], while approximately 40 patients per million population below the age of 60 years develop chronic renal failure which requires dialysis[19,20]. Put another way, more than half of the patients who develop chronic renal failure each year cannot be offered life-saving treatment.

There have been many studies into the cost of haemodialysis, the best researched was by Buxton and West[21]. On a 1975 costing they estimated that the cost of hospital dialysis is £6100 p.a. while home dialysis incurs a capital cost of £5900, which includes equipment, home adaptation and training and a maintenance cost of £4200 p.a. There are no published figures for the cost of transplantation in the United Kingdom, but judging from European and North American experience, it is almost certainly less expensive than the cost of hospital dialysis for one year[22]. This estimate includes failed transplants returning to dialysis.

The disadvantage of transplantation is the necessity for long-term immunosuppressive therapy with its risks of infection, malignancy and steroidal side effects. Thus infection accounts for one-third of deaths following transplantation. This compares unfavourably with haemodialysis, where only one-fifth of patients die as a result of infection[14]. Moreover, patients on chronic immunosuppression are at a greater risk of developing malignancy, particularly lymphomas and sarcomas. The advent[23] of cyclosporin A, an effective yet less toxic immunosuppressive agent, and the finding that it may not be necessary to give immunosuppressive therapy indefinitely[24] offer the hope that these risks may be reduced in the future.

It can be concluded that renal transplantation when successful offers an improved quality of life. It is less expensive than maintenance dialysis and enables more patients to be treated on the existing budget. Moreover, results for renal transplantation, both in terms of patient and graft survival can be expected to improve if patients are adequately prepared for surgery by a period of maintenance dialysis and if the supply of cadaveric kidneys improves in number and quality.

(III) SELECTION OF THE KIDNEY DONOR

(1) The human donor: living or dead?

There are two sources of kidneys for transplantation: the living or cadaveric donor. A kidney transplanted from a live related donor remains the best treatment for chronic renal failure with a graft survival of about 70% at 1 year[25]. This success is thought to reflect matching of non-HLA factors. In view of the risks of the operation and the chance that the remaining kidney might be damaged by disease or injury, live donation is restricted to parents or siblings whose compatibility loci closely match those of the recipient. These donors deserve careful explanation. They should be told that the operation carries a risk to life in the order of 1 in 1000, but that postoperatively they will have a normal life expectancy. They must be carefully screened for occult renal disease, vascular disease and extracerebral malignancy. Preoperatively, they require an intravenous urogram and renal arteriography. This may uncover anomalies which make the operation technically impractical. Unfortunately only 10–15% of uraemic patients have a suitably matched relative who is prepared to donate a kidney. Hence, the greatest potential source of kidneys remains the brain-dead donor. Every brain-dead patient with normal renal function should be regarded as a potential donor. Children below 1 year are unsuitable because the small size of their renal vessels makes operation technically impractical. Similarly, adults over 60 years are seldom suitable because of the likelihood of extensive atheroma.

(2) Causes of brain death

The causes of brain death are head injury, spontaneous subarachnoid haemorrhage, cerebral tumour, acute self-poisoning and cardiac arrest. Patients with self-poisoning can only be considered as donors when the offending drug has been eliminated and is no longer contributing to the clinical picture. In practice the majority of kidneys are obtained from patients with spontaneous subarachnoid haemorrhage or head injury and very few from the remaining categories. At Whiston, the policy of admitting all cases of subarachnoid haemorrhage with coma to the intensive care unit has resulted in a threefold increase in kidneys supplied for donation. Patients who are unsuitable as potential donors fall into four groups:

(1) Proven extracerebral malignancy.
(2) Systemic infections (e.g. bacteraemia); bacteriuria without systemic infection is usually acceptable.
(3) Primary renal disease (e.g. pyelonephritis, glomerulonephritis).
(4) Other diseases where renal involvement is likely (e.g. diabetes, hypertension, atheroma, autoimmune disease).

(3) Diagnosis of brain death

Brain death occurs when there is irreversible damage to the cortex and the brain stem. Spontaneous respirations will then cease and unless the lungs are ventilated artificially, hypoxic cardiac arrest will occur. While ventilation is maintained, the heart, kidneys and liver may continue to function for hours or days. It is now well established that once the diagnosis of brain death has been made the patient is dead whether or not the function of other organs is maintained by artificial means[6]. This knowledge has enabled organs to be removed from brain-dead, heart-beating donors, thus minimizing ischaemia. The diagnosis of brain death is made on ventilator-dependent subjects using a series of simple bedside tests. There are three clinical situations in which the tests for brain death may be falsely positive and which must always be excluded before the diagnosis is confirmed. These are severe hypothermia, drug poisoning, particularly with barbiturates and, lastly, severe metabolic disturbances, particularly hypoglycaemia. At the time of testing the core temperature must exceed 35 °C and there must be absolute certainty that the clinical state is not attributable to poisoning or hypoglycaemia. For cadaveric organ transplantation, the UK Conference has recommended that brain death should be diagnosed by two doctors independent of the transplant team, both of whom should have expertise in this field[25,26].

The tests which must be performed to confirm brain death are as follows:

(1)   There must be no response when the pupils are examined with a bright light in a darkened room. Pupil size is irrelevant although they will commonly be dilated.

(2)   There must be no response to corneal stimulation with cotton wool.

(3)   There must be no response to the presence of the endotracheal tube nor any evidence of cough when suction is applied to the trachea.

(4)   There must be no eye movements when 20 ml of ice-cold water are injected into each ear, clear access to the drums having been established.

(5)   There must be no response to painful stimuli applied to the head and neck, for example, supraorbital pressure and firm pinching of the ear lobes.

(6)   Spontaneous breathing must be absent during hypercapnia; this may be tested in either of two ways:
      (a) the ventilator is disconnected and a 2 litre reservoir bag filled with oxygen is substituted. Oxygen is stopped and the pressure valve closed. The bag is then squeezed four times a minute for 3 minutes. Assisted ventilation is stopped and the bag is observed for respiratory movements, which must be absent for 5 minutes. Cardiac contractions cause movement of the bag synchronous with the heart beat and should not be confused with respiratory movements.
      (b) Arterial carbon dioxide pressure ($PaCO_2$) is measured. If this is below 4.8 kPa (36 mmHg) alveolar ventilation is reduced to attain normocapnia, while oxygen concentration is increased to prevent hypoxaemia. Table 10.2 gives the predicted ventilator settings required to achieve normocapnia. After 15 minutes the $PaCO_2$ is measured again to confirm normocapnia. The patient

221

Table 10.2 Ventilator settings predicted to attain normocapnia at 12 respirations/ min (values were obtained from nomogram constructed by Radford and assume normal basal metabolic rate and fixed dead space)

Body weight (kg)	Tidal volume (ml)	Minute volume (l)	Oxygen to be added to inspiratory circuit (l/min)
20	200	2.4	1.5
40	350	4.2	2.0
60	450	5.4	2.5
70	500	6.0	3.0
80	575	6.9	3.5
100	700	8.4	4.0

is then disconnected from the ventilator and oxygen delivered at 2 l/min through a fine cannula introduced into the trachea. The patient's chest is observed for 5 minutes during which there must be no spontaneous respiratory movements.

If all the criteria are satisfied, brain death is confirmed and there is no need to repeat the tests. If any test gives an equivocal result, then patient treatment must be continued and the tests repeated at 4 hourly intervals. It will be noted that electroencephalography is not required to confirm the diagnosis and may be misleading[27]. Purely spinal reflexes may persist and do not preclude the diagnosis. Both doctors confirming brain death are required to record their observations in the patient's case notes, which may be subsequently scrutinized by a coroner.

(4) Transplantation and the law

The United Kingdom has no precise legal framework for organ donation. Provision for the transplantation of organs[28] is made in the Human Tissues Act (1961). This provides that the person lawfully in possession of the body may authorize the removal of organs for transplantation under the following circumstances: (1) where the deceased person has made a declaration in writing (or orally in the presence of two witnesses) expressing a wish that his organs be used for this purpose; (2) after making such reasonable enquiry as may be practicable, the doctor has no reason to believe that the deceased has objected to the use of his body and that the surviving spouse or any surviving relative does not object. Difficulties have arisen in the legal interpretation of two points: (a) who is the person 'lawfully in possession of the body?' (b) what constitutes making 'such reasonable enquiry as may be practicable?' When death occurs in hospital, the appropriate National Health Service Authority is lawfully in possession of the body until it is claimed by relatives or executors. If the deceased is carrying an appropriately worded and signed donor card, the hospital administrator may therefore give consent for organ removal without approval of the relatives. In all other instances, the permission of a close relative should be obtained and enquiry made into the possible disapproval of other members of the family. In view of the continued need for public support, most doctors would agree that the kidneys should not be removed in cases of doubt.

Proposals have been made to alter the law, particularly to a 'contracting out' system, which is widely accepted on the Continent. Such a system puts the onus on each person to make his intentions clear during life if he does not wish his organs to be used for transplantation. In the absence of such a request, doctors may remove organs after death without the need for further enquiries. Since it is the medical profession and not the public which is largely responsible for the shortage of cadaveric kidneys, it is widely felt that such a change in the law is probably unnecessary.

(IV) PROGRAMME OF PATIENT CARE

The single most reliable index of good renal function is the urinary output. Ideally, this should be in excess of 90 ml/hour. To achieve this figure one must ensure that the kidney remains well perfused with oxygenated blood. The two most important aspects of donor care are therefore (i) maintenance of pulmonary gas exchange and (ii) maintenance of the circulation[29]. The bladder is catheterized and a urinometer used to measure output.

(1) Pulmonary gas exchange

When brain death is diagnosed, patients are already ventilator-dependent. Intermittent positive pressure ventilation (IPPV) must continue up to the time of donor nephrectomy and may be given by any type or make of ventilator. Following the diagnosis of brain death, the machine must be adjusted to avoid extreme hypocapnia and a high airway pressure, which may reduce cardiac output. Extreme hypocapnia causes vasoconstriction with resulting oliguria. The machine must therefore be set at a low tidal volume and airway pressure. Table 10.2 illustrates a series of typical values for tidal volume and minute volume against body weight designed to achieve normocapnia and a low airway pressure[30]. Oxygen must be added to the inspiratory circuit to avoid hypoxaemia. The final column of Table 10.2

shows the amounts of oxygen which should be added to achieve an inspired oxygen concentration of about 60%. Complete saturation of arterial blood can be expected with this figure. If IPPV causes hypotension, a subatmospheric (negative) phase may be introduced into the respiratory cycle. This has the effect of increasing venous return to the heart with consequent rise in cardiac output and blood pressure.

(2) Maintaining the circulation

Treatment is aimed at maintaining the blood pressure and urine output. At Whiston this aspect of donor care is facilitated by the use of a flow chart

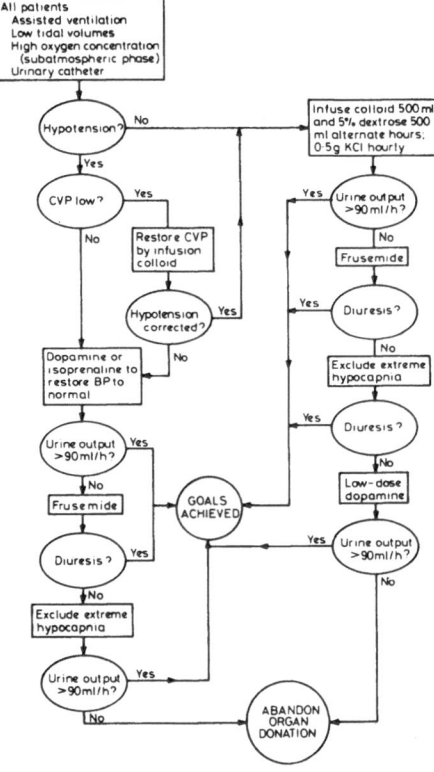

Figure 10.1 Flow diagram showing methods to maintain circulation and urine flow. Reproduced from *British Medical Journal*, **1**, 1316–19 (1979), by kind permission of the Editor.

(Figure 10.1). Thus, when the subject is normotensive, a peripheral vein is cannulated and 500 ml of colloid (Haemaccel or Gelofusine) and 500 ml of 5% dextrose, each with 0.5 g of added potassium chloride, are infused hourly. Frequently, this is all that is required to achieve a good urinary output.

Oliguria

Exceptionally, a normotensive subject will remain oliguric. In this case the right hand branch of Figure 10.1 describes three manoeuvres which should be tried in sequence. Firstly a powerful loop diuretic such as frusemide (furosemide USP) 80 mg may be given. If this fails to achieve a diuretic within 20 minutes, hypocapnia should be excluded by measuring $PaCO_2$. Hypocapnia is corrected by introducing an additional dead space into the ventilator circuit between the endotracheal tube and the ventilator hoses. Finally, a continuous infusion of dopamine in low doses can be given to stimulate urine formation. Dopamine is a direct-acting sympathomimetic agent with effects on both α- and β-adrenergic receptors. A dose of 2–5 μg kg^{-1}min^{-1}, increases renal and mesenteric blood flow, resulting in increased urine production. At doses above 5 μg kg^{-1}min^{-1}, it acts directly on the heart increasing cardiac output without altering myocardial oxygen consumption or heart rate. When the dose exceeds 10 μg/kg^{-1}min^{-1}, peripheral vasoconstriction occurs. This may lead to a paradoxical decrease in urine formation. Consequently at high doses, dopamine must be combined with a vasodilator such as nitroprusside. Dopamine may be administered through an infusion pump or by using a paediatric burette.

Hypotension

Hypotension is a common problem following brain death and its management is dealt with in the left hand branch of the flow diagram. The causes of hypotension in this situation are: hypovolaemia secondary to neurogenic peripheral vasodilation; 'pump' failure due to myocardial necrosis associated with spontaneous subarachnoid haemorrhage[31]; direct myocardial damage from trauma. Distinguishing the cause of hypotension is important and the distinction is made by measuring the central venous pressure (CVP). Normal values for CVP are shown in Table 10.2. A low CVP means hypovolaemia and is an indication for the rapid infusion of colloid. Restoring the CVP to normal may be all that is required to correct the blood pressure and urine formation. Persistent hypotension with a normal or high CVP indicates 'pump' failure which should be treated by continuous infusion of an inotropic agent. The use of dopamine in high dosage is one possibility which has already been discussed. An alternative drug is isoprenaline (isoprotenerol USP) which is a sympathomimetic agent acting exclusively on β-adrenergic receptors[32]. It acts directly on the heart increasing cardiac output and heart rate. Unlike dopamine it causes peripheral vasodilation in high doses and can therefore be used alone. One disadvantage of isoprenaline is its tendency to produce ventricular dysrhythmias and the e.c.g. needs to be monitored continuously. If ventricular tachycardia occurs, the drug must be stopped immediately but can be restarted at a lower dose 5 minutes later. Infusion is commenced at a dose of 2 μg/min and increased slowly until the desired effect is achieved. When the blood pressure has been restored by the use of an inotropic agent, urine production may restart. If oliguria persists, a diuretic should be given and arterial blood gases measured to exclude hypocapnia. Very rarely, urinary output remains poor despite all the above measures. In these cases organ donation must be abandoned.

(3) Preparing for donation

The protocol for kidney donation requires the co-ordination of several steps taken in chronological order. This aspect of management is facilitated by a flow diagram (Figure 10.2), which prevents errors and helps to simplify the procedure. The flow diagram is largely self-explanatory but further comment is required on the following points.

(a) Investigations

Once brain death has been confirmed in a potential kidney donor, blood samples are taken for estimation of blood urea, blood group and hepatitis B antigen (HbsAg). HbsAg positive donors are unacceptable. A further 10 ml of heparinized blood and 10 ml of clotted blood are set aside for later tissue-typing. If the request for donation is granted then these samples are dispatched by taxi to the regional tissue-typing centre and the appropriate technician is informed by telephone. A catheter specimen of urine should be taken at the same time to screen for infection. Positive results may influence later management of the recipient and should be forwarded to the transplant unit.

(b) Consent

The interview with the relatives is conducted by the clinician in charge of the unit, by his deputy if qualified for more than 5 years, or by the transplant surgeon. Verbal consent is legally satisfactory so long as a witness, usually a registered nurse, is present at the interview. A record of the interview must be entered into the donor's case notes and signed by both the clinician and the witness.

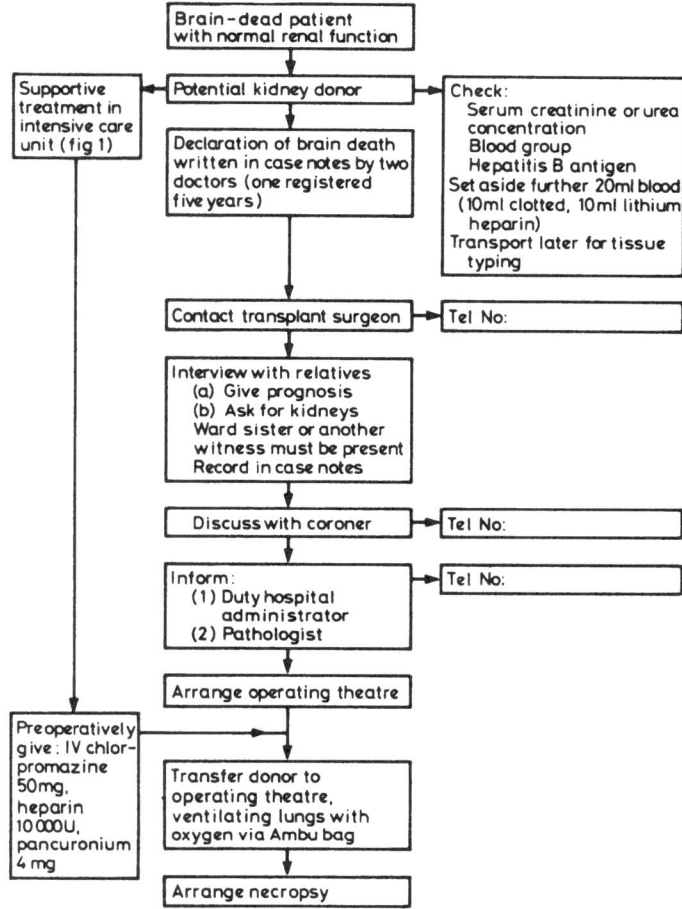

Figure 10.2 Flow diagram giving protocol for kidney donation. Reproduced from *British Medical Journal,* **1**, 1316–19 (1979), by kind permission of the Editor

(c) Coroner or procurator fiscal

Two rules apply. Firstly, in cases where death is likely to be the subject of criminal proceedings, donation must not be considered. Secondly, in cases where death has been unnatural and may be the subject of an inquest, permission for donation must be obtained from the coroner's officer. In all other instances procedure varies between different localities. Our policy is to contact the coroner's officer in all cases, irrespective of circumstances, in order to maintain good working relationships.

(d) Drugs

Donor pretreatment with a wide variety of drugs has been advocated for two reasons. Firstly, to improve the tolerance of the kidney to ischaemia. Secondly, to alter the immune response of the recipient to the donor graft. The more commonly used drugs are listed in Table 10.3. Although heparin is widely used prior to donor nephrectomy to prevent intrarenal coagulation, its role is unproven. Phenoxybenzamine and chlorpromazine are both powerful α-adrenergic blocking agents which are given to prevent renal vasoconstriction from acidosis and operative handling[33]. Chlorpromazine is thought to have an additional role in stabilizing cell membranes and therefore inhibiting the release of toxic lysozomal enzymes[34]. The second group of drugs comprises steroids and cytotoxic agents. There is some evidence to suggest that high doses of methyl prednisolone and cyclophosphamide given 5 hours prior to nephrectomy reduce the immunogenicity of the donor by eliminating 'passenger' leukocytes[35]. This leads to fewer episodes of early rejection. Our practice is to give chlorpromazine 50 mg and heparin 10 000 units intravenously 30 minutes before the expected time of nephrectomy and to give phenoxybenzamine 100 mg and pancuronium 4 mg intravenously immediately before surgery. Phenoxybenzamine is now available under special licence and is supplied by the transplant surgeon. Pancuronium is given to prevent muscular contractions at laparotomy which can distress the nursing staff.

Table 10.3 Drugs commonly used in donor pretreatment

Name of drug	Action
Heparin	prevents intrarenal coagulation
Phenoxybenzamine	α-blockade prevents renal vasoconstriction
Chlorpromazine	α-blockade, cell membrane stabilizer
Cyclophosphamide	immunosuppression
Methyl prednisolone	immunosuppression, cell membrane stabilizer

(VI) RESULTS

The results of transplantation from centres throughout the world are uniform and they are shown in Table 10.1. Whiston Hospital supplied 34 kidneys for transplantation in the 5 years up to February 1979. Six of these were not used by reason of anatomical abnormality or unsuspected renal pathology. Among the 28 transplanted kidneys, there was only one case of primary failure (3%) and 80% of grafts were functioning after 2 years. There were no deaths attributable to transplantation. These figures are considerably better than other published series which claim a primary failure rate of 17% and a graft survival figure of approximately 50% at 1 year[36]. Primary failure means that the kidneys fail to function from the time of transplantation. Its cause is controversial. Two major arguments exist, one claiming that the kidneys are irreversibly damaged by ischaemia prior to transplantation[37] and the other claiming that failure to function represents an acute rejection episode[38]. Our results support the view that failure is physiological rather than immunological. With correct management of the brain-dead kidney donor, the incidence of primary failure could be markedly reduced.

Conclusion

Cadaveric renal transplantation has become a successful and well established treatment for patients with chronic renal failure. It can match maintenance dialysis in terms of cost and patient survival. Moreover, the quality of life is vastly improved following a successful transplant. Despite these benefits and the potential availability of donors, supply constantly fails to meet the need. It is the attitude of the medical profession and not of the public that is responsible for the shortfall, an illogical attitude elegantly summarized by Sir George Young, MP: 'Doctors seem very willing to act when their patient is a potential recipient of a kidney, because it is their patient who is ill. They seem far less willing to act when their patient is a potential donor, because he has died. This is an illogical position for the medical profession to be in because there is a recipient only when there is a donor and equal initiative is required in both cases'.[39]

ACKNOWLEDGEMENTS

Figures 10.1 and 10.2 and Table 10.2 are reproduced by permission of the editor of the *British Medical Journal*.

References

1. Hume, D. M., Merril, J. P., Miller, B. F. and Thorn, G. W. (1955). Experiences with renal homotransplantation in the human: report of nine cases. *J. Clin. Invest.*, **34**, 327

2. Murray, J. E., Merril, J. P., Dammin, G. J., Dealy, J. B., Walter, C. W., Brooke, M. S. and Wilson, R. E. (1960). Study on transplantation immunity after total body irradiation: clinical and experimental investigation. *Surgery*, **48**, 272

3. Merril, J. P., Murray, J. E., Harrison, J. H. and Guild, W. R. (1956). Successful homotransplantation of human kidney between identical twins. *J. Am. Med. Assoc.*, **160**, 277

4. Schwartz, R. S. and Damashek, W. (1960). The effects of 6-mercaptopurine on homograft reactions. *J. Clin. Invest.*, **39**, 952

5. Diagnosis of death. (1979). *Br. Med. J.*, **1**, 332; *Lancet*, **1**, 261

6. Diagnosis of brain death. A paper endorsed by the Conference of Royal Colleges and Faculties of the United Kingdom. (1976). *Lancet*, **2**, 1069; *Br. Med. J.*, **2**, 1187

7. Luksza, A. R. (1979). Brain-dead kidney donor: selection, care and administration. *Br. Med. J.*, **1**, 1316

8. British Transplantation Society Report (1975). *Br. Med. J.*, **1**, 251

9. Slapak, M. (1979). Is my patient a potential donor for kidney transplantation? *Br. J. Hosp. Med.*, **21**, 627

10. Nelson, S. D. and Tovey, G. M. (1974). National Organ and distribution Service. *Br. Med. J.*, **1**, 622

11. Office of Population Censuses and Surveys, Series DH4 (1976). *Mortality Statistics, 1974.* (London: HMSO)

12. Moores, B., Clarke, G., Lewis, B. R. and Mallick, N. P. (1976). Public attitudes towards kidney transplantation. *Br. Med. J.*, **1**, 629

13. Gurland, H. J., Brunner, F. P., Dehn, V. H., Harlen, H., Parsons, F. M. and Scharer, K. (1973). Combined report on regular dialysis and transplantation in Europe, III, 1972. Dialysis, Transplantation and Nephrology. *Proc. Eur. Dial. Transplant Assoc.*, **10**, 17

14. Mathew, T. H., Vikraman, P., Johnson, W., Morris, P. J., Marshall, V. C., Hill, A. V. L., McOmish, D. and Kincaid-Smith, P. (1975). Integrated programme of dialysis and renal transplantation. *Lancet*, **2**, 137

15. Gurland, J. H., Brunner, F. P., Chantler, C., Jacobs, C., Scharer, K., Selwood, N. H., Spies, G. and Wing, A. J. (1976). Combined report on regular dialysis and transplantation in Europe, vi, 1975. *Transpl. Assoc.*, **13**, 3

16. Simmons, R. G. (1978). Social and psychological adjustment of adult post-transplant patients. In Friedman, E. A. (ed.). *Strategy in Renal Failure*, pp. 463–482. (New York: Wiley Medical)

17. Henry, J. A. (1978). Haemodialysis and transplantation – a personal experience. In Anderton, J. L., Parsons, F. M., and Jones D. E. (eds.). *Living with Renal Failure.* pp. 215–221. (Lancaster: MTP Press)

18. Leading article (1977). Kidneys from cadavers. *Br. Med. J.*, **1**, 188

19. Pendreigh, D. M., Heasman, M. A., Howitt, L. F., Kennedy, A. C., MacDougall, A. I., Macleod, M., Robson, J. S. and Stewart, W. K. (1972). Survey of chronic renal failure in Scotland. *Lancet*, **1**, 304

20. Branch, R. A., Clark, G. W., Cochrane, A. L., Henry-Jones, J. and Scarborough, H. (1971). Incidence of uraemia and requirements for maintenance haemodialysis. *Br. Med. J.*, **1**, 249

21. Buxton, M. J. and West, R. R. (1975). Cost benefit analysis of long-term

haemodialysis for chronic renal failure. *Br. Med. J.*, **2**, 376
22. Park, D. M. (1978). The economics of treating chronic renal failure. In Anderson, J. L., Parsons, F. M. and Jones, D. E. (eds.). *Living with Renal Failure*, pp. 51–65. (Lancaster: MTP Press)
23. Leading article (1979). Cyclosporin A. *Lancet*, **2**, 779
24. Padova, F. D., Merandi, E., Mazzei, D., Quarto di Palo, F., Baldini, L., Briandi, G. and Polli, E. E. (1979). Is long-term immunosuppressive treatment necessary to maintain good kidney graft function? *Br. Med. J.*, **2**, 421
25. Parsons, F. M., Brunner, F. P., Burk, H. C., Grazer, W., Gurland, H. J., Harlen H., Scharer, K. and Spies, G. W. (1975). Statistical report. *Proc. Eur. Dial. Transplant Assoc.*, **2**, 3
26. Department of Health and Social Security (1969). *Advice from Advisory Group on Transplantation Problems on the question of amending the Human Tissues Act 1961. Cmnd 4106*. (MacLennan Report) (London: HMSO)
27. Mohandas, A. and Chou, S. N. (1971). Brain death: a clinical and pathological study. *J. Neurosurg.*, **35**, 211
28. Human Tissues Act 1961. (London: HMSO)
29. Jones, E. S. and Wright, D. M. (1978). Cardiac arrest and shock. In *Essential Intensive Care*, pp. 163–196. (Lancaster: MTP Press)
30. Radford, E. P. (1955). Ventilation standards for use in artificial respiration. *J. Appl. Physiol.*, **7**, 451
31. Conor, R. C. R. (1969). Myocardial damage secondary to brain lesions. *Am. Ht. J.*, **78**, 145
32. Martindale, W. (1977). *The Extra Pharmacopoeia*, 27th Ed. (London: Pharmaceutical Press)
33. Bell, P. R. F., Quinn, R. O. and Calman, K. C. (1974). Donor pretreatment and organ preservation. *Transplant. Proc.*, **6**, 245
34. Turner, M. D., Hicks, F. R. and Hicks J. B. (1969). The use of metabolic inhibitors in hypothermic kidney storage. *J. Surg. Res.*, **9**, 665
35. Guttman, R. D., Beaudoin, J. G. and Moorhouse, D. D. (1973). Reduction of immunogenicity of human cadaver renal allografts by donor pretreatment. *Transplant. Proc.*, **5**, 663
36. 13th Report of Human Renal Transplant Registry (1977). *Transplant. Proc.*, **9**, 9
37. British Transplantation Society Report (1975). *Br. Med. J.*, **1**, 251
38. Hamilton, D. N. M. and Briggs, J. D. (1975). Kidneys for transplantation. *Lancet*, **2**, 461
39. Young, G. (1978). *Hansard 945*. 3rd March. Col. 888

11
Chest injuries

MALCOLM WRIGHT

Chest trauma frequently presents at a hospital without thoracic specialists and it thus becomes the responsibility of physicians and anaesthetists working in intensive care to manage the patient. Since in about 90% of cases, treatment is possible without resort to operation, it follows that a majority of patients will never need to be moved to a thoracic surgical centre. Thus the general intensive care unit in most hospitals has become the centre of expertise for the management of chest injuries. The pattern of chest injuries varies worldwide. In Europe and Australasia there is a substantial predominance of non-penetrating chest injury but in the United States there is a high incidence of penetrating chest injury due to the frequent resort to the knife and the gun as a means of settling disputes. This chapter is based on 8 years experience in both the United Kingdom and Australia.

(I) RESUSCITATION

(1) Airway

The importance of maintaining a satisfactory airway cannot be overemphasized; firstly, in order to ensure good oxygenation of vital tissues and, secondly, because a partially obstructed airway will result in violent respiratory excursions with worsening of chest wall instability, pain and shock. It is sometimes argued that early protection of the airway by endotracheal intubation commits the patient to management which may, with hindsight, be seen to have been overinterventive. This may be true, and it is also true that in very large centres with substantial nursing and medical resources it may be possible to manage 'conservatively' many patients who might otherwise be ventilated. But if it is decided to manage a patient without endotracheal intubation, it should be clearly understood by the whole team that IPPV is avoided or postponed because improvement is anticipated in a few hours. In all other respects, 'conservative' management is demanding in the extreme in terms of nursing and medical attention. In our large referral centre we see far more problems resulting from well meant attempts to avoid airway support than from unwarranted intubation. Although it is theoretically possible to manage a patient with an oral or nasal endotracheal tube without controlling ventilation, in practice the inevitable coughing, gagging and overall disturbance that this entails is unacceptable and once intubated it is usual to start IPPV, at least until assessment is complete. Certain injuries make airway support by intubation of the trachea mandatory and in these patients IPPV should be started without delay (Table 11.1). If a patient with marginal chest injury requires surgery and anaesthesia it is wise to continue IPPV at the end of the procedure especially if a laparotomy or thoracotomy has been carried out.

Table 11.1 Indications for tracheal intubation

Coma – all causes, including alcohol or drugs
Confusional state requiring sedation
Faciomaxillary, oral or pharyngeal trauma
Vomiting
Bleeding from within the airway
Absent or weak cough (including weak cough due to spinal injury)
Apparent or incipient respiratory failure
Cyanosis on oxygen
Massive associated injuries
Imminent general anaesthesia

---

(2) Oxygen therapy

Tissue hypoxia is invariably harmful and administration of oxygen throughout the period of resuscitation is of critical importance. Failure to correct cyanosis by oxygen delivered by mask is an indication for immediate endotracheal intubation and ventilation. Even if cyanosis can be corrected by oxygen there may still be significant venous admixture and it is therefore important to monitor progress by arterial blood gas measurements and calculation of the alveolar–arterial oxygen difference. Initially the risks of hypoxia greatly outweigh the risks of pulmonary oxygen toxicity, but as the situation stabilizes the oxygen therapy must be adjusted to maintain a normal arterial oxygen. Very high PaO_2 levels are not only unnecessary but may be a further insult to an already damaged lung.

(3) Intravenous infusions

If there is significant blood loss, measurement of the CVP is essential for monitoring resuscitation. It is easy to identify haemorrhage associated with intrathoracic injury but the blood loss into the injured chest wall occurs gradually and is deceptive so that the patient's blood volume may remain suboptimal for several hours. This is accompanied by oliguria and the temptation to administer diuretics rather than investigate the problem by CVP measurement should be resisted. Despite substantial research into intravenous infusions for resuscitation there is no consensus regarding the best material to use[1]. In the absence of unequivocal guidelines we have adopted the following 'rule of thumb' in the early fluid resuscitation of adult patients suffering concealed haemorrhage as a result of thoracic and other injuries: (i) immediate infusion of 1 litre of saline or other isotonic electrolyte solution, (ii) under CVP control, up to 1 litre of plasma protein solution is administered, (iii) when available, blood is given to maintain the CVP at an optimal level and good tissue perfusion as judged by the temperature and colour of the periphery and the spontaneous production of urine. Further transfusion policy is dependent upon the nature and severity of other injuries. An i.v. drip line cannot keep pace with massive bleeding from a large pulmonary or abdominal blood vessel. As soon as it is apparent that haemorrhage is continuing, operation should be undertaken as surgical arrest of bleeding is the only effective measure. Delay will only result in the patient's blood being progressively exchanged for banked blood with all the risks of massive transfusion (Chapter 6). Although unwise fluid therapy has been incriminated in the genesis of ARDS[2] and in the worsening of the effects of lung contusions[3], it is also true that persisting shock, hypoperfusion and acidosis are also involved in the genesis of both ARDS and acute renal failure. There is therefore no case for withholding fluid therapy justified by haemodynamic criteria. Haemodynamic data obtained by the use of a Swan–Ganz catheter can be of great value in optimizing fluid therapy (Chapter 6). This procedure can be time-consuming and must not be allowed to delay other phases of resuscitation.

(II) INTRATHORACIC

(1) Heart

Penetrating injuries of the heart, usually caused by stab or gunshot wounds, are not invariably fatal and recovery is possible in a majority following surgery. The heart wounds are often relatively minor and cardiac tamponade is the needless cause of death in some patients. Treatment consists of resuscitation, pericardiocentesis and immediate thoracotomy[8].

Blunt injury to the heart can cause three types of lesion: cardiac rupture, myocardial contusion, or tears of internal structures.

(a) Cardiac rupture

Following rupture of an atrium the patient may survive long enough for operative repair[10,11]. Late rupture of the heart may complicate myocardial contusion.

(b) Myocardial contusion

Myocardial contusion has been recognized for many years[12] and is reported as occurring in from 15 to 70% of accident cases. Contusion is recognized as one of the common complicating features of chest injury and also one of the most readily missed[4]. The signs and e.c.g. changes are like those of myocardial infarction, although coronary angiography has shown that ventricular dysfunction can occur without damage to major coronary arteries. Severe depression of myocardial function can occur, accompanied by elevated cardiac enzyme levels. There are no specific features to differentiate myocardial contusion from infarction. Management is along the same lines as for myocardial infarction. Thus rest, oxygen, diuretics, e.c.g. monitoring and anti-arrhythmic therapy may be required. Surgery and anaesthesia should be avoided.

(c) Intracardiac damage

A variety of intracardiac lesions have been described. Usually the victims die in hospital, but a bruit should alert one to the possibility of a valve lesion or rupture of the interventricular septum.

235

(2) The pericardium

The pericardium may be torn in association with rupture of the diaphragm. Pericardial wounds usually occur as a result of a penetrating injury but two major threats to life then occur. Firstly, the heart may herniate through the tear, causing severe embarrassment to cardiac function. Secondly, pericardial tamponade may occur from the accumulation of blood in the pericardium. In either of these situations there is no place for conservative management or prolonged observation. Pericardiocentesis should be regarded as a holding manoeuvre until operative exploration enables a full assessment to be made of cardiac and pericardial damage. Additional advantages of surgery are that clots may be removed from the pericardium and unsuspected wounds of the heart treated. During resuscitation there is evidence that plasma infusions combined with isoprenaline or dopamine may be valuable in preparing the patient for operation[14].

(3) Aorta

This results from a rapid deceleration injury but is not always immediately fatal. The early course can be benign because a haematoma around the vessel arrests initial bleeding[9]. Suspicion should be aroused by the circumstances of the injury and by the finding of a wide mediastinum on a chest

Table 11.2 Causes of a wide mediastinum on a chest X-ray

(1) *Technical*
Patient supine
Anteroposterior view
Rotation
Film taken in expiration

(2) *Pathological*
Aortic rupture
Vertebral injury with mediastinal haematoma
Mediastinal venous bleeding
Lymphatic extravasation
Anterior mediastinal haematoma
Collapse of right upper lobe
Rupture of oesophagus
Pericardial collection of fluid
Atrial rupture

(3) *Iatrogenic*
Misplaced central venous catheter causing loculated fluid in mediastinal
pleural space

radiograph. Unfortunately, this is only one cause of mediastinal widening which is itself a common and non-specific finding following chest trauma (Table 11.2). Diagnosis can only be established by angiography which should be carried out promptly in suspected cases. There is no safe conservative treatment for an aortic rupture even though the false aneurysm can remain intact for hours, days or weeks. The definitive treatment is surgical repair using cardiopulmonary bypass.

(4) Airways and lungs

Breaches of small airways and minor tears of lung tissue must be very common as judged by the frequent finding of significant air leaks. These persist for a day or two and then settle without further trouble. The end result of all leaks is the loss of air from the airways into either the thoracic cavity or the tissues as tissue emphysema.

(a) Tissue emphysema

The accumulation of air into the soft tissues may be rapid and alarming, but is an essentially benign although inconvenient condition. The chest radiograph will show air outlining the muscles of the shoulder girdle, in particular the pectoral muscles are usually conspicuous. There is no satisfactory treatment, but further accumulation may be reduced or prevented by avoiding a build-up of air under pressure. An endotracheal tube may prevent pressure build-up in the trachea during coughing and if the patient is on a ventilator, gagging and struggling should be prevented. Pneumothorax should be drained and it should be ensured that the side holes of the drainage catheter do not lie within the chest wall, as this provides a direct air conduit from the pleural cavity to the chest wall tissues. Mediastinal and pericardial air are frequently seen on the chest film and are attended by alarming noises on auscultation. Mediastinal emphysema may denote rupture of a major airway.

(b) Pneumothorax

Traumatic pneumothorax is a very frequent finding. Drainage is essential if it is under tension as cardiac filling is severely compromised. In minor injuries a small collection can be left alone, but when the patient is to be treated by IPPV, then all collections of air should be drained, as the risk of tension is high. If the lungs are stiff due to oedema and contusion, complete collapse will not occur and serious tension effects can develop in association

237

with a small pneumothorax. A portable chest film taken with the patient supine will show a partial pneumothorax as a round dark shadow overlying the lower lung and not as an apical collection. Before draining such a collection it is wise to make sure that it is not a dilated stomach herniating through a ruptured diaphragm.

(c) Trachea and bronchus

Complete rupture of the trachea with wide separation of the portions is incompatible with survival as death from asphyxia is inevitable; fortunately such an occurrence is rare. More commonly, the continuity of the airway is maintained, at least for a time. Severe mediastinal and neck emphysema is then seen. Early death from asphyxia will occur if the tear is not recognized and repaired promptly. Until surgery is imminent, IPPV should be withheld if possible, as it can worsen the mediastinal emphysema. Rupture of a main bronchus behaves in the same way and is treated along similar lines, including immediate thoracotomy. Peripheral bronchial ruptures are relatively common. Suspicion should be aroused by the finding of persistent air leak and collapse of related lobe. Diagnosis is by means of flexible bronchoscopy. Small leaks may heal spontaneously but if treated expectantly a follow-up is necessary to detect late stenosis with lung sepsis distal to it. For a persistent tear, thoracotomy with resection of a lobe may be required.

(d) Lung contusion

Lung contusion or bruising of the lung has been studied extensively for many decades. The spectrum of pathology ranges from diffuse injury to the lung seen in blast injury, to the more localized lesion which merges into the lung haematoma. The important features of lung contusion are firstly that it causes progressive and life-threatening respiratory failure and, secondly, considerable resolution can occur with time and therefore treatment is justified.

Blast injury has been recognized as a cause of respiratory failure since World War I. Zuckermann[16] established that the pressure wave from an explosion damages the lung by the impact on the chest wall. More localized contusions can be caused experimentally by non-penetrating explosions against the chest wall. It is probable that the rapid deceleration of the human thorax in motor vehicle collisions is responsible for the lung contusions seen in this situation. There is no reason why a seat belt should protect against such an injury since, no matter how firmly held the thoracic cavity, the intrathoracic contents are still free to impact against the chest wall.

238

Within a few hours of contusion there is haemorrhage into alveoli, although alveolar walls remain intact. Later, organization takes place and resolution usually follows within 10 days. In the accident victim, serial radiographs are the best method of assessing progress. The earliest sign is a hazy opacity which extends and opacifies over the next few hours. The effects of contusions should not be underestimated and the degree of damage to the chest wall does not correlate with the severity of the lung contusion. Indeed some of the most severe or fatal contusions are seen in patients whose bony chest wall has resisted the impact without fracture. In both experimental animals and in man, excessive i.v. infusions can worsen the contusion, the contused portion of the lung becoming selectively more oedematous. For this reason, infusions in patients with chest trauma should be monitored by the CVP or PAWP in order to minimize the risk of overload.

The management is inseparable from the management of chest wall injury with which it is intimately associated. The principles are relief of pain, drainage of intrapleural air and fluid and encouragement of inflation of collapsed or underventilated alveoli. Excessive fluid infusions should be avoided. Prophylactic antibiotics are unnecessary in the previously healthy individual. Methyl prednisolone in high dose has been reported to reduce the size of the contusion and the weight of a contused lobe in experimental animals[17].

(e) Lung haematoma

This lesion may be seen as a round or oval opacity within the lung substance. No specific treatment is required and resolution by resorption or rupture into a bronchus with haemoptysis is the usual course. Unless the haematoma is very large, or bleeding continues, no operative intervention is required.

(III) CHEST WALL

The dominant cause of morbidity in chest wall injury is pain. Pain control by one means or another remains the fulcrum upon which the overall management rests. Pain is the cause of inadequate respiratory excursions and poor coughing, which in turn leads to retention of secretions and collapse of lung tissues. Attempts to control pain beyond a certain point by powerful analgesics can reduce ventilation and further abolish coughing, as well as causing excessive somnolence and lack of co-operation by the patient. This was the treatment used for many years in the severe cases. In retrospect, the results were unsatisfactory until the application of ventilator treatment[18,19]. Reports from many centres have confirmed the value of IPPV which has now become the standard against which new or alternative measures are judged.

(1) Classification

It is important to assess the patient's injuries and use some sort of classification in order to inform clinicians and nurses of the likely course and prognosis and to assign appropriate treatment. Most injuries defy rigid categorization but a breakdown into three groups of mild, moderate and severe is widely used. This classification is based on the ventilatory capacity[20] and reduced to elegant simplicity by Moore[21].

Grade I   Mild $\begin{cases} \text{can ventilate} \\ \text{can cough} \end{cases}$

Grade II   Moderate $\begin{cases} \text{can ventilate} \\ \text{cannot cough} \end{cases}$

Grade III Severe $\begin{cases} \text{cannot ventilate} \\ \text{cannot cough} \end{cases}$

It is important to recognize that patients in the moderate grade are in an unstable ventilatory state.

Obviously the situation is not simple. Extrathoracic trauma may severely compromise a patient who, on ventilatory criteria alone, justifies classification as mild. Despite this disadvantage a profile does emerge with implications for management (Table 11.3).

(2) Grade I (Mild)

In this group, pain control is based on simple analgesics (aspirin and paracetamol) and regional analgesia. Narcotics are used sparingly in the daytime and liberally at night. Myocardial contusion is excluded, all unnecessary encumbrances such as drips and catheters are removed, and early mobilization is then undertaken. Where the resources permit, the patient is kept in the ICU during this time. A disadvantage of narcotic analgesics in this group is their tendency to cause somnolence and giddiness in the ambulant patient.

Table 11.3 Major clinical features and modes of management of the three classes of closed chest injury

Clinical features	Grade I	Grade II	Grade III
Chest wall injury	minor flail	obvious flail	severe flail
Lung injury	minimal	contused	contused
Other injury	moderate peripheral	extensive limb damage	laparotomy visceral injury
General condition	stable	unstable	unstable
Gastrointestinal function	mobile gut	ileus	ileus
Head injury	absent	minor	significant
Patient co-operation	good	poor or inhibited	absent
Spinal injury	absent	usually absent	often present
Pre-existing lung disease	absent	present	present
Mode of treatment			
Airway support	not required	may need tracheostomy	will need tracheostomy
Ventilator	not needed	not needed	always used
Mobility	ambulant if feasible	bedfast	bedfast
Physiotherapy	active	active	passive
Analgesia	simple oral IC blocks; narcotics at night	narcotic; IC blocks; thoracic extradural	narcotics; extradural

This is especially so in the early stages, which is when mobilization is particularly beneficial. For this reason we explain to the patient that he will be given oral analgesics and regional blocks and then attempt aggressive mobilization. The aim is to carry out vigorous exercise of those parts of the body which do not cause pain (e.g. walking, moving about the bed). The exercise increases ventilation and results in expansion of poorly ventilated lung. Simple analgesics should not be under-rated in alleviating the pain of rib injuries provided that they are given with sufficient frequency, for example, 2-hourly using aspirin and paracetamol alternatively. Physiotherapy is directed at mobilizing and expanding the underlying lung. In this context we have found the use of an incentive spirometer to be invaluable (Triflo II – Cheseborough Ponds Inc. No. 5 – 7173). By means of audible and visual indices of ventilatory achievement this simple device enables both therapist and patient to assess progress objectively. Premixed nitrous oxide and oxygen (Entonox) has a place as an adjunct to physiotherapy and in supplementing regional analgesia during painful procedures such as the insertion of chest drains. Three points need emphasis. Firstly, this is an active policy

241

and requires the same complement of staff as does IPPV except in the particular case that continuous observation for apnoea is not essential. Secondly, there must be thorough explanation to the patient if his full co-operation is to be maintained. Finally, adequate narcotic analgesia must be given to obtain a good night's sleep and prevent deterioration in morale which will inevitably accompany sleep deprivation.

(3) Grade II (Moderate)

Patients assigned to Grade II are in a grey zone. They should be regarded as unstable and are assigned to this class with the firm intention of continuous assessment. Failure to progress to Grade I automatically implies reclassification to Grade III and the use of IPPV or other intervention.

The natural history of chest injuries is for deterioration to occur during the first 24–48 hours as flail segments become more mobile, lung contusions consolidate and lung infection develops. Some patients in this grade can, surprisingly, be successfully managed by resuscitation, pain control, airway care and oxygen therapy without IPPV. Occasionally an early tracheostomy enables tracheal suction to be performed easily and, because of the ease of starting IPPV, it is possible to use narcotic analgesia more liberally. The use of IPPV in this grade should not be regarded as a failure of judgment.

Patients in this category are ideal for the use of continuous narcotic infusions which avoid the peaks of disabling pain and troughs of somnolence and nausea which characterize the use of intermittent injections. One regime consists of morphine in a suitable diluent given at a rate of 1–2 mg per hour and infused by pump. A loading dose of 2–3 mg of morphine may be given.

In some centres, notably Oxford[20] and Adelaide[22], large numbers of these patients have been managed using thoracic epidural analgesia as the major method of pain control. An impressive feature of this technique is that respiratory function can be adequate in the presence of a mobile flail segment once pain control has been achieved. In many cases the need for IPPV has been avoided but the controversial aspect lies in the inevitable development of a depressed chest wall segment, amounting in some cases to a 'traumatic thoracoplasty'. The long-term results of this are not known, but disability could result because of the known development of late respiratory failure associated with both therapeutic thoracoplasty[18] and severe scoliosis[34]. My view is that significant chest wall deformity should not be accepted lightly in the younger patient. We have therefore only used this technique on a few patients, when it provided excellent analgesia.

(4) Grade III (Severe)

Patients in this group can neither ventilate nor cough adequately. A tracheostomy may assist in removal of secretions but it will not improve ventilation. The combination of shallow breathing caused by pain, diminished lung compliance due to contusion, collapse and retention of secretions, and ventilatory failure due to an unstable chest wall create a lethal situation which can only be retrieved by using IPPV. For the maximum benefit to be obtained, the patient should not be permitted to 'earn' his ventilator therapy by sliding to the brink of cardio–respiratory collapse. By the time this stage is reached the systemic effects of hypoxia and shock will cause lowered resistance to infection, renal failure and mental confusion.

(a) Control of ventilation

Most patients requiring IPPV will have a powerful though inadequate respiratory drive, manifested by rapid, jerky and shallow breathing. For this reason abolition of respiratory drive is initially required and this is achieved by using large doses of muscle relaxants and narcotics. Later, the drugs can be altered when trial and error show that the patient can tolerate the ventilator and synchronize his respirations with it. Paradoxically, it is the patient whose lungs are improving who finds it easier to comply with the ventilator. Sudden deterioration in the control of IPPV frequently means that additional lung pathology has developed, e.g. infection or collapse. A common error is to interpret struggling as an indication for weaning from the machine. In fact, quite the reverse is true; the patient who is ready to be weaned from the ventilator is usually quiet and compliant. Once established on a ventilator the patient is never left unattended, electronic alarm notwithstanding. It is no security to reason that if relaxants are not used, then the patient will be safe. Effective doses of narcotics may easily lead to apnoea and will be just as lethal as relaxants should a ventilator disconnection occur. After 3 or 4 days relaxants can usually be discontinued and control maintained by narcotic analgesics alone. In this unit we use morphine, papaveretum or phenoperidine. Usually all three are prescribed, the nursing staff choosing a drug or combination of drugs which give the best results. Long-acting drugs like diazepam and some phenothiazines are also effective but lack analgesic activity and, because of their prolonged action, can make weaning difficult. An important benefit of this treatment is lost unless pain is fully controlled. In particular, narcotics are given prior to physiotherapy.

It is possible to achieve excellent results by the use of any ventilator capable of generating sufficient pressure to ventilate lungs which may be lacking in compliance as a result of contusion or aspiration. If a pressure cycled machine is used, then its major limitation must be taken into account: a reduced compliance will result in a fall in tidal volume at a preset pressure. In other words, those patients in whom inflation of damaged lung is most critical are those in whom inflation is most likely to be compromised. Provided that tidal volume is measured repeatedly and the pressure limit is frequently re-set, a pressure cycled machine can give good results. Despite the technical feasibility of satisfactory results by using pressure cycled machines, the tendency in large units has been to use a volume-pre-set time-cycled machine to guarantee constant lung inflation. The greater complexity and expense of these machines are justified by their reliability and ease of operation by the nurse, who is then freed to nurse the patient rather than the ventilator. Our own choice has been the Bennet MA 1, which is electronically controlled. This make has proved to be outstandingly reliable during a total of over 300 000 hours of operation.

(b) Monitoring

Regular recordings of pulse, blood pressure, urine output and peripheral perfusion are made. When indicated, CVP measurements are made. Once stable, a daily chest film and blood gas estimation should suffice, but while the patient is unstable, these tests need to be carried out more frequently. The development of a tension pneumothorax is an ever present threat, and junior medical staff must be made aware of the need for immediate drainage should this occur. Physical signs may be minimal or absent especially if the pneumothorax is bilateral. E.c.g. monitoring is usual, but may be suspended in the convalescent case.

(c) Nutrition

In a large number of cases, ventilator treatment of the crushed chest is prolonged. In the uncomplicated case, energy requirements are raised by about 25% and with complications such as abdominal trauma, this figure[23] can rise to 70%. The successful management of these patients requires a policy of adequate nutritional support capable of supplying 5000 kcal/day (20 000 kJ/day). Furthermore, not more than 48 hours should elapse before starting such a regime. During the first 24 hours the intravenous route is required for resuscitation or anaesthesia rather than nutrition, and during this period the gastrointestinal tract is rarely functioning to allow tube feeding. After this time either nasogastric or intravenous feeding should be started and the energy intake increased over a few days so that, by the fifth day, a full protein and calorie intake is achieved. Failure to attend to this aspect of treatment will lead to progressive loss of muscle with weakness of

244

respiratory, postural and locomotor muscles, defective repair of tissues and immuno-incompetence (Chapter 2). At best malnutrition will prolong re-habilitation, at worst the patient will die from infection. Ileus occurs frequently in the paralysed and ventilated patient but mainly resolves when the patient can tolerate IPPV without much sedation. Nutrition, which in-cludes the appropriate fluid therapy, is monitored clinically and by an external balance for water, sodium and potassium. When calculating the fluid balance, it is important to take account of the 'invisible intake' caused by accelerated catabolism. A positive balance could predispose to pul-monary oedema and infection. In this unit we routinely proceed to i.v. feeding at 48 hours rather than wait for ileus to resolve.

Many commercial tube feeds are available (e.g. Triosorbon (BDH), Isocal (Mead Johnson), Complan (Glaxo)) and the protein or energy con-tent of these may be adjusted to individual needs by the addition of a glucose polymer (Caloreen), soya protein or eggs. Some patients tolerate nasogastric feeding better when given a continuous slow drip via a fine bore nasogastric tube (Clinifeed) than as intermittent boluses. Occasionally, metoclopramide i.v. is necessary to promote gastric emptying.

(d) Infection control

Table 11.4 shows methods of controlling infection. The majority of patients undergoing IPPV for chest trauma will develop some degree of chest in-fection. As a general rule this infection will cause more severe effects when there is pre-existing lung disease, malnutrition or pulmonary oedema. The

Table 11.4 Infection control in chest injuries

Maximize patient resistance
  Early complete resuscitation
  Nutrition
  Avoid steroids
  Avoid saline excess

Control environmental factors
  Effective control policy
  Handwashing
  Ventilator cleansing
  Bed spacing
  Gloving for tracheal toilet

Antibiotic policy
  Early detection of infection
  Prompt appropriate antibiotic treatment

management must take account of these risk factors if antibiotic therapy is to be effective. In particular, daily chest radiographs and fluid balance charts must be carefully assessed. Cultures and microscopic examination of the tracheal aspirate should be made daily but antibiotics withheld until there is evidence of infection.

The latter is recognized by identifying pathogens in the aspirate together with radiographic evidence of consolidation or when two of the following changes occur: fever in excess of 38.5°C, glucose intolerance, a white cell count above 11×10^9/litre. If a laparotomy has taken place then antibiotics should be given[24]. Which antibiotics are used depends on the results of culture, but in many cases blind therapy must be initiated. It has been shown that cultures of gastric contents can provide a valuable early identification of the likely pathogen[25]. Ampicillin alone is virtually useless as a sole antimicrobial agent despite its efficacy against *Haemophilus* and *Escherichia spp*. Inevitably superinfection with *Klebsiella* will occur and for this reason the writer uses gentamicin and ampicillin. If *Pseudomonas* is found, then combined therapy with an aminoglycoside and ticarcillin is given. The high sodium load required by a full course of ticarcillin (or carbenicillin) must be taken into account in these patients in whom sodium retention is already a problem[26]. Those individuals with pre-existing chronic bronchitis should start on antibiotics at the time of admission.

(e) Early rehabilitation

Prolonged IPPV is mentally and physically debilitating to the patient and exhausting to his family. Once good control of ventilation has been gained then rehabilitation should start. Relaxants should be discontinued as soon as control can be achieved without them, in order to minimize muscle wasting from lack of tone and immobility. The patient's position is altered in stages, first to sitting and eventually to standing whilst still on IPPV. This programme permits a greater range of physical and mental activities as well as avoiding postural hypotension. If the arms are functional, the patient is encouraged to lift himself about the bed. Pencil and paper are essential to allow him to write messages whilst aphonic from the tracheostomy. Mental activity of all kinds should be encouraged. Many patients get used to a cuffed tracheostomy and can enjoy soft foods and favourite drinks by mouth. Family visiting is essential. Provided extrathoracic injuries allow, the aim of early rehabilitation is for the patient to be mobile and almost ready to leave hospital as soon as IPPV can be stopped.

(f) Weaning from IPPV

Minor chest wall injuries are stable enough and comfortable enough for IPPV to be discontinued after 5–7 days. Large painful and unstable injuries may require 3 or more weeks of IPPV, especially if they are complicated by pre-existing chronic lung disease. Weaning from the ventilator will only succeed when certain conditions are met. The chest wall must be stable and comfortable enough to permit effective coughing. Any chest infection must be under control. Blood gases on the ventilator must permit a safe margin of deterioration during the weaning process. Failure to observe these conditions will result in failed weaning and very likely a serious complication such as bacteraemia or hypoxic cardiac arrest. In this unit IMV is the preferred method of weaning (Chapter 7). The rate of the ventilator is gradually reduced over hours or days and the patient takes extra breaths from a reservoir in the ventilator circuit. The method is simple and causes minimal distress to the patient. New ventilators usually incorporate IMV facilities. Old machines can be adapted by the use of a disposable IMV attachment (Hudson IMV Manifold No. 1654). The other method of weaning is to 'train' the patient to breathe for progressively longer and longer periods without ventilatory support. Starting with 30 seconds every half hour, the intervals are extended until the patient is comfortable without ventilatory support for several hours at a time. Whichever technique is used, the golden rule is that the patient must never become exhausted during weaning. To permit this to happen is to run the real risk of syncope or cardiac arrest as well as the inevitable sacrifice of the patient's confidence. The myth of the patient who becomes emotionally dependent on a ventilator is exactly that – a myth. A small group of patients have extreme difficulty coming off ventilators due to severe lung disease, either pre-existing emphysema or ARDS. If a patient really has reached the end of his pulmonary reserve, then the situation is almost hopeless. For a few, perseverence and gradual weaning over many days may be rewarded by partial recovery of lung function over the next few weeks.

(g) Internal fixation of the chest wall

Operative treatment of chest wall instability is an attractive concept but one which has never gained widespread popularity. Excellent results reported by Moore[21] suggest that the technique of chest wall stabilization by wiring or intramedullary nailing has been unjustly neglected. IPPV is not invariably avoided, however. Sternal fractures can be very unstable and give rise to marked chest wall mobility, and internal fixation may be especially valuable for this injury.

(IV) EXTRATHORACIC INJURIES

Injuries of sufficient violence to cause significant thoracic injury frequently cause damage to other structures. Such damage may pass unnoticed during the ventilatory emergency and it is important to search actively for other injuries as soon as possible. Intra-abdominal injuries may be hard to detect in a patient when communication is impaired by intubation and IPPV. Despite this disadvantage of immediate IPPV, I believe that it should never be withheld for fear of masking physical signs. Accurate diagnostic methods do exist to detect injury without the patient's co-operation. Some patterns of injury occur sufficiently often to warrant individual attention.

(1) Diaphragm

Rupture of the diaphragm is frequently missed[4]. Suspicion is aroused by a history of trauma likely to cause such an injury and the diagnosis may be clarified by serial X-rays in the erect position, fluoroscopy and by contrast radiology. A large basal air collection on the left may represent a herniated stomach. The important points about this injury are that: (a) it occurs fairly frequently, (b) it is readily missed and becomes asymptomatic and, (c) it can become life-threatening at any time by reason of strangulation of abdominal viscera.

(2) Abdominal viscera

It would be a serious omission to describe the management of chest trauma without including the common abdominal injuries which occur regularly, as their management is critical to good results. The clinician treating closed chest injuries conservatively must be conversant with the diagnostic methods employed. Plain X-rays of the abdomen are examined for free gas before peritoneal lavage is used to detect intraperitoneal blood. Peritoneal lavage simply consists of introducing 500–1000 ml of saline or dialysis fluid into the abdomen via a fine cannula. The returning fluid is examined for blood. In the search for ruptured abdominal viscera these two manoeuvres should be carried out routinely unless the abdomen is absolutely above suspicion. If the results are not totally reassuring then early laparotomy should be performed to search for rupture of the spleen or liver, mesenteric trauma or bowel rupture. The consequences of such a laparotomy are small[5] but the consequences of a missed intra-abdominal injury can be lethal. Should the patient be maintained on a ventilator for several days by reason of the chest injury then an early but negative laparotomy can be very reassuring should ileus develop in the first few days. A confusing factor in the assessment of a patient with a chest injury is the occurrence of abdominal pain and guarding associated with fractures of the lower ribs and possibly due to referred pain. A kidney may be ruptured or avulsed without there being peritoneal bleeding. In the case of avulsion there need be no haematuria. The diagnosis of renal injury is by means of IVP, performed in the unit if necessary. Traumatic pancreatitis may be initially asymptomatic. Later, ileus, fever, leukocytosis and a raised serum amylase will suggest the diagnosis. It is often accompanied by a coagulopathy and gastric erosions.

Because many patients will need several days of IPPV, it is defensible to recommend an exploratory laparotomy when intra-abdominal damage is suspected but not confirmed. In our own series one third of patients came to laparotomy and a life-threatening intra-abdominal injury was found in 80%. This laparotomy can also provide an opportunity to search for rupture of the diaphragm. Following a laparotomy, the pain and spasm in the abdominal wall militate against effective spontaneous respiration and it is my policy to leave such patients intubated and ventilated postoperatively, at least until the discomfort of the abdominal incision has settled down.

(3) Spinal injury

Injuries of the upper ribs, especially when accompanied by fractures of the clavicle or scapula, should prompt a careful search for cervical spine injury, as the force causing these fractures may also break the neck (Chapter 12). Fractures of the middle ribs may divert attention from the very real possibility of a thoracic spine injury. It cannot be overstated how easy it is to overlook such an injury as bleeding into the mediastinum may obscure the bony injury. Occasionally a degree of chest wall paradox may be seen which cannot be wholly explained by the chest injury. The possibility of paralysis of part of the chest wall as a result of spinal injury should be borne in mind. In particular, the paradox is very striking when the paralysis is unilateral – the whole chest wall on that side appears flail.

(4) Larynx

If misdiagnosed or missed, minor laryngeal damage may lead to permanent laryngeal dysfunction with voice changes or obstruction. Studies at this hospital[6] suggest that laryngeal damage may be overlooked readily in those patients who are comatose on admission and also have a tracheostomy. Major laryngeal damage is a life-threatening emergency as complete airway obstruction may occur at any moment. Suspicion should be aroused by bruising about the neck, loss of normal laryngeal outline on palpation and extensive surgical emphysema[7]. Laryngeal damage warrants immediate assessment by direct laryngoscopy by an experienced surgeon. Examination using a Macintosh intubating laryngoscope is not satisfactory as it does not give an adequate view of laryngeal structures.

(V) RESULTS OF TREATMENT

The management of chest injuries remains a challenge to the intensive care team and an exercise in the deployment of the resources of nursing, physiotherapy, clinical microbiology and medical care. Our experience has confirmed the findings in other centres, namely that deaths are rarely due to the chest injury (Table 11.5). Of the patients who died in our unit, the largest group had head injuries and the next largest in number were old and had pre-existing chronic disease. The effects of abdominal trauma came next and, lastly, the deaths due to the chest injury. The mortality in the patients who underwent laparotomy was virtually the same as in those who did not require such treatment.

Table 11.5 Cause of death

Number of patients treated	155	
Cause of death		
Brain injury	7	
Pre-existing morbidity	9	
Abdominal injury	4	
Chest injury	2	
Total	22	(14.2%)

References

1. Shoemaker, W. C. and Hauser, C. J. (1979). Critique of crystalloid versus colloid therapy in shock and shock lung. *Crit. Care Med.*, **7**, 117
2. Wilson, R. F. and Sibbald, W. J. (1976). Acute respiratory failure. *Crit. Care Med.*, **4**, 79
3. Moseley, R. V., Vernick, J. J. and Doty, D. B. (1970). Response to blunt chest injury: a new experimental model. *J. Trauma*, **10**, 682
4. Blair, E., Topuzlu, C. and Davis J. H. (1971). Delayed or missed diagnosis in blunt chest trauma. *J. Trauma*, **11**, 129
5. Relihan, M. and Litwin, M. S. (1973). Morbidity and mortality associated with flail chest injury: a review of 85 cases. *J. Trauma*, **13**, 663
6. Black, R. J. (1979). *Laryngeal Trauma* (In preparation)
7. Larson, D. L. and Cohn, A. M. (1976). Management of acute laryngeal injury: a critical review. *J. Trauma*, **16**, 858

8. Beall, A. C., Patrick, T. A., Okies, J. E., Bricker, D. L. and de Bakey, M. E. (1972). Penetrating wounds of the heart: changing patterns of surgical management. *J. Trauma*, **12**, 468
9. Sutorius, D. J., Schreiber, J. T. and Helmsworth, J. A. (1973). Traumatic disruption of the thoracic aorta. *J. Trauma*, **13**, 583
10. Noon, C. P., Boulafendis, D. and Beall, A. C. (1971). Rupture of the heart secondary to blunt trauma. *J. Trauma*, **11**, 122
11. O'Sullivan, M. J., Spagna, P. M., Bellinger, S. B. and Doohen D. J. (1972). Rupture of the right atrium secondary to blunt trauma. *J. Trauma*, **12**, 208
12. Barber, H. (1940). Contusion of the myocardium. *Br. Med. J.*, **3**, 520
13. Katz, S., Gimmon (Goldschmidt) Z., Lewis, B. S. and Applebaum, A. (1979). Coronary angiography after traumatic myocardial contusion. *J. Trauma*, **19**, 126
14. Shoemaker, W. C., *et al.* (1973). Haemodynamic monitoring for physiological evaluation diagnosis and therapy of acute haemopericardial tamponade from penetrating wounds. *J. Trauma*, **13**, 36
15. Bertelsen, S. and Howitz, P. (1972). Injuries of the trachea and bronchi. *Thorax*, **27**, 188
16. Zuckerman, S. (1940). Experimental study of blast injuries to the lungs. *Lancet*, **2**, 219
17. Franz, J. L., Richardson, J., Grover, F. L. and Trinkle, J. K. (1974). Effects of methylprednisolone sodium succinate on experimental pulmonary contusion. *J. Thorac. Cardiovasc. Surg.*, **68**, 842
18. Avery, E. A., Morch, E. T., Head, J. R. and Benson, D. W. (1955). Severe crushing injuries of the chest: a new method of treatment. *Q. Bull. Northwest. Univ. Med. Sch.*, **39**, 301
19. Windsor, H. X. and Dwyer, B. (1961). The crushed chest. *Thorax*, **16**, 3
20. Lloyd, J. W., Crampton Smith, A. and O'Connor, B. T. (1965). Classification of chest injuries as an aid to treatment *Br. Med. J.*, **1**, 1518
21. Moore, B. P. (1977). In Williams, W. G. and Smith, R. E. (eds.). *Trauma of the Chest*, pp. 1–7. (Bristol: John Wright)
22. Worthley, L. I. (1976). Chest wall trauma. Presented at the *49th General Scientific Meeting of the Royal Australian College of Surgeons*, May 8–13, Adelaide
23. Wilmore, D. W. (1977). *The Metabolic Management of the Critically Ill.*, p. 36. (New York: Plenum Medical).
24. Atherton, S. T., Wright, D. M., White, D. J. and Jones, E. S. (1977). An antibiotic policy for bacterial and other infections after thoracic and other injuries. *Thorax*, **32**, 596
25. Atherton, S. T. and White, D. J. (1978). Stomach as source of bacteria colonising the respiratory tract during artificial ventilation. *Lancet*, **2**, 968
26. Gett, P. M., Jones, E. S. and Shepherd, G. F. (1971). Pulmonary oedema associated with sodium retention during ventilator treatment. *Br. J. Anaesth.*, **43**, 460

Reference books

Keen, G. (1975). *Chest Injuries*. (Bristol: John Wright)

Blaisdell, F. W. and Lewis, F. R. (1977). *Respiratory Distress Syndrome of Shock and Trauma*. (Philadelphia: W. B. Saunders Company)

12
Spinal cord injuries

BILL DAVIES

Injury to the vertebral column results in varying degrees of paralysis which is a 'disease' characteristic of urban mechanized society in the latter half of the 20th century. The frequency with which the injury is reported varies from society to society, but there seems to be little doubt that the numbers are increasing in urbanized communities. Gehrig and Michaelis[1] reported an incidence of 15 new cases per million of population per year. Sutton[2] reported 15–20 per million of population per year, while White and Yashon[3] estimated the incidence in the USA to be 50 new cases per million each year. In Queensland the incidence in 1978/79 was 38 per million of population per year, which is an increase of 23 above Sutton's estimate for the same region in 1973. The figure for Queensland is an underestimate because it does not include those who die at the site of the accident, or who are not referred to a spinal injuries unit. It is quite certain that many cases of fatal spinal cord damage are unrecognized, and this must affect the statistics of such injuries. The road traffic accident remains the major cause of trauma to the spinal cord (Figure 12.1). In Queensland the proportion of road traffic accidents involving motor cycles is increasing year by year, because the motor cycle is a cheap and efficient form of transport. In contrast, it is evident that with restrictions in some countries on the availability of fuel and the use of motor cars for leisure, the rising costs of motoring and the severe penalties imposed for drinking and driving, the incidence of spinal cord injuries from motor car accidents decreases.

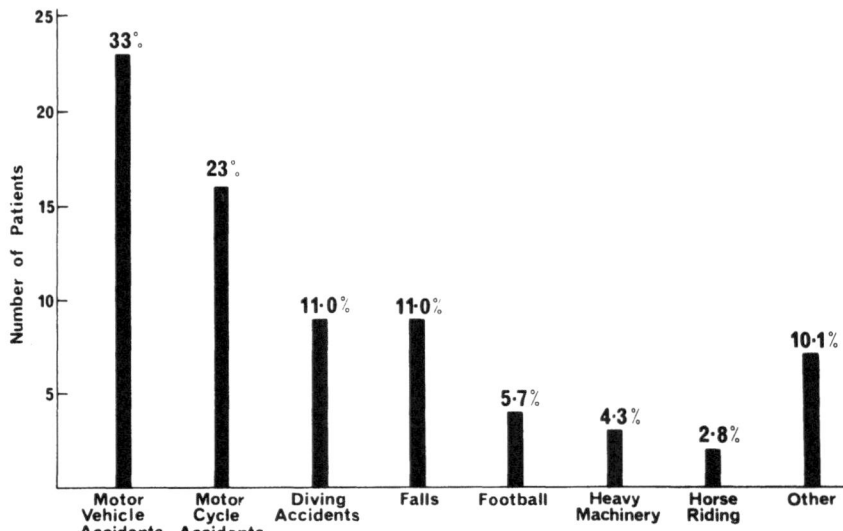

Figure 12.1 The major causes of spinal cord injury; road traffic accidents represent the major subgroups

(I) ORGANIZATION OF THE SERVICE

The concept of a comprehensive regional spinal injuries service to meet the needs of a fixed population had its origins in Stoke Mandeville under the guidance of the late Sir Ludwig Guttman towards the end of World War II. It was considered that a comprehensive specialized service would increase the efficiency of the various disciplines required to manage such patients. The simultaneous management of all systems, rather than their management in sequence has led to reductions in the death rate, the complications and consequently the cost. Comparisons of costs between 'system' and 'non-system' management have produced strong support for the 'systems' approach[4-6]. It is important that the spinal injuries unit is part of a major general hospital with easy and rapid access to all specialized services. An especially close liaison should be maintained with the ICU. This is because 15–20% of all new cases of spinal injury require a period of treatment in the ICU and there is a slight upward trend in this number. It is speculated that this increase may be a result of an increasing severity of motor vehicle accidents, combined with improving standards of first aid and resuscitation at

254

the site of the accident. Also the number of motor cycle accidents has increased and in those with spinal cord damage the site is commonly thoraco-lumbar; of these 23% have chest injuries requiring intensive care.

(II) DIAGNOSIS

The diagnosis of spinal cord damage is usually easy. Situations in which diagnosis is difficult are: in the unconscious patient; in patients with minimal or no spinal cord damage, when, because of unstable vertebral fractures, poor handling or inappropriate movement may worsen existing damage or injure the previously normal spinal cord. It is not uncommon to overlook spinal cord damage in patients who are unconscious or have other injuries that overshadow the less evident spinal cord damage. Hence, in all head injuries one should suspect that there may be concurrent injury to the spinal cord. The clinical signs of spinal cord damage can then be confirmed by a radiological survey of the spinal column. In the unconscious patient the signs that alert the clinician to the possibility of spinal cord damage are absent deep tendon jerks, abnormal pattern of breathing, priapism and urinary retention, and unequal and irregular pupils. The unconscious patient without a spinal cord lesion usually has deep tendon reflexes. If the spinal cord has been damaged, spinal shock is immediate and the patient is areflexic below the level of the lesion. The cause of this suppressed reflex activity below the level of the lesion cannot readily be explained. Nonetheless, absent deep tendon reflexes in an unconscious patient should prompt careful examination and an X-ray survey of the spine for damage.

The pattern of respiratory excursion in the tetraplegic is specific. Examination of the breathing pattern in patients with severe trauma is mandatory to exclude chest wall trauma and flail segments. In the tetraplegic patient the paradoxic movement of the chest wall and abdomen is evident due to the paralysis of intercostal muscles, while the diaphragm remains in action. Asymmetric lesions of the spinal cord may affect the respiratory excursions asymmetrically. In those lesions further down the spine an increasing number of intercostal muscles come into play and in those with lesions below T_{11}, all the intercostals are functional.

Partial or full priapism occurs specifically in spinal cord injury, and should lead to a careful examination of the spine. If some time has elapsed between the accident and examination, there may be a palpable bladder (Figure 12.2). Irregular or unequal pupils are relatively common in patients with cervical lesions. This results from division of the sympathetic tracts and unilateral or bilateral Horner's syndrome can often cause concern in patients who have had head injuries. The existence of a Horner's syndrome should prompt further examination for possible cervical spinal cord damage.

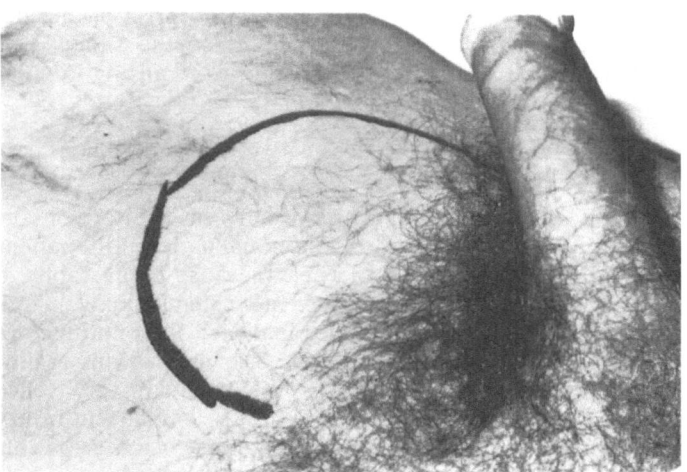

Figure 12.2 Priapism in a patient with significant spinal cord injury, and unconscious from a head injury. Note the outline of the over-distended bladder

Fractures of the spine which cause minimal or no spinal cord damage are easily missed, especially in the unconscious or partially conscious patient. In a patient with an unstable fracture without spinal cord damage, it is important to identify vertebral damage to avoid possible injury to the spinal cord during management and transportation. Inability to micturate should draw attention to the possibility of spinal cord damage. An inability to void urine is not uncommonly the only sign of minimal cord damage. Fractures of the upper third of the thoracic spine can occasionally present without spinal cord damage, and manifest themselves only as a widening of the upper mediastinal shadow. in the antero-posterior view. The latter is due to paravertebral haematoma which develops around the fractured vertebrae.

Case history

A 22 year old man was found in his overturned motor vehicle deeply unconscious. A widened upper mediastinal shadow was noted in the antero-posterior X-ray view of his chest (Figure 12.3). A traumatic aneurysm of the thoracic aorta was considered likely, and aortography was proposed. In the meantime, the patient passed into an irritable phase. Initially, he was able to move his lower limbs, but quickly developed a flaccid paralysis of the legs and lower trunk. X-rays of the thoracic spine in the AP and lateral views were then taken revealing compression fractures of $T_{5, 6 \text{and} 7}$ (Figures 12.4 and 12.5). After appropriate treatment of the fractures by immobilization and

256

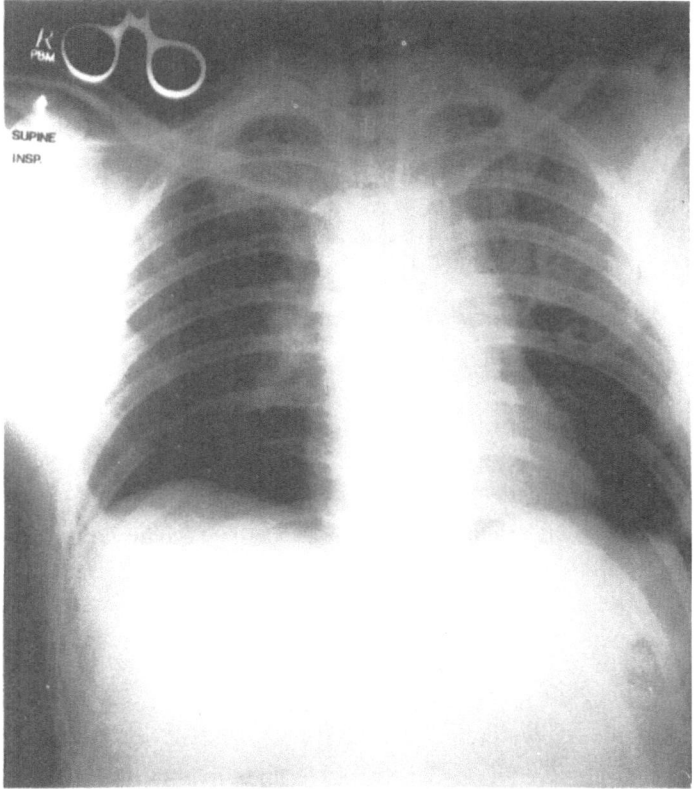

Figure 12.3 Antero-posterior X-ray view of the chest showing widening of the upper mediastinum

the avoidance of unneccesary movement, there was significant recovery of function but not to normality. In this case the mediastinal widening was due to a paravertebral haematoma following fractures of the bodies of $T_{5, 6 \text{and} 7}$. A lateral view of the spine in the region in question would have led to appropriate measures being taken to avoid undue movement at the fracture site and thus prevent permanent disability from the spinal cord damage.

257

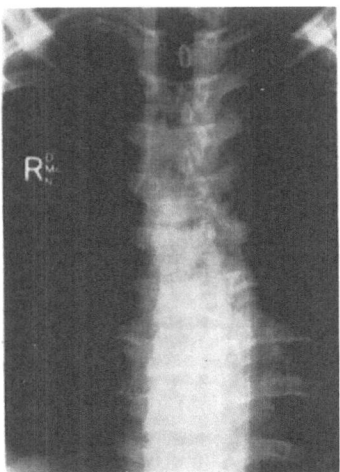

Figure 12.4   The antero-posterior view shows malalignment of $T_{5,6and7}$ with lateral compression of T_6 on the right side. There is also a slight scoliosis, convex to the left

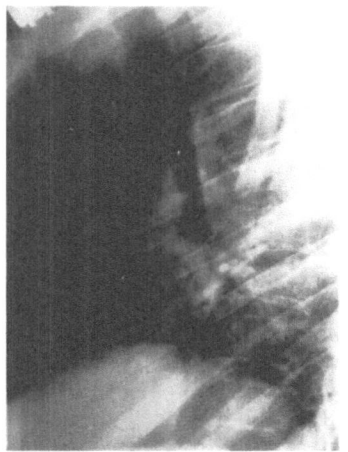

Figure 12.5   The lateral view of the thoracic spine shows significant compression of the bodies of $T_{5,6and7}$

(III) CRITERIA FOR INTENSIVE CARE

It is imperative that there should be a close working relationship between the spinal injuries and intensive care units at all levels. The two units should be close together to facilitate the transfer of patients and movement of staff. While a patient with a spinal injury is in the ICU, his primary problem is the one which dictated his admission. This is usually a chest injury, and the staff of the spinal injuries unit then assist as required in the ICU, particularly with patient handling. The converse should also apply, when staff from the ICU are called on to advise and assist in the spinal injuries unit. In particular, patients who are discharged from the ICU with tracheostomy tubes *in situ* should be cared for in the spinal injuries unit, but help should be readily available from the ICU staff.

By far the most frequent indication for admission to the ICU is a chest injury with imminent or established respiratory failure. More than 90% of all patients with spinal cord damage who are admitted to the ICU of this hospital have, as their primary indication for admission, respiratory insufficiency due to lung contusion. The majority of these patients have thoracic or thoraco-lumbar spinal cord injuries. Of 82 consecutive thoraco-lumbar injuries admitted under the care of this unit, 19 (23%) required admission to intensive care. Of 92 consecutive cervical injuries, 2 (2.1%) were admitted to the ICU. Of 174 consecutive patients 21 (12%) were admitted to the ICU with respiratory failure[7]. Overall, 16.2% of patients required intensive care. Patients who required IPPV comprised 50% of those with chest injuries and the average duration of IPPV was 6.3 days.

Other indications for admission were relatively infrequent: head injury, multiple injuries, vascular injury, inhalation lung damage, burns, and post-operative. Tetraplegics who have undergone surgery or manipulation for cervical dislocation under relaxant general anaesthesia are often sent to the ICU for the first 12–24 hours for post-operative care.

The factors, which influence the decision to start intensive care in other diseases, also apply to those with spinal cord damage. In this group, however, additional factors have to be considered; these are age and the prognosis. The majority of these patients are under 25 years of age, which inevitably influences the clinician towards active intervention, and the use of support systems. During World War I, 90% of all patients with spinal cord injury died within one year of the injury[8]. In this unit the death rate within one year in 1977/78 was 2.7% of all cases. While it is still difficult to give firm prognoses as regards longevity, the indications are that the majority of paraplegic patients can expect to live out a life span which is close to normal. A tetraplegic with added risk factors, such as susceptibility to serious chest infections, has a life span shortened by approximately 15 years, provided that he receives adequate care. The older patient who becomes completely tetraplegic later in life has a much worse prognosis.

259

Those injured at 45 years of age and over have a reducing life expectancy, so that at the age of 60 years few survive for one year[10]. The prognosis in terms of useful recovery of function is often germane to the ultimate decision as to whether or not to proceed with radical treatment, such as intensive care and IPPV. About 80% of all incomplete lesions achieve some form of useful recovery, while only 10–15% of all complete lesions achieve any recovery of function at all. With existing techniques of management and rehabilitation, a relatively high proportion of patients eventually return to physical independence and a reasonably satisfying quality of life. From this unit, 74% become fully independent in or out of a wheelchair, 20% partly dependent, and 6% totally dependent. When dealing with respiratory failure in high tetraplegic patients, one is inevitably confronted with a patient with inadequately functioning diaphragms and lung disease. The prospect of intubating these patients and eventually reaching the situation of a grossly paralysed tetraplegic who cannot survive without permanent assisted ventilation is real and daunting. The impact of this situation upon the patient, his family, the medical staff, hospital and society, is immense. The physician required to make this decision finds himself in one of the most serious clinical dilemmas in medicine. The problem that he faces carries practical, philosophical and ethical consequences. In making the decision whether or not to start IPPV in the high tetraplegic patient (that is lesions at C_4 and above), all the factors mentioned above must be considered. In the end the clinician is forced to make value judgments as to what action would be considered in the best interests of that patient, his family and society as a whole. Having assumed the responsibility for care of this patient, the responsibility for making such a decision cannot be offloaded.

(IV) MANAGEMENT

Perhaps the most valuable dictum on the good management of spinal cord injuries would be that of early referral to the nearest spinal injuries unit. The method of transport usually will depend upon the distance to be covered. Experience suggests that road transport is appropriate over distances up to 300–350 km. Over greater distances the use of aircraft is more appropriate. If an aircraft, pressurized or non-pressurized, is used, it is imperative to prepare the patient for safe travel. Dysbarism must be avoided, e.g. in patients with lung trauma and pneumothoraces, or impaired gas exchange in the lungs[11]. In Queensland, where great distances are the rule, the helicopter is reserved for retrieval from inaccessible areas, otherwise fixed wing aircraft and motor vehicles are used. The simultaneous management of all affected systems is mandatory if serious complications are to be avoided. In this chapter these systems are described in a sequence but it should be emphasized that in practice the management is directed at all systems in concert. Thus treatment concerns the simultaneous maintenance and management of the fracture or fracture-dislocation, the spinal cord, cardiovascular system, respiratory system, urinary tract, gastrointestinal tract, skin, maintenance of body temperature, and musculoskeletal system.

(1) The fracture or fracture dislocation

Management of the spinal bony damage follows the standard premises of orthopaedic surgery: reduce and realign, maintain. The controversy between the operative and non-operative management of spinal fractures and fracture-dislocations has continued for many years. It is not the aim of this chapter to argue either case, apart from stating our own position, which is for conservative management in all but a very few specific instances[12-15,51].

(a) Cervical injuries

In cervical injuries without facet dislocation we use skull traction for maintenance and immobilization. When unilateral or bilateral posterior facet dislocations are present, early and rapid reduction is required. The available methods include: (a) manipulation under relaxant general anaesthesia with image intensifier control[16,17], (b) graded traction using skull tongs, (c) open reduction when conservation methods fail. Some centres use open reduction as a first line of treatment.

In neck injuries the maintenance of the reduced fracture or dislocation in good position is effected by skull traction using various types of beds: Stryker wedge turning frame, orthopaedic bed with Balkan frame, Egerton Stoke Mandeville tilting and turning bed. The Stryker frame cannot be used in the following relatively common situations: (a) in patients with endotracheal tube treated by IPPV, since the tube may dislodge when the patient is prone and death result, (b) when there is chest injury and the prone position further reduces the respiratory reserve, (c) in those with facial damage who cannot tolerate the face support, (d) in those with limb fractures requiring traction. In most of the above situations the Egerton Stoke Mandeville tilting and turning bed adequately meets the need (Figure 12.6).

(b) Thoraco–lumbar injuries

This unit adopts the method of postural reduction, by extension of the patient over a foam bolster at the fracture site. In a very small group with specific indications (e.g. pure dislocation without posterior facet fracture),

261

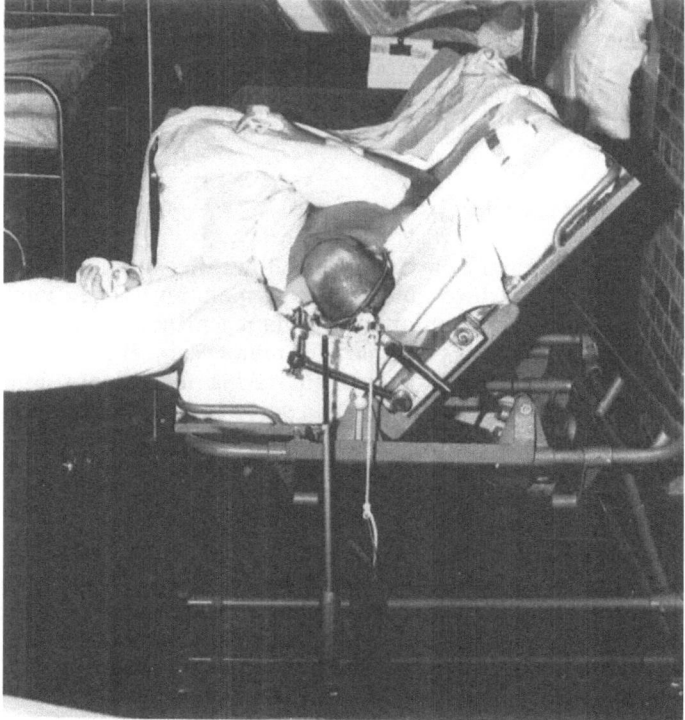

Figure 12.6 The Egerton Stoke Mandeville tilting and turning bed used for skull traction in the side position

open reduction and instrumentation with Harrington rods is required. The Egerton tilting and turning bed is quite effective for this purpose (Figure 12.7). The controversy continues between the protagonists of conservatism[18], and the supporters of early surgical intervention[19].

(2) The spinal cord

Surgical or medical procedures aimed directly at the spinal cord have no beneficial effects. In most countries laminectomy has fallen into disrepute[20]. Midline myelotomy, rhizotomy, hypothermia, steroids, urea therapy, antifibrinolytic therapy, antiserotonins, α-methyl tyrosine therapy, reserpine and numerous other forms of treatment are experimental and the results inconclusive or discouraging[21]. The use of hyperbaric oxygen therapy as a possible treatment of spinal cord injury was suggested by Kelly[22], and

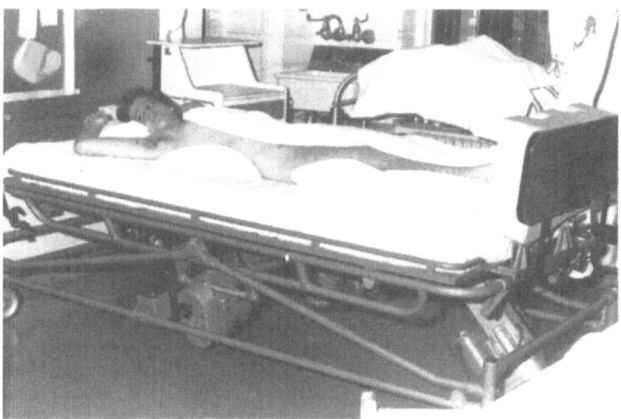

Figure 12.7 Hyperextension of a thoraco-lumbar fracture–dislocation over a foam bolster using an Egerton tilting and turning bed

further investigated by Yeo[23] in paraplegic sheep. Yeo[24] has now extended this treatment to clinical practice but the results have yet to be evaluated conclusively.

There is evidence that spinal cord ischaemia continues for 24 hours after the definitive damage. In the experimental animal model, Sandler and Tator[25] demonstrated continuing ischaemia and impaired blood flow in the grey matter and these processes extended beyond the site of compression. Bingham and co-workers[26] demonstrated a severe reduction in grey matter perfusion which persisted for long periods following contusion. These results are the basis for using hyperbaric oxygen to increase tissue oxygen tension in the damaged cord. They also emphasize the need to start treatment at the earliest moment. Experience has shown that the recovery rate from incomplete tetraplegia is sharply curtailed by such systemic disturbances as pulmonary embolism or infection. When these are treated the recovery continues at the same rate as before the disturbance. It follows that it is important to support all systems as soon as possible, in particular the cardiorespiratory system, in order to maintain the optimum delivery of oxygen to the damaged cord.

When overviewed, the definitive treatment of the damaged spinal cord can be reduced to three basic components: (1) earliest possible referral to the nearest spinal injuries unit, (2) early reduction and realignment of the neural canal, (3) aggressive support of all disordered systems, especially the maintenance of oxygen delivery to the tissues, particularly the spinal cord.

(3) Cardiovascular system

The sympathetic innervation of the heart arises from the neural segments C_5 to T_5[27]. Destruction of the spinal cord above T_5 severs the connections of the heart with the sympathetic system. Progressively more fibres are divided with higher lesions, until total loss occurs at C_5. While separating the heart from sympathetic activity, section of the sympathetic tract also isolates the blood vessels from sympathetic connections. As a result of this interruption there is a significant reduction of vasomotor tone, an increase in volume of the vascular compartment, and a resultant fall of blood pressure. It is quite common for patients to present in casualty after cervical spinal injuries with a systolic blood pressure between 80 and 90 mmHg but without a tachycardia. This hypotension should be carefully differentiated from the hypotension of other causes, and particularly blood loss. It is not necessary to transfuse vigorously to elevate the blood pressure to higher levels. The cardiac output is unchanged or reduced, and if challenged by a fluid load, the heart cannot respond normally by increasing its rate, stroke volume and cardiac output[28].

The pulmonary artery pressure and pulmonary artery wedge pressure (PAWP) are variably affected, but tend to be normal or elevated. The abnormal vascular tone and vascular volume combined with these pressures result in variable central venous pressure measurements, which often neither reflect the true blood volume nor cardiovascular status. Because of the elevated PAWP with relatively low systemic blood pressures, there is a distinct risk of causing pulmonary oedema when giving fluids intravenously. Consequently, intravenous replacement of fluids should be carried out with circumspection in the tetraplegic. In the sympathetomized tetraplegic patient pulmonary artery pressure and PAWP will increase during IPPV especially with positive end-expiratory pressure (PEEP). Thus the problems associated with i.v. fluids are magnified during IPPV with PEEP.

Although the sympathetic fibres to the heart are interrupted, the parasympathetic fibres running in the vagus remain intact and continue to function without the opposing influence of the sympathetic system. Welply[29] demonstrated reflex bradycardia during tracheal aspiration sometimes leading to cardiac asystole. This only occurred in patients in spinal shock who were also hypoxic during suction. They attributed the bradycardia to a vasovagal reflex unopposed by sympathetic action. These episodes can be prevented by atropine and indicate the need to avoid hypoxia, even though transient, and the need for great care during any manoeuvre which causes vagal stimulation. Occasionally these episodes continue with great frequency and for some reason are associated with turning the patient. In this situation the use of oral sustained-release isoprenaline has been found to be very successful.

264

Following the period of spinal shock there is a gradual return of reflex activity in all systems, which is divorced from supraspinal control if the lesion is complete. There is also some return of sympathetic tone. The tendency to hypotension when assuming the vertical or sitting position persists, but is not marked as in early phases. Similarly, in the tetraplegic the propensity to vaso-vagal asystole diminishes considerably.

(4) Respiratory system

The intercostal muscles are innervated by the neurological segments T_2 to T_{11}. Hence lesions above T_{11} cause increasingly extensive intercostal paralysis which impairs the mechanics of volume breathing. In the patient with chest injuries there are a number of problems posed by the vertebral and spinal cord damage which make management of the patient considerably more difficult than in those without spinal lesions.

(1)   The immobilization and positioning of the fracture to effect its reduction and then maintain that reduction, make respiratory care particularly difficult. The optimum position for fracture reduction is not that for the efficient action of the respiratory muscles. Similarly, there is little latitude for the positioning required for chest physiotherapy.

(2)   Intercostal paralysis and abdominal muscle paralysis reduce the respiratory reserve and efficiency of coughing. In lower thoracic spinal injuries, the FVC falls to about half the normal value and to one third of the expected value in cervical lesions[30,31]. In the acutely injured patient, and especially in the tetraplegic patient, intensive chest physiotherapy around the clock is essential. Nursing staff should be taught how to splint the diaphragm in order to assist coughing at times when the physiotherapist is not available.

(3)   Lung damage from aspiration of gastric contents is a special risk in patients with spinal cord injury. A high proportion have a paralytic ileus which is dealt with below. The combination of supine posture, impaired consciousness because of a head injury, paralytic ileus and poor cough power make these patients particularly prone to the lethal complication of aspiration lung damage. It is particularly important to prepare for this exigency when transporting patients. If there is any risk of the patient vomiting, the stomach should be emptied with a nasogastric tube and kept so by intermittent or continuous aspiration. Analgesics and sedatives must be used judiciously.

Concurrent chest injury is quite common, occurring in 2% of all cervical injuries and 23% of thoraco-lumbar injuries admitted to this unit. It is not surprising that there is a high incidence of chest injury associated with fractures of the thoracic spine because the forces combine flexion and rotation. At the instant of impact the ribs protect the spine and offer strong resistance to deformation of the thorax. An increasing force causes multiple rib fractures and then the spine itself fractures. In the process the underlying lung is contused. The rib fractures are usually widespread enough to allow flail movement to occur. This type of injury is most common in those who have been thrown onto the point of one shoulder, e.g. from a motor cycle. Chest damage is the rule in those crushed under heavy machinery when the mechanism is pure flexion of the thoracic spine. Early diagnosis of lung involvement is of major importance because rapid deterioration can occur at any time within the first 7–10 days. The presence of a lung contusion should be continuously suspect. The history is important, bearing in mind the site of spinal injury, the mechanism of injury and the presence of chest wall damage. Activity of accessory muscles of respiration is always an ominous sign of impending respiratory failure.

Haemothoraces are almost always present when the chest is injured and are occasionally missed in supine X-rays. They should be regarded as larger than the X-ray suggests, since it requires at least 1.0 l of blood in the pleural

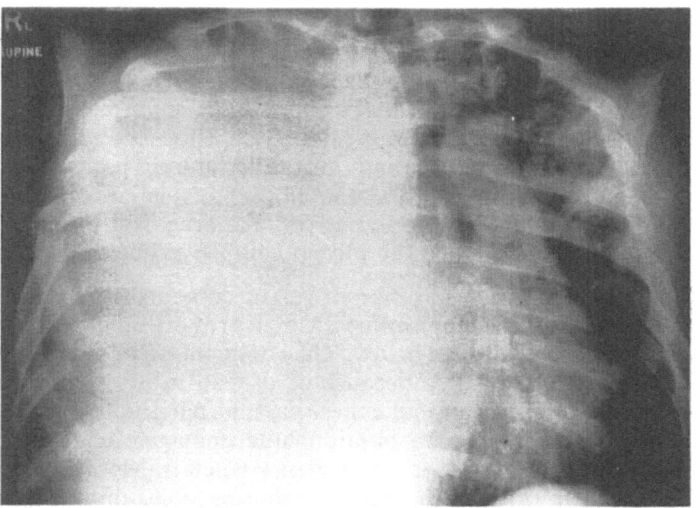

Figure 12.8   Right haemothorax with multiple rib fractures. 2.5 l of blood were aspirated through a chest drain. The patient was not distressed and the PaO_2 was 7.9 kPa (59 mm Hg) and $PaCO_2$ was 4.7 kPa (35 mm Hg). The PaO_2 rapidly returned to 10.6 kPa (80 mm Hg) after aspiration, and there was no recurrence

cavity to show a separation of the lung margin from the parietal pleura in the supine antero-posterior view. Haemothoraces collect from any or all of three sites: fractured ribs, leakage from a paravertebral haematoma, the surface of contused lungs. The compression of the lung by intrapleural blood does not significantly embarrass respiratory function unless the haemothorax is very large (Figure 12.8). It is not usual to have haemothoraces without concurrent lung contusions. The existence of lung contusions with evidence of interstitial oedema signals the need for admission to the ICU. The decision to admit to the ICU or to start IPPV is foremost a clinical one. The decision is supported by laboratory investigations. Factors influencing the decision to use IPPV are: (1) the history of the injury including the circumstances and the mechanism. (2) the presence of respiratory distress, the activity of accessory respiratory muscles, tachypnoea and flaring of the external nares, (3) X-ray changes showing haemothoraces and shadowing in the lung fields due to interstitial oedema, (4) the presence of chest wall damage, fractured ribs, or flail segments, (5) the development of fatigue or exhaustion, (6) following laparotomy virtually every case with lung contusions will require IPPV.

Arterial gas analysis is a valuable adjunct in the diagnosis and management of respiratory failure. It should, however, remain an adjunct to clinical judgment confirming a preconceived clinical decision. In 53 consecutive cases of lung contusion reviewed in this unit the initial PaO_2 and PaO_2 when breathing air was low, and the $P(A-a)O_2$ was high (Table 12.1). The initial PaO_2 was consistently low and was a useful alerting sign of hypoxaemic failure. When breathing 40%, PaO_2 rose but only to 11.9 kPa (89.5 mmHg) indicating an increased venous admixture. The practice of using rigid values, e.g. PaO_2 less than 8.0 kPa (60 mmHg), $PaCO_2$ greater than 6.5 kPa (49 mmHg) for the diagnosis of respiratory failure[32] is fraught with risk, as an elevation of the $PaCO_2$ occurs late in these patients. We maintain that early diagnosis is absolutely essential and 'if ventilatory assistance in critically ill and injured patients is delayed until there is obvious clinical evidence of respiratory failure, many of these patients will die'[33]. The high $P(A-a)O_2$ is an essential feature of the syndrome of ARDS, i.e. impaired alveolar gas exchange, ventilation perfusion imbalance, and reduced lung compliance. Gas exchange is further aggravated by paralysis of the intercostal muscle and the supine posture due either to skull traction or hyperextension. The radiographic features of interstitial oedema followed by alveolar oedema become evident at an advanced stage of the syndrome (Figure 12.9).

Treatment is aggressive with a policy of starting IPPV early rather than late. The policy of management is: control the primary process, do not overhydrate, resort to ventilation early using PEEP, and monitor the blood gases regularly. Of course, this applies to the management of all posttraumatic respiratory failure. However, the management is particularly

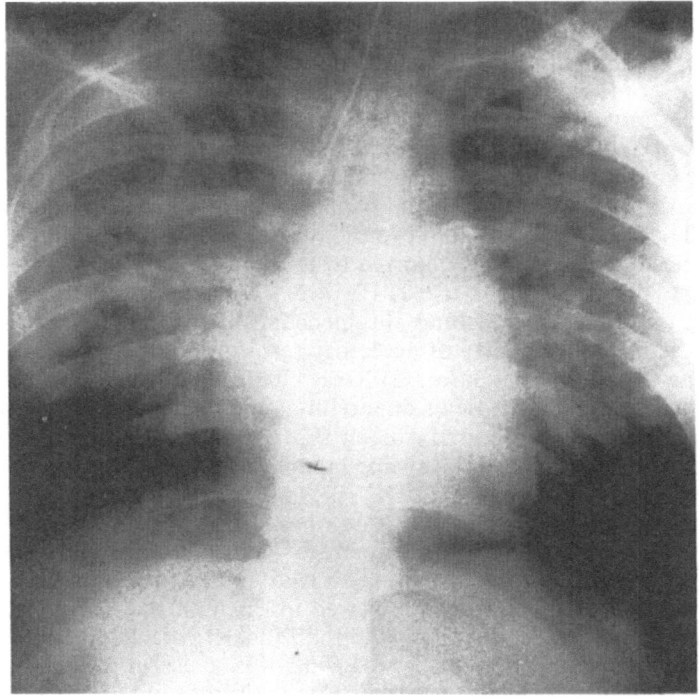

Figure 12.9 Flexion compression injury of T_4 on T_5 with lung contusions, bilateral haemothoraces and pulmonary oedema

Table 12.1 Mean arterial gas values and oxygen gradient breathing air of 40% oxygen

FIO_2%	PaO_2 (kPa) (mmHg)	$PaCO_2$ (kPa) (mmHg)	$P(A-a)O_2$ (kPa) (mmHg)
21	7.8 58.7	4.6 34.7	7.1 53.4
40	11.9 89.5	4.6 34.6	19.3 145.3

difficult in spinal injuries. In lesions above T_5 the risk of inducing pulmonary oedema is always present as already described. This risk is further increased in lung trauma when the lung water is already increased and pulmonary oedema is an inherent risk. The death rate in this series of 53 was 11.3%. Of those who recovered, two had some residual impairment of lung

268

function, one with reduced vital capacity and one with pulmonary hypertension from multiple pulmonary emboli. The average duration of IPPV was 12 days.

(5) Anaesthesia

Special problems apply in the anaesthesia of patients with spinal cord injuries, particularly in the acute phase and especially in tetraplegia. The risks and difficulties encountered during intubation of patients with cervical fractures while at the same time causing minimal movement of the fracture are evident, but can be surmounted with care and skill.

There is a real probability of sudden hyperkalaemia and fatal cardiac arrhythmias with the use of suxamethonium in newly injured patients[34]. The period during which the drug is unsafe extends from the third day for approximately 6 months after the injury. Since the actual times are not well defined, but the risk of hyperkalaemia is definite, then muscle relaxants other than suxamethonium should be used during this period.

(6) Urinary tract

During the period of spinal shock the bladder remains atonic and areflexic. Reflex activity returns at about the same time as the deep tendon jerks but this may not come about for up to 2 months. While the bulbocavernosus and superficial anal reflexes often return much earlier than the deep tendon reflexes, bladder reflex activity, for unknown reasons, does not parallel them.

From the outset the bladder must be drained artificially, either by an indwelling catheter or by the intermittent catheter technique. Intermittent catheterization, with control of fluid intake to avoid damaging overdistension of the bladder, was first proposed and practised by Sir Ludwig Guttman in 1947. This method is now commonly used to eliminate infection [35,36] and urethral complications[52] and to expedite the return of reflex detrusor activity[38]. It should be assumed that all patients thought to have spinal cord damage have neurogenic bladders until proved otherwise. Intermittent catheterization cannot be safely used while intravenous infusions are in progress. This is virtually always the case in the intensive care situation when we use the inlying Foley bag catheter. The inlying catheter, whether the Foley catheter or other type, should be of small calibre, preferably No. 16 French. The balloon should be as small as possible, preferably 5 ml. This minimizes the irritation from the balloon and reduces the amount of stretch of the external urethral sphincter. The latter is known to set up reflexes within the detrusor muscle of the bladder and inhibits the

269

return of reflex activity after spinal shock[39]. It must be realised that this seemingly innocuous piece of equipment must never be used in a cavalier fashion. The inlying urethral catheter is perhaps the most serious and ubiquitous reservoir of cross-infection in any hospital. In an ICU many patients have catheter drainage and require varied antibiotics. The result is a permanent source of pathogens whose resistance to the whole spectrum of antibiotics is continuously modified. All ICUs are now familiar with resistant strains of *Pseudomonas, Klebsiella* and even *E. coli*.

The major complications of catheter drainage which need to be avoided are: (a) overdistension, (b) infection, (c) anatomical damage.

(a) Overdistension

In the experimental animal, overdistension of the bladder may cause disruption of nexuses between muscle cells and the deposition of collagen leading to detrusor fibrosis and impaired contractility[39,40]. Experience suggests that this can also happen in the neutrogenic human bladder which begins to show adverse effects at volumes above 500 ml. Following overdistension there is a real risk of local and systemic infection and a delay in the return of reflex detrusor activity. This is accompanied by an increase in the number of cases which require bladder neck surgery in order to remove the catheter. Thus, an occluded urinary catheter should be changed immediately. Catheter irrigation is only used to diagnose an occluded catheter, and if the diagnosis is made the catheter must be changed even if the irrigation renders the catheter patent. Blocked catheters which have been cleared by irrigation almost invariably reblock and eventually result in overdistension and damage.

(b) Infection

Every indwelling urethral catheter must eventually become infected. They can, however, be maintained bacteriologically sterile for quite long periods – up to 12 weeks by absolute adherence to extremely stringent techniques of insertion and maintenance. High standards of care result in a reduction in the following: the frequency of infections of the bladder, kidneys and blood, the need for bladder neck surgery, the reservoir of cross-infecting pathogens, the incidence of multiple infections, and the number of antibiotic-resistant pathogens.

Infection is controlled by the following factors:

    (a)   Drainage is strictly closed, using a suitable collecting reservoir which is never disconnected from the catheter except under strictly controlled circumstances[37].

270

(b)   The collected urine is disinfected by adding a disinfectant, e.g. a synthetic phenol, to the bag.

(c)   Rigidly controlled and standardized methods of catheterization are used, observing all the basic tenets of surgical sterility[41]. This includes the installation of a disinfectant lubricant into the urethra before catheterization and the installation of a suitable disinfectant or antibiotic after passage of the catheter, e.g. 50 ml of 1 in 5000 chlorhexidine or an antibiotic such as neomycin 1% solution[42]. Our own experience with chlorhexidine 1 in 5000 in a volume of 50 ml has been satisfactory and rarely caused a chemical cystitis.

(d)   Daily toilet and dressing of the penis are carried out three times daily, using chlorhexidine cream to reduce the entry of organisms from the fossa navicularis along the sterile exudate that forms between the catheter and the urethral mucosa.

(e)   Frequent perineal toilets are carried out using suitable disinfectants such as alcoholic Hibitane hand lotion.

The use of suprapubic drainage by a silicone elastomer catheter, inserted through the lower abdominal wall and fitted with a body seal (silastic cysto-cath), may be a valuable alternative[43], provided the rigid methods are employed. Our own experience suggests that inert urethral catheters (silastic, silicone, etc.) should be changed much more frequently to reduce the risk of infection and the accumulation of debris and egg shell calculi.

The use of systemic antibiotics to convert an infected urine culture to a sterile one in patients who have inlying urethral catheters is to be deplored because it quickly converts sensitive organisms to resistant ones and paves the way for multiple infections. If systemic infection develops, it must be treated vigorously along standard lines. There is no benefit from attempting to eliminate established infection from the bladder with antibiotics unless there is systemic dissemination or upper tract involvement. These bladder infections are quickly eliminated by starting intermittent catheterization, at which time appropriate antibiotics can be commenced. In the interim, heavy bladder infections can be controlled by irrigation, using saline solution, chlorhexidine 1 in 5000 solution and topical antibiotics such as neomycin, polymyxin and bacitracin. The last practice may well be questioned on the basis of antibiotic resistance.

(c) Anatomical damage

The incidence of anatomical abnormalities such as penoscrotal diverticula, false passages and urethral strictures can be virtually eliminated by good catheter care and infection control techniques. Similarly it is certain that if infection can be eliminated, the incidence of vesico-ureteric reflux diminishes proportionately. In many units the urethral catheter in the male is strapped to the abdomen in the belief that this reduces the incidence of penoscrotal diverticula. This practice is carried out in this unit and appears to be successful although there is no statistical evidence to support this.

To summarize, the bladder management aims to: reduce or eliminate infection, avoid detrusor damage as well as facilitate the return of reflex bladder activity, thus making it possible to remove the catheter, reduce cross-infection by a process of 'internal isolation' consisting of closed drainage and disinfection.

(7) Gastrointestinal tract

Most patients with serious spinal injury have no sense of abdominal pain and the possibility of intra-abdominal visceral damage must be considered in every patient. The fact that they have no bowel sounds may be accounted for by the fact that 20% have a paralytic ileus. Patients may experience a form of visceral abdominal pain which is hard to describe and this makes the diagnosis of visceral rupture extremely difficult. The practice of peritoneal lavage to identify intra-peritoneal blood is often of value. However, in many cases, particularly in fractures of the lumbar spine, blood from a paravertebral haematoma leaks into the peritoneum, and the return from peritoneal lavage is blood stained. In these instances an exploratory laparotomy is the only course of action.

Abnormalities of gastrointestinal motility are quite common in patients with spinal cord damage. They can present as paralytic ileus with a distended and silent abdomen. More often, there are abnormal bowel sounds with a disco-ordinative ileus and progressive distension. Approximately 20% of all cases in this unit are so diagnosed. Acute gastric dilation is far less common, but must not go undiagnosed or untreated by nasogastric aspiration and intravenous fluid replacement. The complications of both these conditions are: (1) vomiting and aspiration lung damage, (2) elevation of the diaphragm by gas filled loops of gut which impede respiration, and (3) dehydration and electrolyte imbalance. These problems settle within 4–7 days, after which the patient can be graduated through increasing fluids to solids. Special attention should be given to these problems when contemplating air transport. Vomiting is difficult to manage in a supine patient with a spinal injury. Furthermore, even in pressurized aircraft, gas in the gut expands, further increasing the hazard of vomiting and aspiration as well as impairing the action of the diaphragm. The incidence of haemorrhage from stress ulcers is variably estimated from 5% to 22%[44]. The lesions usually appear as multiple superficial erosions on the greater curvature of the stomach but are also described in the lower oesophagus and duodenun. Generally, these are anticipated and prevented by the use of antacids given regularly via the nasogastric tube.

The rectum must be evacuated approximately 4 days after injury by using suppositories, and if these are unsuccessful, by manual evacuation. This is followed by a regime of regular evacuations, 3 days per week using oral aperients and rectal suppositories. Eventually a pattern of reflex evacuations develops and faecal incontinence is almost entirely prevented. It is emphasized that the regime must start early and continue regularly, otherwise the colon and rectum become overloaded and overstretched and do not regain the capability to empty reflexly at a given stimulus.

(8) Fluid and electrolyte balance

Fluid and electrolyte balance is maintained according to the principles which apply to any major trauma (Chapter 1). There is early and very severe muscle wasting which cannot as yet be controlled. If a prolonged period of intensive care is required during which solid food cannot be eaten, then a high protein fluid is indicated. This is administered via a nasogastric tube, and is usually necessary in those patients who require an extended period of IPPV.

(9) Body temperature

Impairment of blood vessel control and the absence of the capacity to sweat below the level of a complete lesion eliminate the normal mechanism of heat conservation and elimination. In the tetraplegic, the major part of his body surface is unable to control temperature and there is a continuing risk of hypothermia. This is particularly likely in operating theatres and recovery rooms. The converse is also true, and air conditioning is necessary to avoid hyperthermia in hot environments[45]. In the ICU the rectal temperature should be monitored continuously and body heat conserved.

(10) Thromboembolism

Venous thrombosis in the calf, femoral, pelvic and iliac veins is common. Just how common has been controversial for a long time. Estimates range from 12.5%[46] to 100%[47]. The incidence of clinical pulmonary embolism varies from 5%[48] to 20%[46]. Most significant pulmonary emboli originate from femoral, pelvic and iliac veins. It is evident from experience that clinical signs of venous thrombosis may be absent. Consequently the diag-

273

nosis of pulmonary embolism remains difficult, and requires a high degree of suspicion. Ancillary diagnostic tests such as e.c.g., arterial blood gases, enzyme studies, and X-rays are notoriously unreliable. The logistics of moving patients with spinal injuries, especially those on skull traction, are quite prohibitive. Thus, the decision to use the more valuable diagnostic procedures, lung scan and pulmonary angiography, along with venography, must be made in the light of the risks involved in moving these patients. The diagnosis of deep venous thrombosis in the acute phase is essentially a clinical one, aided by ultrasound. Prevention of deep venous thrombosis is practised using standard methods: twice daily passive movements of all limbs, calf and thigh massage at each turn of the patient throughout the 24 hours, subcutaneous calcium heparin given twice daily in a dosage of 6250 units[46], and the use of 'antiembolism' compression stockings. A higher dose of subcutaneous calcium heparin (7500 units 12 hourly) was recommended by Casas et al[48].

Pulmonary embolism is treated on standard lines, using continuous intravenous infusions of heparin, changing to an oral anticoagulant after approximately 1 week. In this unit the incidence of pulmonary embolism diagnosed on clinical grounds was approximately 15%. There have been two deaths from massive pulmonary emboli out of 450 consecutive patients. All deaths on this unit have had the pulmonary vessels examined at a coroner's autopsy and this figure can thus be regarded as accurate. Two patients required streptokinase therapy, one of whom subsequently developed pulmonary hypertension from multiple small emboli. Thus, venous thrombosis and pulmonary embolism remain a continuing diagnostic problem in all patients sustaining spinal injuries. There is a multiplicity of presentations of small emboli which often precede larger ones. Chest pain is by no means always present. Sometimes there is transient dyspnoea, fever, tachycardia or confusional state, shoulder tip pain, localized pleural friction rub, and leukocytosis.

The variable presentation together with impaired sensation in the thorax, and absent signs of deep venous thrombosis make the diagnosis of small pulmonary emboli quite difficult.

(11) The skin, muscles and joints

These tissues quite properly receive a great deal of attention in an ICU, but too often there is scant attention to the maintenance of paralysed limbs. Nursing techniques and bed design for spinal cord injuries are largely developed around the care of the skin and the relief of pressure while maintaining fractures in good position. Regular 2-hourly skin checks and patient turning are routine. The skin must be kept clean and dry and all sources of pressure, no matter how small, avoided. Rubbing the back, particularly

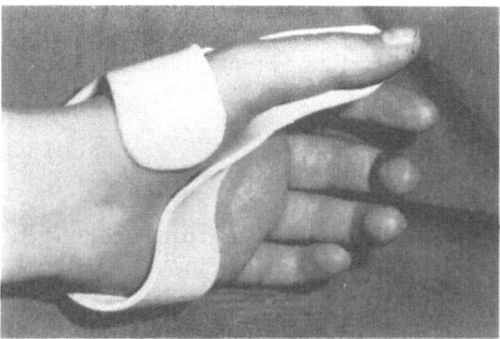

Figure 12.10 'Orthoplast' short opponens splint in the paralysed hand with one functioning wrist extensor and no finger function. This splint moulds the thumb into opposition with the paralysed index finger

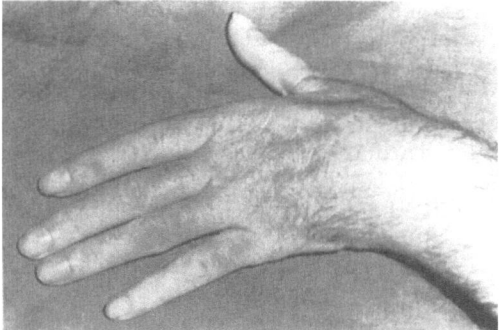

Figure 12.11 The hand of a tetraplegic with the fingers fixed in extension and the wrist fixed in ulnar deviation. The patient's hand had lain flat without splintage during several weeks of IPPV. In spite of a great deal of treatment the hand remained useless because of fixed contractures

with alcohol, presumably to increase resistance to the development of pressure sores, is traditional but little else.

The occupational therapist and physiotherapist should be involved from the first day. The occupational therapist is particularly concerned with the paralysed hand. This involves the design and manufacture of serial hand splints in order to reduce oedema, avoid contractures, and mould the hand into a functional limb which is cosmetically acceptable (Figure 12.10). Neglect of serial splinting, even for relatively short periods of time, can lead to deformities and contractures in non-functional positions (Figure 12.11). In a similar way, physiotherapy with passive movement and massage of the

275

limbs from the first day is designed to maintain muscle length and joint range and mobility. This prepares for any neurological recovery that may occur at a later date, and facilitates rehabilitation whether recovery occurs or not.

(V) CRITERIA FOR READMISSION

Patients with spinal paralysis may need to be readmitted to the ICU for various reasons, the commonest being respiratory failure in the tetraplegic. All the tenets of care previously described then apply.

(1) Autonomic dysreflexia

After spinal shock has passed off, reflex activity returns. In complete lesions this reflex activity is uncontrolled by the supraspinal centres. In particular, the phenomenon of autonomic dysreflexia or hyperreflexia becomes evident in lesions above T_5, and is more marked in higher lesions in the neck[39,49]. This condition is episodic and characterized by severe pounding headache, rapidly progressive and severe hypertension, sweating, flushing and pilo-erection in the areas innervated by segments above the level of the cord lesion, and bradycardia.

It can be triggered off by any noxious stimulus below the level of the lesion, but particularly by distension of a hollow viscus, notably the bladder, e.g. when a catheter becomes occluded. The stimulus of distension provokes mass reflex vasospasm throughout the sympathetic fibres below the spinal cord lesion. The resulting paroxysm of hypertension is recorded in the carotid body and relayed to the vasomotor centre. From here sympathetic vasodilator, sweating, and pilo-erector impulses pass via the cord to all segments above the cord lesion where they are arrested by that lesion. Hence, there is sweating, flushing and pilo-erection above the level of the cord lesion. Intracranial vasodilation associated with the severely elevated blood pressure accounts for the headache. Vagal impulses, unopposed by sympathetic impulses to the heart, cause the bradycardia. The syndrome is potentially lethal and even young patients can develop a stroke if the hypertension is not controlled. Treatment requires rapid removal of the causative stimulus, e.g. by changing an occluded urethral catheter and decompressing the bladder. When the causative stimulus cannot readily be removed the hypertensive crisis is treated by standard methods.

Many tetraplegic patients have extremely hyperactive reflexes and are troubled by headaches due to autonomic dysreflexia at what would be regarded as normal bladder volumes and even during reflex voiding. In such patients instrumentation, e.g. cystoscopy, can be hazardous, and the patient may have to be prepared medically before the procedure. α-adrenergic blockers such as phenoxybenzamine in quite large doses (up to 60 mg per day) are quite effective in controlling the symptoms and the hypertension. The bladder spasm, which is actually a part of the dysreflexia, and is accompanied by hypertension, can hinder instrumentation. It can be controlled by anticholinergic drugs such as Pro-Banthine, penthienate bromide (Monodral), tricyclic antidepressants or combinations of these. A useful additional drug is oral salbutamol which stimulates β-adrenergic endings in the bladder which appear to promote relaxation of the detrusor muscle[50]. It is often necessary to prepare a patient for bladder instrumentation or surgery with these drugs to reduce the risks of accompanying autonomic dysreflexia.

(2) Acute abdomen

The acute abdomen in patients with spinal paralysis, and in particular the high paraplegic and tetraplegic in which abdominal sensation is lost, poses a very real problem. Many of these patients eventually reach the ICU because of late diagnosis of intra-abdominal emergencies. Because a large number of patients with spinal paralysis are young, they have retained their appendices. Thus appendicitis often poses a very real problem of diagnosis, especially from urinary tract infection. Localizing signs are difficult to elicit. Occasionally there is a form of visceral pain which patients can describe, but it is rarely localized. There is often a change in the pattern of their skeletal muscle spasticity. The increase may, in fact, localize over the involved organ, e.g. the appendix. The increase in tone may be confined to one side of the body, e.g. the right leg, in appendicitis. Very often one is left with the description of a vague feeling of generalized illness associated with fever and a leukocytosis. It should be remembered that the tetraplegic has an unpredictable febrile response to infection and may not have a fever commensurate with the degree of infection. Similarly, the heart rate may be limited by damage to the sympathetic tracts. In these instances, it is often necessary to resort to laparotomy on the basis of suspicion, when in the unparalysed patient management would be expectant.

Conclusion

The management of patients with severe spinal cord injury taxes any system of critical care, especially its nursing staff. When the assistance of the ICU is required the management problems can become massive. Apart from the pure logistics of handling the spinal damage along with the associated injuries, difficult decisions have to be made by the medical staff. When deciding how far to go with intensive support systems and invasive techniques of management, the decision maker is forced to look to the future and every option he takes often carries with it a value judgment. It has to be remembered that a significant number of patients make a neurological recovery and life expectancies are now approaching the norm. The general negative view of spinal paralysis should be modified by the fact that, although spinal paralysis is indeed one of the most severe disabilities that can be suffered by man, its sufferers also have the greatest potential for survival in a productive and reasonably comfortable way. This is because the condition does not progress, the intelligence is spared and the long-term complications of spinal paralysis are all predictable and avoidable by relatively simple measures.

The relationship between the ICU and the spinal injuries unit must be a close one. The spinal injuries unit must realise that the immediate life-threatening problems of its patients are the responsibility of the ICU, and the spinal injuries unit has a supportive role, dealing with the fracture and paralysis, and must be prepared to give advice and resources to that end. The reverse must also apply when the spinal injuries unit requires the assistance of the ICU. As with all interdisciplinary relationships, this particular one will founder if not based upon the final common denominators which cannot be legislated – common sense, common goals and mutual respect.

References

1. Gehrig, R. and Michaelis, L. S. (1968). Statistics of acute paraplegia and tetraplegia on a national scale. *Paraplegia*, **6**, 93
2. Sutton, N. G. (1973). *Spinal Cord Injuries.* (London: Butterworth)
3. White, R. J. and Yashon, D. (1973). Dorsal and lumbar cord injuries. In Youmans, J. R. (ed.). *Neurosurgery II*, pp. 1085–1088. (Philadelphia: Saunders)
4. Charles, E. D., Van Matre, J. G. and Meller III, J. M. (1974). Spinal cord injury – A cost benefit analysis of alternate treatment modals. *Paraplegia*, **12**, 222
5. Hamilton, B. B., Rath, G. J., Meyer, P. R. and Rosen, J. S. (1976). A basis evaluation framework for spinal injury care systems. *Paraplegia*, **14**, 87
6. Charles, E. D., Fine, P. R., Stover, S. L., Wood, T., Lott, A. F. and Kronenfeld, J. (1978). The costs of spinal cord injury. *Paraplegia*, **15**, 311
7. Davies, W. E., Wright, M., Hill, V. (1976). Respiratory Failure associated with Spinal Cord Injury. *Proceedings of the Far East and South Pacific Spinal Cord Conference*, pp. 47–54
8. Jacobs, S. C. and Kaufman, J. M. (1978). Complications of permanent bladder catheter drainage in spinal cord injury patients. *J. Urol.*, **119**, 740
9. Watson, N. (1976). Pattern of spinal cord injury in the elderly. *Paraplegia*, **14**, 36

10. Hardy, A. G. (1976). Survival periods in traumatic tetraplegia. *Paraplegia*, **14**, 41
11. Oxer, H. F. (1975). Aeromedical evacuation of the seriously ill. *Br. Med. J.*, **3**, 692
12. Munro, D. (1961). Treatment of fractures and dislocations of the cervical spine complicated by cervical cord and root injuries. A comparative study of fusion versus non-fusion therapy. *N. Engl. J. Med.*, **264**, 573
13. Guttman, Sir Ludwig (1973). *Spinal Cord Injuries Comprehensive Management and Research*, pp. 345–358. (Oxford: Blackwell)
14. Bedbrook, G. M. (1976). Injuries of the thoraco–lumbar spine with neurological symptoms. In Vinken, P. J. and Bruyn, G. W. (eds.). *Handbook of Clinical Neurology*, pp. 437–466. (Amsterdam: Elsevier-North Holland)
15. Braakman, R. and Penning,' L. (1976). Injuries of the cervical spine. In Vinken, P. J. and Bruyn, G. W. (eds.). *Handbook of Clinical Neurology*, pp. 227–380. (Amsterdam: Elsevier-North Holland)
16. Evans, D. (1969). Reduction of cervical dislocations. *J. Bone Jt. Surg.*, **43B**, 552
17. Burke, D. C. and Berryman, K. (1971). The place of closed manipulation in the management of flexion-rotation dislocations of the cervical spine. *J. Bone Jt. Surg.*, **53B**, 165
18. Guttman, Sir Ludwig (1976). The conservative management of closed injuries of the vertebral column resulting in damage to the spinal cord and spinal roots. In Vinken, P. J. and Bruyn, G. W. (eds.). *Handbook of Clinical Neurology*, pp. 285–306. (Amsterdam: Elsevier-North Holland)
19. Dickson, J. H., Harrington, P. R. and Erwin, W. D. (1977). Results of reduction and stabilization of the severely fractured thoracic and lumbar spine. *J. Bone Jt. Surg.*, **59A**, 143
20. Morgan, T. H., Wharton, G. W. and Austin, G. N. (1970). The results of laminectomy in patients with incomplete spinal cord injuries. *J. Bone Jt. Surg.*, **52A**, 822
21. Osterholm, J. L. (1974). The pathophysiological response to spinal cord injury. *J. Neurosurg.*, **40**, 5
22. Kelly, D. L., Lassiter, K. R. L. and Vongsvivul, A. *et al.* (1972). Effects of hyperbaric oxygenation and tissue oxygen studies in experimental paraplegia. *J. Neurosurg.*, **36**, 425
23. Yeo, J. D., McKenzie, B., Hinwood, B. and Kidman, A. (1976). Treatment of paraplegic sheep with hyperbaric oxygen – a preliminary report. *Med. J. Aust.*, **1**, 538
24. Yeo, J. D., Lowry, C. and McKenzie, B. (1978). Preliminary report on ten patients with spinal cord injuries treated with hyperbaric oxygen. *Med. J. Aust.*, **2**, 572
25. Sandler, A. N. and Tator, C. H. (1976). Effect of acute spinal cord compression injury on regional spinal cord blood flow in primates. *J. Neurosurg.*, **45**, 660
26. Bingham, G. W., Goldman, H., Friedman, S. J., Murphy, S., Yashon, D. and Hunt, W. E. (1975). Blood flow in normal and injured monkey spinal cord. *J. Neurosurg.*, **43**, 162
27. Ranson, S. W. and Clark, S. I. (1959). *The Anatomy of the Nervous System,*

its Development and Function. p. 158 (Philadelphia: Saunders)

28. Troll, G. F. and Dohrmann, G. J. (1975). Anaesthesia of the spinal cord injured patient: cardiovascular problems and their management. *Paraplegia*, **13**, 162

29. Welply, N. C., Mathias, C. J. and Frankel, H. L. (1975). Circulatory reflexes in tetraplegics during artificial ventilation and general anaesthesia. *Paraplegia*, **13**, 172

30. Ohry, A., Molho, M. and Rosin, R. (1975). Alterations of pulmonary function in spinal cord injured patients. *Paraplegia*, **13**, 101

31. Forner, J. V., Llombart, R. L. and Valledor, M. C. V. (1977). The flow volume loop in tetraplegia. *Paraplegia*, **15**, 245

32. Gibbons, J., James, O. and Quacil, A. (1973). Management of 130 cases of chest injury with respiratory failure. *Br. J. Anaesth.*, **45**, 1130

33. Wilson, R. F. and Sibbald, W. J. (1976). Acute respiratory failure. *Crit. Care Med.*, **4**, 78

34. Snow, J. C., Kripke, B. J., Sessions, G. P. and Fink, A. J. (1973). Cardiovascular collapse following succinylcholine in a paraplegia patient. *Paraplegia*, **11**, 199

35. Pearman, J. W. (1976). Urological follow-up of 99 spinal cord injured patients initially managed by intermittent catheterisation. *Br. J. Urol.*, **48**, 297

36. Shapiro, S. R., Santamaria, A. and Harrison, J. H. (1974). Catheter associated urinary tract infections: incidence and a new approach to prevention. *J. Urol.*, **112**, 659

37. Pearman, J. W. and Cox, L. A. (1972). The Shenton Park urodrain – a urine collection bag for continuous closed drainage of an indwelling catheter. *Paraplegia*, **10**, 161

38. Lindan, R. and Bellamy, V. (1971). The use of intermittent catheterisation in a bladder training program. Preliminary report. *J. Chronic Dis.*, **24**, 727

39. Pearman, J. W. and England, E. J. (1973). *The Urological Management of the Patient following Spinal Cord Injury.* (Springfield: Charles C. Thomas)

40. Lloyd-Davies, R. W., Clark, A. E., Prout, W. E., Shuttleworth, K. E. D. and Tighe, J. R. (1970). The effects of stretching of the rabbit bladder. *Invest. Urol.*, **8**, 145

41. Lindan, R. (1969). The prevention of ascending catheter-induced infections of the urinary tract. *J. Chronic Dis.*, **12**, 321

42. Clark, L. W. (1973). Neomycin in the prevention of post-catheterisation Bacteruria. *Med. J. Aust.*, **1**, 1034

43. Morton, D. C. (1973). Suprapubic bladder drainage following gynaecological surgery. *Med. J. Aust.*, **2**, 928

44. Nuseibeh, I. M. (1976). Stress ulceration in spinal injuries. In Vinkey, P. J. and Bruyn, G. W. (eds.). *Handbook of Clinical Neurology*, pp. 351–353 (Amsterdam: Elsevier-North Holland)

45. Johnson, R. H. (1976). Temperature regulation in spinal cord injuries. In Vinken, P. J. and Bruyn, G. W. (eds.). *Handbook of Clinical Neurology*, pp. 355–376. (Amsterdam: Elsevier-North Holland)

46. Watson, N., (1978). Anticoagulant therapy in the prevention of venous thrombosis and pulmonary embolism in the spinal cord injury. *Paraplegia*, **16**, 265

47. Todd, J. W., Fusbie, J. H., Rossier, A. B., Adams, M. D., Alo, A. V.,

Armenia, R. J., Sasahara, A. A. and Two, D. E. (1976). Deep venous thrombosis in acute spinal cord injury: a comparison of 125 I fibrinogen by scanning, impedance plethysmography and venography. *Paraplegia*, **14**, 50

48. Casas, E. R., Sanchez, M. P., Arias, C. R. and Masip, J. P. (1978). Prophylaxis of venous thrombosis and pulmonary embolism in patients with acute traumatic spinal cord lesions. *Paraplegia*, **15**, 209

49. Kursh, E. D., Freehafer, A. and Persky, L. (1977). Complications of autonomic dysreflexia. *J. Urol.*, **118**, 70

50. Khanna, O. P. (1976). Disorders of micturition, neuropharmacologic basis and results of drug therapy. *Urology*, **3**, 316

51. Davies, W. E., Morris, J. H. and Hill, V. (1980). An analysis of conservative (non-surgical) management of thorocolumbar fractures and fracture-dislocations with neural damage. *J. Bone Jt. Surg.*, 62A, **8**, 1324

52. Ferlit, C. F., Canning, J. R., Lloyd, F. A., Cross, R. R. and Brewer, R. (1975). Experience with intermittent catheterisation in chronic spinal cord injury patients. *J. Urol.*, **144**, 234

13
Acute myocardial infarction

THOMAS PORTS, DAVID HESS AND KANU CHATTERJEE

Acute myocardial infarction is the major cause of death in most western continents. In the United States it is estimated that about 1 400 000 myocardial infarctions occur each year. Annually over 675 000 die in this country from the complications of coronary artery disease. Major advances have been made over the last decade which continue to reduce the mortality associated with acute myocardial infarction.

The establishment of coronary care units which provide continuous electrocardiographic monitoring and advances in antiarrhythmic drug therapy have resulted in a reduction in mortality from serious arrhythmias. The development of balloon-tip flotation catheters has allowed for relatively safe, continuous bedside haemodynamic monitoring in critically ill patients with acute myocardial infarction. The ability to identify haemodynamic abnormalities at the bedside has greatly facilitated our management of the low output syndrome complicating myocardial infarction.

In this chapter we review the three major goals of therapy in the acute phase of myocardial infarction: prevention and treatment of serious arrhythmias and conduction disturbances, correction of haemodynamic abnormalities, and preservation of ischaemic myocardium.

(I) ARRHYTHMIAS AND CONDUCTION DISTURBANCES

Experience gained in the last 15 years from coronary care units has resulted in a better understanding of the natural history, prognosis, and treatment of disorders of impulse formation and conduction. It is estimated that between 75 and 95% of patients with acute myocardial infarctions have cardiac arrhythmias and between 11 and 21% have atrioventricular (AV) or ventricular conduction abnormalities[1-9]. The early recognition and successful treatment of tachyarrhythmias, in particular ventricular tachycardia and ventricular fibrillation, has been responsible in most part for the reported reduction in mortality of hospitalized patients with acute myocardial infarction[10-12]. However, early and proper management of patients with bradyarrhythmias and conduction disturbances may also affect survival[13,14]. It is the purpose of this section to review the present treatment of disorders of impulse formation and conduction.

(1) Ventricular arrhythmias

The most common and potentially the most serious arrhythmic complication of acute myocardial infarction is ventricular premature contractions, with an incidence of 40–80%[15-17]. The clinical significance of this arrhythmia rests in the potential for the development of ventricular tachycardia, flutter, or fibrillation. Originally, it was thought that frequent (greater than 6/minute), early, multifocal, and runs of premature ventricular contractions (greater than 2 beats in a row) predisposed the patient to ventricular tachycardia or ventricular fibrillation[4,15,18-21]. However, recent studies have shown that late coupled premature ventricular contractions trigger ventricular tachyarrhythmias[22]. In addition, in 25–40% of cases, no premonitory arrhythmias are noted prior to the occurrence of ventricular fibrillation[23-25]. Consequently, many clinicians argued that prophylactic antiarrhythmic therapy should be used in all patients with acute myocardial infarction. Subsequent justification of the efficacy of prophylactic antiarrhythmic therapy in patients with acute myocardial infarction was provided by Lie et al.[26] in a double-blind randomized study of 212 patients hospitalized within 6 hours of the onset of symptoms. 107 patients were treated with a 100 mg intravenous (i.v.) bolus of lignocaine followed by a 3 mg/min lignocaine infusion, while a comparable control group was treated with an infusion of dextrose and water. No episodes of ventricular fibrillation were observed in the treated group while nine patients in the control group experienced ventricular fibrillation, four of which occurred without premonitory arrhythmias. 15% of the treated patients had drug side-effects and approximately one third of the treated patients continued to have warning dysrhythmias despite the continuous lignocaine infusion. It appears therefore that the goal of lignocaine prophylaxis is to achieve and maintain therapeutic serum drug levels and that this level may not necessarily suppress all ventricular ectopy. Several regimens have been

283

suggested to attain therapeutic lignocaine levels rapidly, and at the present we recommend a protocol adapted from Wyman *et al.*[27]: 1 mg/kg i.v. bolus of lignocaine is infused over 1 minute followed immediately by a 2 mg/minute i.v. infusion. A 50 mg i.v. bolus is given every 5–10 minutes for three additional doses. This loading schedule should be adjusted appropriately for the body weight, liver function, and the degree of cardiac failure. The infusion is continued for 48 hours and is usually not increased for warning arrhythmias. Because of lignocaine's β-decay half-life of 120–200 minutes[28], it may be discontinued abruptly at 48 hours if no ongoing ischaemia or ventricular ectopy is present. Although some reports are available on the use of newer antiarrhythmics (disopyramide, aprindine, and bretylium tosylate) as prophylactic agents in acute myocardial infarction, none of these studies have contained large numbers of patients or proved efficacy over that of lignocaine[29-33]. At the present time their use should be limited to special circumstances as discussed below.

When it occurs, ventricular tachycardia may be treated with either drugs or direct current cardioversion depending upon the patient's haemodynamic status. Lignocaine is usually effective in treating and/or preventing the recurrence of ventricular tachycardia encountered in the early hospital phase of acute myocardial infarction[34]. However, ventricular tachycardia resistant to lignocaine occurs in approximately 10–15% of these patients and additional therapy is required[35,36]. Prior to and coincident with the use of antiarrythmic drugs, every effort should be made to correct congestive heart failure, hypotension, electrolyte abnormalities or ongoing ischaemia. We use i.v. procainamide as the second choice drug. Our protocol includes the use of procainamide at 50 mg/minute i.v. until either 600–700 mg of the drug has been infused, the blood pressure falls below 90 systolic, or the QRS duration widens by 50% or more[37]. This initial loading dose will produce serum levels of 4.0–6.0 μg/ml and if it is effective in terminating ventricular tachycardia or preventing its recurrence, a 2–4 mg/minute i.v infusion is begun[35]. If the arrhythmia is not controlled, an additional 500–1400 mg of procainamide may be given i.v. at the same rate with the same noted precautions. With this latter protocol, the serum levels can be increased to 8–18 μg/ml[38]. Although these higher dosages have not been evaluated for the treatment of ventricular tachycardia in the setting of acute myocardial infarction, high serum procainamide levels are often required for control of recurrent ventricular tachycardia in patients with coronary artery disease[38].

Ventricular tachycardia refractory to the above measures pose a grave clinical problem. It has been our general experience that quinidine will not be helpful if procainamide in the above dosages has been unsuccessful in controlling the arrhythmia. In addition, intramuscular quinidine may be poorly absorbed if peripheral perfusion is compromised, and i.v. quinidine has a high incidence of hypotensive reactions. Diphenylhydantoin

(Dilantin) appears most useful in cases where digitalis toxicity is a contributing factor to the ventricular tachycardia or in which the baseline QT interval is prolonged[39]. Its advantage is that it can be administered i.v. and blood levels are readily available to aid in dose titration. Bigger *et al.*[40] reported that phenytoin plasma levels within the range of 2–18 μg/ml suppressed ectopic ventricular rhythms in 22 of 24 (91%) patients. Levels between 10 and 18 μg/ml were required in 16 of the 22 successfully treated patients. An additional eight patients with ventricular tachycardia were successfully treated but not included because plasma drug levels were not available. Based on this data, the objective of phenytoin therapy should be to rapidly achieve and maintain plasma levels between 10 and 20 μg/ml. Drug failure exists when ventricular tachycardia persists or occurs despite adequate drug levels. Proper phenytoin loading incorporates the drug's two-compartment pharmacokinetics and its half-life of 22 hours[41]. We currently infuse phenytoin at a maximum rate of 50 mg/minute i.v. for an initial dose of 350 mg. This results in an average plasma level of 10 μg/ml for approximately 20 minutes. If this initial dose successfully controls the ventricular arrhythmia, an additional 650 mg (total loading dose of 1000 mg) is infused over the next one hour period at a rate of 100 mg/10 minutes. If the initial 350 mg infusion does not result in arrhythmia control, the additional 650 mg of phenytoin can be infused at 50 mg/minute while the patient is monitored for neurotoxicity and hypotension. The transition to chronic phenytoin therapy is accomplished by giving 500 mg orally or by slow i.v. infusion (100 mg/10 minutes) on the subsequent day[42]. Daily doses thereafter will vary from 300–400 mg depending on the patient's body weight, liver function, and the plasma level required[42].

Although several studies have shown that disopyramide can prophylactically suppress ventricular arrhythmias in the setting of acute myocardial infarction[29-31], none report its effectiveness in controlling recurrent or refractory ventricular tachycardia. Hence, its use in these settings is empiric at the present time, but disopyramide does offer the clinician another type I antiarrhythmic agent from which to choose and tailor therapy. Because of disopyramide's negative inotropic properties it is contraindicated in patients with congestive heart failure[43,44]. In a similar manner, propranolol has an undefined position in the treatment of refractory ventricular arrhythmias in the patient with an acute myocardial infarction. Although ventricular arrhythmias secondary to catecholamine excess may respond to propranolol[45,46] studies to evaluate the anti-arrhythmic effectiveness of propranolol during the hospital phase of acute myocardial infarction have been directed at delineating propranolol's prophylactic efficacy[47,48]. These studies revealed that in a controlled double-blind protocol, propranolol, in dosages of 20 mg orally every 6 hours, did not affect the incidence of ventricular arrhythmias in patients with acute myocardial infarction. Since these studies did not assess the efficacy of high dose propranolol in the treatment of refractory life-threatening arrhythmias, it should not be dismissed as a possible antiarrhythmic agent. Propranolol does have the advantages of being available in a parenteral form and of possibly improving ongoing ischaemia[49]. At present, we employ propranolol in a dose of 0.15–0.20 mg/kg given at a maximum rate of 1.0 mg/min i.v. in patients whose ventricular tachycardia is refractory to lignocaine and procainamide and who present with no or mild evidence of congestive heart failure. When given orally for maintenance therapy the dose of propranolol required to achieve an equivalent effect may be 8–10 times the i.v. dose[49]. This results primarily from the drug's first pass metabolism by the liver after being absorbed from the gastrointestinal tract following oral administration.

Bretylium tosylate has also shown promise in treating episodes of refractory ventricular tachycardia in the setting of acute myocardial infarction. Several uncontrolled clinical series have been published and report that approximately 60–70% of patients with ventricular tachycardia refractory to conventional antiarrhythmics responded to bretylium therapy in dosages of 5 mg/kg i.v. or i.m.[50-52]. Maintenance therapy was provided by a 3–5 mg/kg dose given i.m. every 6–8 hours, or by a constant i.v. infusion of 2–4 mg/min. Long-term therapy with bretylium tosylate has been limited by the drug's undesirable side-effect of orthostatic hypotension.

Occasionally, ventricular tachycardia may be preceded by brady-arrhythmias in the setting of acute myocardial infarction[53]. Since the dispersion of repolarization is greater with longer cycle length in the setting of myocardial ischaemia, such bradyarrhythmias may produce a milieu for initiation of ventricular tachycardia[54]. Treatment of ventricular tachycardia preceded by bradyarrhythmias requires an increase in the basic heart rate, and if such increases cannot be maintained by atropine, ventricular pacing at proper rates may be beneficial. In general, ventricular ectopy unrelated to bradycardia will not be suppressed by right ventricular pacing. A temporary ventricular pacemaker can on occasion be used to overdrive ventricular tachycardia, when the rate of the ventricular tachycardia is reasonably slow, less than 170[55]. However, such overdrive manoeuvres may result in worsening ischaemia or overdrive acceleration resulting in ventricular fibrillation[56]. Pacing modalities should only be employed by those experienced in its use. We therefore recommend that ventricular pacing be used only when bradycardia results in ventricular irritability and the brady-arrhythmia is unresponsive to standard pharmacological treatment. If ventricular tachycardia is recurrent despite maximum antiarrhythmic therapy, a trial of ventricular overdrive pacing may be warranted in some patients. Figure 13.1 illustrates in a flow diagram form our general approach to the patient with recurrent ventricular tachycardia in the setting of acute myocardial infarction. The specifics of the indicated drug therapy on the diagram are explained in detail in the above text.

Although most forms of ventricular tachycardia encountered in the setting of acute myocardial infarction are considered life threatening, the appearance of an accelerated idioventricular rhythm (slow ventricular tachycardia) is generally considered benign[57,58]. This type of arrhythmia is characterized electrocardiographically by wide bizarre QRS complexes occurring in short paroxysms of 3–30 complexes at rates varying from 70–110 beats/min. The first QRS complex of the arrhythmia is commonly a fusion beat because of the long coupling interval of the ectopic complex. Accelerated idioventricular rhythms occur in 9–23% of patients with acute myocardial infarction, and may be associated with a bradyarrhythmia, i.e. a slow heart rate allows for the escape of a ventricular or fascicular rhythm[59,60]. Norris et al. reported 94 cases of accelerated idioventricular rhythm in 1000 monitored patients with acute myocardial infarction, and noted it was twice as common in patients with inferior myocardial infarction than in those with anterior infarction[60]. Whereas 52% of patients with ventricular tachycardia in the study group had associated ventricular fibrillation, Norris et al. found that only 12% of patients with accelerated idioventricular rhythm had an episode of ventricular fibrillation. Furthermore, they stated that the hospital mortality for patients with accelerated idioventricular rhythm was no different than the expected mortality in their coronary care unit (18%). Hence, accelerated idioventricular rhythms are usually benign self-limited arrhythmias that rarely compromise left ventricular function, and do not require routine suppressive treatment. We currently recommend treatment of idioventricular rhythms when haemodynamic compromise results from either: (1) acceleration of the idioventricular rhythm (rates >120 beats/min) or (2) loss of the atrial kick without a concomitant acceleration of the idioventricular rhythm. In the first instance both lignocaine and type I antiarrhythmic agents have been reported to be effective in terminating the arrhythmia[60]. In the latter case, atropine may suppress the arrhythmia by increasing the underlying sinus rate[60,61]. An initial atropine dose of 0.5 mg will have a similar effect on the sinus rate as larger doses with a lower incidence of major adverse side-effects (sustained sinus tachycardia, ventricular tachycardia or toxic psychosis)[61]. On occasion additional doses of 0.5 mg may be required to maintain an adequate sinus rate. With this protocol, Scheinman et al.[61] successfully treated 13 of 14 episodes of idioventricular rhythm encountered in their coronary care unit.

When ventricular fibrillation is encountered, direct current cardioversion is the most effective means of therapy. However, recent publications are in disagreement over the optimal energy level required for defibrillation[62]. Tacker et al.[63-65] in a combined retrospective clinical trial and experimental rabbit study found that '300 watt seconds of maximum energy delivered by commercial defibrillators was insufficient to convert 35% of subjects

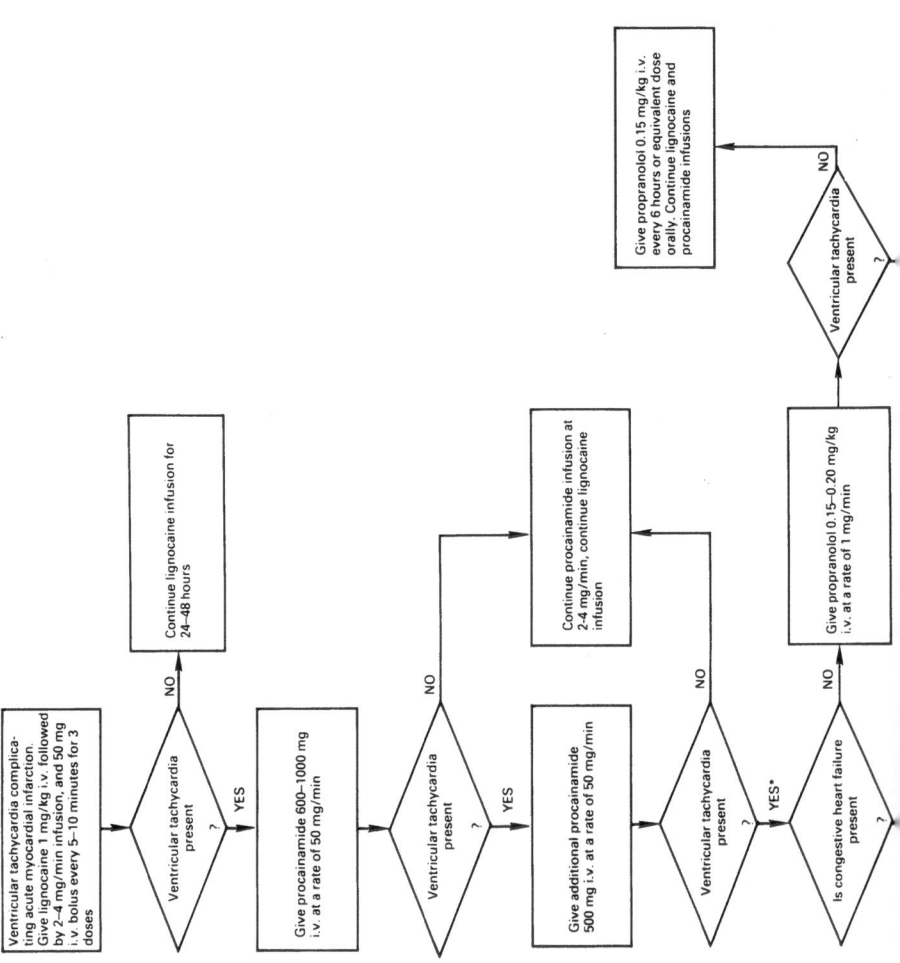

Figure 13.1 Treatment of ventricular tachycardia in acute myocardial infarction

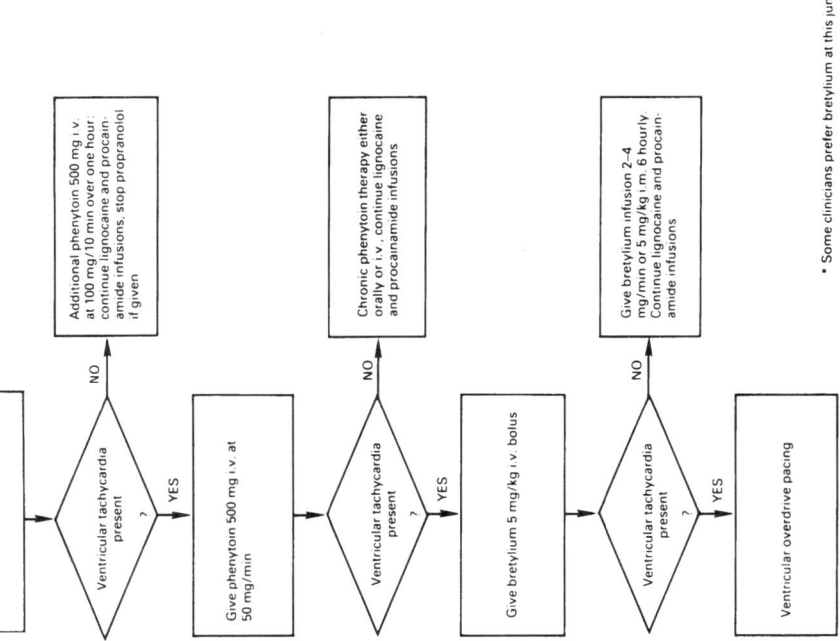

* Some clinicians prefer bretylium at this juncture

Additional phenytoin 500 mg i.v. at 100 mg/10 min over one hour; continue lignocaine and procainamide infusions; stop propranolol if given

Ventricular tachycardia present ?

NO

YES

Give phenytoin 500 mg i.v. at 50 mg/min

Chronic phenytoin therapy either orally or i.v.; continue lignocaine and procainamide infusions

Ventricular tachycardia present ?

NO

YES

Give bretylium 5 mg/kg i.v. bolus

Give bretylium infusion 2–4 mg/min or 5 mg/kg i.m. 6 hourly. Continue lignocaine and procainamide infusions

Ventricular tachycardia present ?

NO

YES

Ventricular overdrive pacing

289

weighing greater than 50 kg and was ineffective in 60% of patients weighing 90–100 kg'. Based on this data, several investigators advocated employment of equipment capable of providing 500–1000 J (watt seconds) of stored energy. The use of higher energy is not without risk in that animal studies have demonstrated that the higher energy levels are associated with greater myocardial damage and increased post-defibrillation arrhythmias[66–68].

In 1977 and 1978, Pantridge and associates published their experience employing 200 J of stored energy in attempted countershock of 233 episodes of ventricular fibrillation in 120 patients[69,70]. In 199 incidences (85%) a single shock was successful, and 95% of episodes were successfully converted by up to three 200 J shocks. In the few patients who were refractory to 200 J shocks, a 400 J shock was always successful. In this group, 90% of patients had coronary artery disease, 65% had primary ventricular fibrillation, and 74% of the episodes were present for 2 minutes or less. This experience is similar to Lown's in which 95% of 253 episodes of ventricular fibrillation were consistently converted with 196 J of delivered energy[71]. Within this group, the same energy level was successful in converting 45 out of 46 episodes of ventricular fibrillation in 12 patients weighing an average of 107 kg.

Unsuccessful defibrillation may not be related solely to the body weight and the amount of delivered energy but rather secondary to other factors. Some of these factors have been evaluated in a retrospective clinical study by Kerber et al.[72] in 52 cases of emergency ventricular fibrillation. 38 patients were successfully defibrillated (73%), but only one of two patients weighing greater than 100 kg was successfully defibrillated. When the successfully defibrillated group was compared to those not converted to a stable rhythm, the following factors were found to adversely affect successful defibrillation: (1) prolonged delay before the first defibrillatory shock (7 minutes in the successful group versus 17 minutes in the unsuccessful group), (2) acidosis (pH = 7.36 in the successful group versus 7.23 in the unsuccessful group) and (3) hypoxia ($PaO_2 = 13.3$ kPa (100 mmHg) in the successfully converted group versus $PaO_2 = 5.3$ kPa (40 mmHg in the unsuccessful group). Body weight, energy delivered per body weight, and energy delivered per heart weight were not determinants of successful defibrillation. From this data we recommend that defibrillation be attempted employing 200 J of stored energy and that this be repeated once if initially unsuccessful before employing a higher energy level. In addition, efforts to correct hypoxia, acidosis, and other metabolic abnormalities should be carried out simultaneously.

Despite optimal conditions, resistant ventricular fibrillation is not an uncommon clinical setting encountered by physicians caring for critically ill patients. It was noted to occur in 8% of in-hospital cardiac arrests at one large university teaching hospital, and formed the basis for a clinical study on the effectiveness of bretylium tosylate in resistant ventricular fibrillation[73]. Holder *et al.*[73] reported on 27 cases of ventricular fibrillation which were completely resistant to conventional forms of electrical and pharmacological resuscitative therapy over a 30 minute period. All patients were initially treated during the first 10 minutes with at least two bolus injections of 100 mg of lignocaine, and direct current countershocks with 400 J of stored energy. Over the second 10 minute period, either procainamide, propranolol, or phenytoin was given i.v. and strict attention was given to ventilation and acid–base balance. Despite 20 minutes of sustained closed-chest cardiac massage and the above measures, ventricular fibrillation persisted in all 27 patients. Bretylium tosylate was then given as a single 5 mg/kg i.v. bolus injection and standard resuscitative efforts continued for an additional 15 minutes. In 20 of the 27 patients, electrical cardioversion of the ventricular fibrillation was facilitated (within an average of 10 minutes), with only one and rarely more than two direct current countershocks being required subsequent to the bretylium bolus. More significantly, 12 of these 20 patients survived to leave the hospital. Although complete evaluation in the setting of cardiac arrest is pending, we currently employ bretylium tosylate in a 5 mg/kg i.v. dose for refractory ventricular fibrillation, if standard resuscitative measures do not result in a stable rhythm within 15 to 20 minutes. If the resuscitation is successful, bretylium is administered as a constant infusion at 2–4 mg/minute for an additional 24 hours.

(2) Supraventricular arrhythmias

Although ventricular tachyarrhythmias hold a position of primary importance in acute myocardial infarction, numerous supraventricular tachyarrhythmias occur in this setting. This section will discuss the prognostic implications and therapeutic interventions of these arrhythmias. Sinus tachycardia has an incidence of 8–50%, and transient sinus tachycardia during the early phase of acute myocardial infarction is probably clinically insignificant[1,3,4]. However, persistent sinus tachycardia, i.e. heart rate greater than 100 for more than 24–48 hours, has a very poor prognosis[3,4,74]. Although sinus tachycardia may be secondary to fever, pericarditis, pulmonary embolism, hyperdynamic circulation, or volume depletion, it is usually secondary to increased sympathetic adrenergic drive initiated by left ventricular failure. Whereas the former causes are readily treatable, extensive infarction with congestive heart failure carries a grave prognosis. Thus, sinus tachycardia in the setting of acute myocardial infarction requires no treatment *per se*, but a careful search for and treatment of its cause should be undertaken.

Atrial arrhythmias frequently occur in the setting of acute myocardial infarction. The incidence of atrial premature contractions has been reported to be 30%[1]. Since they may lead to atrial tachycardia, fibrillation, or flutter, some authors recommend treatment of frequent atrial premature contractions (greater than 6/minute) with a type I antiarrhythmic agent[75]. At the present time we do not treat frequent atrial premature contractions unless there is a prior history of atrial tachyarrhythmia. Atrial tachycardia occurs uncommonly during acute myocardial infarction with an incidence of 4–8%, and may be associated with digitalis toxicity or coexisting pulmonary disease[1,4]. The appropriate therapy would then depend on its aetiology, but in cases where digitalis toxicity is not present, digitalis therapy may control the ventricular response by decreasing AV nodal conduction. A type I antiarrhythmic agent (quinidine, procainamide, or disopyramide) may then be employed in an attempt to convert the atrial arrhythmia to a sinus rhythm.

Atrial flutter is a rare arrhythmia in the setting of acute myocardial infarction with a reported incidence of 1–2%[1,3,76]. Because 2:1 AV block usually accompanies atrial flutter, the ventricular rate varies from 150 to 175 beats/minute and often exacerbates ischaemia or precipitates heart failure. Atrial flutter readily responds to low energy direct current cardioversion (25 J or less) and this is the treatment of choice for patients with ongoing ischaemia or haemodynamic compromise[77]. If the clinical situation is non-urgent, digoxin, propranolol, or verapamil intravenously, can be used to enhance AV nodal blockade and slow the ventricular response. If after AV nodal blockade the arrhythmia persists, treatment with a type I antiarrhythmic agent may be utilized in an attempt to terminate the arrhythmia. Because type I drugs often slow the atrial flutter rate, and decrease concealed AV nodal conduction, and hence facilitate AV conduction, they should not be employed without prior treatment with an AV nodal blocking agent for fear that the ventricular response may increase. Although Waldo et al.[78] have shown atrial overdrive pacing to be an effective measure in terminating episodes of atrial flutter in the post-operative open heart patient, its efficacy in the setting of acute myocardial infarction has not been demonstrated. Because atrial flutter does not usually recur after its conversion to sinus rhythm, we currently employ low energy direct current cardioversion in all acute myocardial infarction patients with this rare arrhythmia.

The incidence of atrial fibrillation in the setting of acute myocardial infarction varies from 6 to 16%[1,76]. As with atrial flutter, untreated atrial fibrillation is usually accompanied by a rapid ventricular rate, 120–150 beats/minute, and may precipitate angina, congestive heart failure, or infarct extension[79]. If severe haemodynamic compromise or ongoing ischaemia is present, atrial fibrillation should be treated promptly with direct current cardioversion employing higher energies than those recommended for atrial flutter, i.e. 100–400 J. In most patients, atrial fibrillation can be initially treated with i.v. AV nodal blocking agents such as digoxin or propranolol in order to control the ventricular response. After control has been obtained, a type I agent may be added if conversion to normal sinus rhythm is the objective. Recently, Hagemeijer[80] reported the use of i.v. verapamil in treating atrial fibrillation in the setting of acute myocardial infarction. Eight patients without congestive heart failure who developed sustained (greater than 20 minutes) atrial fibrillation with rapid (greater than 100 beats/minute) ventricular response during the first 72 hours after acute myocardial infarction were treated with 1 mg increments of verapamil at 1 minute intervals to a maximum dose of 20 mg. Therapeutic end points included either a ventricular rate less than 100 beats/min or reversion to normal sinus rhythm. Prior to verapamil therapy, the average ventricular response for the group was approximately 160 beats/min. After an average dose of 12 mg of verapamil, one patient reverted to normal sinus rhythm and the average ventricular response of the remaining seven patients fell to 93 beats/min. After digitalization an additional four patients reverted to normal sinus rhythm. Thus, verapamil appears to be an effective and rapid acting agent in controlling the ventricular rate in atrial fibrillation, but further testing in the setting of acute myocardial infarction, especially in those patients with congestive heart failure, is needed before its safety is established.

Junctional tachyarrhythmias do occur in the setting of acute myocardial infarction but their true incidence is not known[81,82]. Non-paroxysmal AV junctional tachycardia with a rate of 70–130 beats/min occurs with an incidence of approximately 10% and is more commonly associated with acute inferior myocardial infarction[83,84]. Knoecke et al.[84] observed 21 instances of non-paroxysmal junctional tachycardia in 203 consecutive patients with acute myocardial infarction. The arrhythmia itself was usually transient and self-limited, and the clinical course of the patient was dependent on the severity of the infarction. All 13 patients with associated cardiogenic shock expired, whereas eight patients with an uncomplicated infarction survived. Paroxysmal junctional tachycardia is uncommon, but because the rate is usually rapid, 160–220 beats/min, it carries the same clinical significance and treatment recommendations as paroxysmal atrial tachycardia[81,82].

Bradyarrhythmias in the setting of acute myocardial infarction may occur as a result of two separate mechanisms: (1) abnormalities of impulse formation in, or conduction abnormalities out of, the sinoatrial node and (2) failure of atrial impulses to propagate over the conduction system to the ventricles. The clinical course and prognosis of these two types of disorders depends upon the location of the obstructive disease in the coronary circulation and its effect on the conducting system and left ventricular function. Detailed descriptions of the coronary supply to the conducting system of the heart have been reported in several studies, and only the major points will be reiterated[85,86]. The coronary artery that supplies the sinoatrial node originates as a proximal branch of the right coronary artery in 55% of patients and as a proximal branch of the left circumflex coronary artery in 45% of patients[85]. The AV nodal artery arises from the distal right coronary in 90% of patients and as a branch of the left circumflex coronary artery in the remaining 10%[85]. The interventricular septum on the other hand has a dual blood supply. The posterior basal segment of the septum is supplied by the posterior descending coronary artery, usually as a branch of the right coronary artery, while the left anterior descending coronary artery supplies the anterior basal segment and much of the body of the interventricular septum[85]. These two arterial supplies have a rich network of anastomoses within the body of the interventricular septum and thus the effects of occlusive disease of one artery or the other is variable and unpredictable.

The sinus node is normally the dominant cardiac pacemaker. Conduction of the sinus impulse through the atria, AV node, bundle of His, and bundle branches results in ventricular depolarization and myocardial contraction. Alteration of the conduction system by ischaemia or infarction may result in life threatening bradyarrhythmias. Dysfunction of impulse formation within the sinoatrial node during acute myocardial infarction is a frequent cause of bradycardia. If the sinus rate slows sufficiently, an escape rhythm usually located in the AV node or junction becomes manifest[87]. Sinus bradycardia is usually a consequence of inferior wall myocardial infarction and is felt to be secondary either to sinoatrial node ischaemia or infarction, or secondary to reflex cholinergic suppression of sinoatrial nodal activity[88-90]. The incidence of sinus bradycardia ranges from 10 to 30% in monitored patients, and is encountered three times more frequently during inferior myocardial infarctions than with anterior infarctions[3,4,13,76,88]. Sinus bradycardia *per se* is not associated with an increase in mortality but may require treatment if the bradycardia is associated with hypotension, heart failure, ventricular irritability, or extremely slow heart rates[13]. Rotman *et al.* reported ten patients with sinus bradycardia and hypotension who responded promptly to i.v. atropine with an increase in both heart rate and blood pressure[13]. Further maintenance doses of atropine were not required and recurrent episodes of sinus bradycardia occurred in only 20% of patients. Similar results were reported by Scheinman *et al.*[61] in 17 patients with bradycardia (average rate 58 beats/minute) and hypotension (average blood pressure of 77 mmHg systolic) in the setting of acute myocardial infarction. After treatment with atropine, 15 of 17 patients had normalization of both the blood pressure (average post atropine of 115 mmHg systolic) and pulse rate (average post atropine 85 beats/min).

Sinus node dysfunction during acute myocardial infarction may also result in sinus pauses or exit block. Sinus exit block is rare during acute infarction and is usually secondary to digitalis excess or secondary to underlying sinus node disease[13]. Sinus pauses, however, are not uncommon. Rotman *et al.* noted a 4% incidence of sudden pauses in a series of 537 monitored patients with acute myocardial infarction[13]. Of their 20 patients with sinus pauses, five had associated AV block and only two required permanent pacing for recurrent sinus pauses.

(3) AV conduction abnormalities

Failure of a sinus or supraventricular impulse to propagate to the ventricles is the major cause of bradycardia in patients with acute myocardial infarction. Block of impulse conduction may occur at the AV node, bundle of His, or bundle branches of the Purkinjé system. Whenever there is a failure of AV conduction, a pause in the ventricular rhythm occurs until either an escape pacemaker rhythm emerges or normal AV conduction returns. Since the escape rhythm varies from 40–60 beats/minute for the AV nodal pacemakers to 20–30 beats/min for infra-Hisian escape rhythms, clinical sequelae usually depend in part on the site of the emerging pacemaker and more importantly on the rate of the escape rhythm.

Because the AV node and inferior myocardial wall are supplied by branches of the distal right coronary artery, AV nodal block is usually secondary to acute inferior wall infarctions[85,86]. When the AV node is the site of block, progressive prolongation of the PR interval and Wenckebach AV block are usually noted prior to the occurrence of complete AV block[6]. Because of its responsiveness to autonomic tone, AV nodal conduction may be enhanced by β-adrenergic agents such as isoprenaline or vagolytic agents such as atropine, and therefore these drugs may be used to treat AV block. If complete AV block does occur, the escape rhythm usually originates in the AV junction and maintains a ventricular rate of 40–55 beats/minute. In the majority of patients, this rhythm is stable and no haemodynamic consequences result[13]. However, in some patients, this rate may be too slow to maintain adequate peripheral perfusion or may predispose to ventricular arrhythmias[52,53]. In these instances, the escape pacemaker rhythm may be increased by the administration of atropine or low dose isoprenaline if its origin is within the AV junction, whereas escape pacemakers arising below the AV junction may respond to isoprenaline. The use of temporary pacemakers in the setting of inferior myocardial infarction and complete AV block remains somewhat controversial. For those patients in whom the block occurs within the AV node and the escape rhythm appears within the AV junction, we recommend temporary pacing only if one of the following occurs: (1) evidence of left ventricular failure, (2) syncope, (3) angina, (4) ventricular irritability or (5) severe bradycardia unresponsive to drugs[13]. If required, pacing is continued until AV conduction returns to normal, which in some cases may take up to 2 weeks[60].

When AV block occurs in the His–Purkinjé system, its onset is often sudden, and because the escape pacemakers located below the His bundle are slow and unstable, the resultant bradycardia is more marked[91]. These idioventricular escape rhythms have varying responses to the emergency drug administration of isoprenaline and adequate treatment requires immediate placement of a temporary pacemaker. Occasionally, complete AV block within the His–Purkinjé system is heralded by the occurrence of Mobitz type II second degree AV block, defined as constant PR intervals of conducted beats prior to block of a sinus impulse[91,92]. When Mobitz type II block is noted in the setting of acute myocardial infarction, preparation for the prophylactic insertion of a temporary pacemaker should be made. Therefore AV block within the His–Purkinjé system differs significantly from block within the AV node in regards to several important electrophysiological and clinical characteristics. These differences are summarized in Table 13.1.

Table 13.1 Comparison of high degree atrioventricular block in relation to the anatomical site of block in acute myocardial infarction

Characteristic	Block within the AV node	Block within the His-Purkinjé system
Incidence	5–10%	1–3%
Location of infarction	usually inferior infarction	anterior infarction much more common than inferior infarction
Pathology	ischaemia or infarction of the AV node, or cholinergic suppression of AV node	infarction of the interventricular septum and bundle branches
Mortality	20–40%	70–80%
Associated conduction abnormalities	1° AV block, Wenckebach AV block (Mobitz type I)	Mobitz type II AV block
Site of the escape rhythm	AV node or His bundle	below the bundle of His
Rate of the escape rhythm during complete heart block	40–60 beats/min, usually stable rhythm	25–45 beats/min, unstable rhythm with sudden asystole not uncommon
Scalar ECG QRS duration	in 80% of cases QRS $\langle 0.12$ s	in 90% of cases QRS $\rangle 0.12$ s
Haemodynamic consequence of block	patient usually tolerates escape rhythm well	patient tolerates escape rhythm poorly

(4) Bundle branch block complicating acute myocardial infarction

When AV block occurs within the His–Purkinjé system, it is usually associated with the appearance of bundle branch block pattern in the scalar electrocardiogram[91]. Rosenbaum and Hecht have previously reported criteria for defining the presence and type of intraventricular defect from the scalar electrocardiogram[93,94]. Their classification of conduction defects divides the intraventricular conduction system into three fascicles, a right bundle branch, and a left bundle branch with anterior and posterior divisions. Although several investigators have noted an increased risk of complete heart block and sudden death in patients with bundle branch block[7,9], it was not until recently that the clinical significance of bundle branch block complicating acute myocardial infarction was studied on a large scale.

Hindman et al.[91] in a multicentre study reviewed the clinical characteristics of patients with acute myocardial infarction and bundle branch block. Patients who developed bundle branch block after the onset of cardiogenic shock were excluded from their study. In all, 432 patients from five different medical centres were included in the study group and all survivors of the acute event had at least 1 year of follow-up. Hospital mortality was 28% and for those surviving hospitalization the 1 year mortality was 28%. Table 13.2 shows the incidence of the various types of bundle branch block, and the in-hospital mortality for each group of bundle branch block.

Table 13.2 Incidence and hospital mortality in 432 patients with acute myocardial infarction complicated by bundle branch block.*

Type of block	No. of patients	Percent of patients	Hospital mortality %
LBBB	163	38	24
RBBB	48	11	22
RBBB + LAFB	149	34	29
RBBB + LPFB	45	10	38
Alternating BBB	27	6	44
Total	432	100	28

Abbreviations: BBB = bundle branch block, LAFB = left anterior fascicular block, LBBB = left bundle branch block, LPFB = left posterior fascicular block, RBBB = right bundle branch block.

* Adapted from Hindman et al.[91]

Of interest is the fact that 208 patients (48%) maintained normal AV conduction during their acute myocardial infarction and an additional 101 patients (23%) developed at worse first degree AV block. 95 patients (22%) progressed to high degree AV block as defined by either Mobitz type II AV block (7 patients), Mobitz type II AV block progressing to third degree AV block (26 patients) and sudden third degree AV block (62 patients). Over one third of the patients who developed complete AV block during their hospital course did so suddenly without prior first degree or second degree AV block. Thus, as Hindman et al.[91] point out 'an interventricular conduction disturbance may be the only warning of jeopardized AV conduction and impending precipitous complete heart block'. This point is emphasized by one subgroup of 36 patients which included those who had high degree AV block and at worse Killip Class II congestive heart failure. Of 11 deaths (31%) recorded in this group, 10 occurred suddenly as a result of sudden progression to high degree AV block[91,95].

In order to prevent this increase in mortality secondary to sudden unexpected progression to high degree AV block in otherwise stable patients, Hindman et al.[95] analysed the hospital and outpatient courses of their patients in order to identify high risk groups which might benefit from prophylactic temporary and permanent pacemaker placement. As noted above, 95 patients in the study group progressed to high degree AV block. The interaction of the PR interval, type of bundle branch block, and the onset of the bundle branch block appeared to be the three variables most predictive of progression to high degree AV block. For purposes of definition, first degree AV block was defined as a PR interval greater than 0.20 seconds and the type of bundle branch block included (1) bilateral bundle branch block (right bundle branch block and left anterior hemiblock, or right bundle branch block and left posterior hemiblock, or alternating bundle branch block) and (2) bundle branch block (right bundle branch block or left bundle branch block). The onset of bundle branch block was defined as either (a) definitely old – block present on an electrocardiogram antedating infarction, (b) possibly new – block present on first electrocardiogram with infarction but no old electrocardiogram available for comparison, (c) probably new – block present on first electrocardiogram with infarction but absent on electrocardiograms taken within 2 years, and (d) definitely new – block which develops in the hospital documented by serial tracings. Table 13.3 demonstrates the interaction of these variables in predicting progression to high degree AV block. Patients with new bilateral bundle branch block regardless of PR interval are at high risk to progression (31–38%), whereas patients with old bundle branch block regardless of PR interval are at low risk (9–13%). Patients with new bundle branch block and normal PR interval have an 11% risk which increases to 19% if there is associated first degree AV block. Consequently Hindman et al.[95] recommend temporary prophylactic pacemaker insertion in patients in the high risk group of new bilateral bundle branch block but do not recommend this procedure for patients in the low risk group ($\leq 13\%$ risk of progression to high degree AV block). We concur with these recommendations and suggest that physicians weigh the risk at their hospital of temporary pacemaker insertion versus the risk of progression to high degree AV block in deciding a course of action for those patients with intermediate risk. At our institution we currently also insert temporary pacemakers in the groups of patients with new bundle branch block and first degree AV block, or with old bilateral bundle branch block and first degree AV block (intermediate risk of 19–20%).

Table 13.3   Risk of progression to high degree atrioventricular block: influence of PR interval and the type and age of bundle branch block.*

Age	Type of BBB	PR ≤ 0.20 s	PR > 0.20 s
Old	RBBB or LBBB	3/33 (9%)	3/23 (13%)
Old	RBBB + LAFB or RBBB + LPFB or Alternating BBB	2/20 (10%)	3/15 (20%)
New	RBBB or LBBB	10/92 (11%)	12/63 (19%)
New	RBBB + LAFB or RBBB + LPFB or Alternating BBB	36/117 (31%)	26/69 (38%)

Age: Old = Bundle branch block present in previous electrocardiogram, New = bundle branch block not present on previous electrocardiogram or no old electrocardiogram available.
Denominator represents total number of patients within a classification. Numerator represents the number of patients progressing to high degree AV block. Abbreviations: BBB = bundle branch block, LAFB = left anterior fascicular block, LBBB = left bundle branch block, LPFB = left posterior fascicular block, RBBB = right bundle branch block.

* Adapted from Hindman et al.[91,95]

Although patients who develop complete heart block in the setting of acute myocardial infarction and bundle branch block have a high in-hospital mortality (48%), an equal number survive to be discharged and often have reverted to normal AV conduction prior to hospital discharge[91,95]. Until recently, many such patients were discharged without permanent pacemaker insertion, but the combined reports by Atkins, Scanlon, and Waugh in the early 1970s revealed that 17 of 22 such patients experienced either sudden death or recurrent high degree AV block within 1 year[7,8,96]. Hindman et al.[95] confirmed this finding during the follow-up of patients who experienced high degree AV block during acute myocardial infarction complicated by bundle branch block. Of 26 such patients who

299

were discharged with normal AV conduction but no permanent pacemaker, seven had documented recurrent high degree AV block and ten died suddenly. In a group of 29 patients who received permanent pacemakers, the incidence of documented recurrent high degree AV block was 0% whereas sudden death within 1 year occurred in only 10% of patients. Based on this data, Hindman et al.[91,95] recommend that all patients with acute myocardial infarction complicated by bundle branch block and high degree AV block have permanent pacemakers placed prior to hospital discharge, irrespective of whether normal AV conduction has returned. Although we concur with this general approach, several related points should be noted: (1) Hindman et al.[95] did not control for other factors related to sudden death (recurrent angina, congestive heart failure, and complex ventricular ectopic beats, etc.) during the follow-up of the two groups of patients surviving transient high degree AV block. (2) Lie et al.[97] have demonstrated that patients with anterior myocardial infarction and bundle branch block have an increased early mortality secondary to ventricular fibrillation. (3) Despite transient high degree AV block a few patients will have normal AV conduction and resolution of the associated bundle branch block on a subsequent scalar electrocardiogram. The proper management of these patients in regards to permanent pacemaker therapy is not known.

Permanent pacing is not required for patients discharged with normal AV conduction in whom progression to high degree AV block was via a Mobitz type I pattern. Although the absolute number of patients within this group is small, long-term follow-up demonstrated no evidence for an increased incidence of sudden death or recurrence of AV block[95].

(5) Late hospital phase ventricular arrhythmias

The discussion to this point has centred on the various arrhythmias and conduction disturbances encountered in the early stages of acute myocardial infarction. The arrhythmia that has attracted the most attention in the late hospital phase of acute myocardial infarction are premature ventricular contractions. Despite numerous studies, the prognostic significance and treatment of late ventricular arrhythmias in patients surviving acute myocardial infarction remains controversial. Numerous studies have found that certain ventricular ectopic beat characteristics recorded in patients surviving acute myocardial infarction are associated with subsequent cardiac mortality[98-100]. Specifically, complex ventricular ectopic beat patterns including bigeminal, multiform, repetitive, and early ventricular ectopic beats were associated with an increased incidence of sudden death post-infarction[98,99]. However, major problems appear when the above studies are critically reviewed. The Coronary Drug Project study evaluated 2035 men, 3–36 months post infarction with a resting electrocardiogram recording an average of 50 beats/patient. In addition, all men were in functional class I or II with no recent worsening of cardiac symptoms (angina or congestive heart failure). The Project reported that in a 3 year follow-up, sudden death was more frequent in men with frequent, repetitive, and possibly early ventricular ectopics, irrespective of other clinical characteristics such as angina, congestive heart failure and hypotension. This study used a brief period of monitoring (thus capturing only a fraction of the arrhythmias), selected men only, and more importantly, evaluated patients an average of 36 months post infarction. Ruberman et al.[99], in a similar study, evaluated 1739 men with 1 hour of electrocardiogram monitoring at varying time intervals after the last myocardial infarction. 50% of the patients had experienced the last infarction within the 3 months before the monitoring, 30% within 3–8 months prior to monitoring, and the remaining 20% 9 months or more after the last infarction. Patients were followed for up to 4 years with an average follow-up of 2 years. Ruberman's conclusions paralleled those of the Coronary Drug Project, i.e. complex ventricular ectopic patterns were associated with an increased risk of sudden death, whereas simple ventricular ectopic patterns, even when frequent, were not associated with an increased incidence of sudden death. The drawbacks however were also similar. The brief monitoring period, the hiatus from last infarction to monitoring, and the all male population prevents direct application of these conclusions to the post-coronary care of ventricular arrhythmias of patients with acute myocardial infarction.

Perhaps the best data available addressing this problem is provided by Moss et al.[101], in a recently published study of 940 survivors of acute myocardial infarction who underwent a 6 hour period of continuous electrocardiographic monitoring prior to hospital discharge. Patients were followed for an average of 36 months and 98 witnessed cardiac deaths occurred, 55 of which were sudden ($\leq$ 1 hour). Using the same criteria as Ruberman, Moss et al. noted that patients with complex ventricular ectopic beats had an increased likelihood of both sudden and non-sudden cardiac death. Within the complex category a high ventricular ectopic frequency (≥ 20/hour) was not associated with an increased mortality when compared with patients with a low ectopic frequency (≤ 20/hour). When significant clinical parameters were controlled (such as age, history of angina, congestive heart failure, etc.) complex ventricular ectopic beats were noted to have an independent role in the follow-up mortality. In contrast, Moss et al. noted no difference in follow-up mortality rates for those patients with simple ventricular ectopic beats as compared to those with no ventricular ectopic beats.

Although complex ventricular ectopic beats appear to have prognostic importance by themselves, it is difficult to separate them from the other factors associated with an increased likelihood of sudden death. Schulze et al.[102] demonstrated this in a prospective study of 81 patients discharged from the coronary care unit with a diagnosis of acute myocardial infarction. All patients underwent 24 hours of continuous electrocardiographic monitoring prior to discharge and had left ventricular function evaluated by a gated nuclear blood pool scan. Of 45 patients with an ejection fraction less than 40%, 26 had recorded complex ventricular patterns, and 8 of the 26 died suddenly during the follow-up period (mean of 7 months). In the 19 patients with a similar ejection fraction but no complex ectopic patterns there were no recorded sudden deaths. There were no recorded instances of sudden death in the 36 patients with good left ventricular function (ejection fraction ⟩40%) regardless of ventricular ectopic pattern. Hence, Schulze *et al.* concluded that complex ventricular ectopic patterns may have prognostic significance only within certain subgroups of patients.

In spite of the above limitations, we currently obtain continuous 24 hour electrocardiographic recordings on all post infarction patients prior to hospital discharge. Those with complex ventricular ectopic patterns are treated with either propranolol or a type I antiarrhythmic agent. The dose and schedule is adjusted in order to obtain maximum suppression of complex ventricular ectopic beats with a minimum of side-effects. Patients are treated for a period of 6–12 months at which time the need for continued antiarrhythmic therapy is re-assessed by monitoring the electrocardiogram continuously for 24–48 hours after all antiarrhythmic agents have been discontinued. Patients demonstrating persistent complex ventricular ectopic beats are then candidates for continued antiarrhythmic therapy. Although this clinical approach has not been proven effective, we feel it is a reasonable programme if the patient tolerates the prescribed drug without significant toxicity.

In conclusion, it appears that the in-hospital mortality of acute myocardial infarction can be favourably affected by proper recognition and treatment of not only ventricular tachyarrhythmias but also the bradyarrhythmias and conduction disturbances that the clinician encounters.

(II) HAEMODYNAMIC ABNORMALITIES AND THEIR CORRECTION

Continuous electrocardiographic monitoring, improved antiarrhythmic therapy and transvenous cardiac pacing have resulted in a reduction in mortality from primary arrhythmias and conduction disturbances in acute myocardial infarction. As a result, pump failure has emerged as a principal cause of death. In this section we review the techniques of haemodynamic monitoring and the use of haemodynamic parameters by placing patients in subsets for directing therapy of the low output state in acute myocardial infarction.

The most important advance in haemodynamic monitoring has been the introduction by Swan *et al.* of the balloon-tip flotation catheter[103]. These catheters can generally be inserted into the heart via a peripheral vein without fluoroscopy. Inflation of the balloon when the tip of the catheter is within the right atrium and advancing the catheter allows blood flow to carry it into the pulmonary artery. The balloon is deflated when the catheter is within the pulmonary artery and transiently re-inflated as necessary to occlude a branch of the pulmonary artery in order to provide a measurement of the downstream pulmonary artery occluded pressure, or as it is more generally termed, 'pulmonary capillary wedge pressure'.

The pulmonary capillary wedge pressure (PAWP) in most situations is an accurate indirect measure of left atrial pressure (left ventricular filling pressure). With the triple lumen model of flotation catheter with a distal thermistor, cardiac output measurements by thermodilution technique can be obtained[104,105]. Some of the latest models of flotation catheters have right atrial and ventricular electrodes, which may be used for emergency atrial, ventricular or A-V sequential pacing, as well as for intracardiac electrograms useful in the diagnosis of complex arrhythmias[106]. A small calibre intra-arterial catheter, usually inserted into the radial artery for accurate measurement of blood pressure in patients with low output state or shock, is preferred to eliminate the disparity between cuff blood pressure and actual arterial pressure. Thus, all the haemodynamic variables clinically important in the management of these critically ill patients (heart rate, arterial pressure, right and left ventricular filling pressures and cardiac output) are obtainable at the bedside.

The determination of PAWP and cardiac output allows characterization of left ventricular function. One of the most useful ways of utilizing the haemodynamic information available on a patient is the construction of a ventricular function curve, which is illustrated in Figure 13.2. In Figure 13.2 a representation of cardiac performance, a measure of ventricular function such as stroke work, stroke volume or cardiac output, is plotted as a function of some measure of preload, such as PAWP. Cardiac function is defined according to Starling's law of the heart, which states that the strength of cardiac contraction is proportional to myocardial fibre length (or size of ventricular volume) at the onset of contraction. The ventricular function curve has an ascending limb, which flattens out at approximately 15–20 mmHg. Studies on patients with acute infarction and the effects of volume loading and diuresis, suggest that the optimal left ventricular filling pressure is approximately 15–20 mmHg[107,108].

A uniform therapeutic approach is not possible for all patients with myocardial infarction. Cardiac function in patients with acute myocardial infarction is highly variable and may change in a matter of minutes. Cardiac function may range from normal to severely depressed with cardiogenic shock. By classifying patients into various haemodynamic subsets it is possible to formulate a rational approach to therapy. Table 13.4 illustrates one useful subset classification that can be applied to patients with acute myocardial infarction; others equally valuable have been suggested[109].

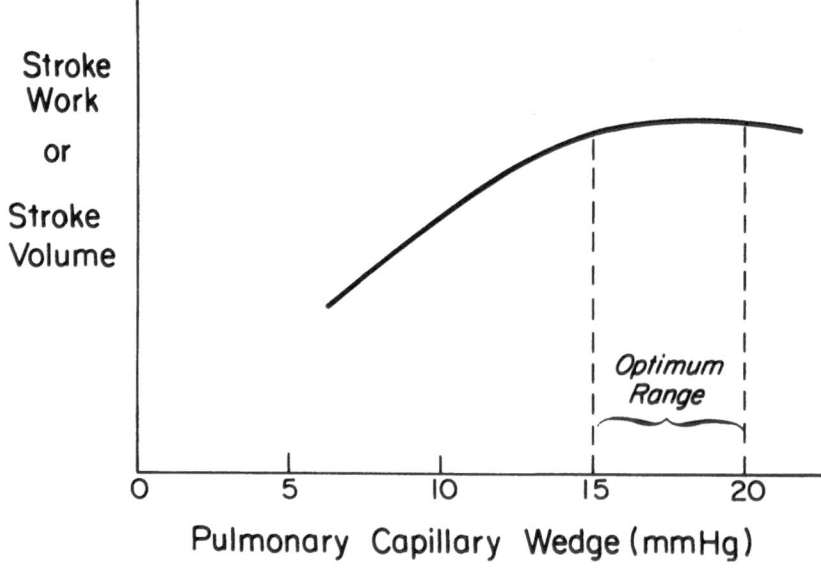

Figure 13.2 Ventricular function curve, constructed as a representation of cardiac performance

(1) Subset 1

Subset 1 represents those patients who have low left ventricular filling pressures and, as a result, low cardiac index and arterial pressure. Frank shock solely as a result of hypovolaemia is an uncommon complication of acute myocardial infarction. When encountered it is seen in those patients with severe diaphoresis and vomiting or in those patients who have received diuretics and/or nitrates. Patients with a low output state resulting from hypovolaemia need intravenous volume administration to raise their left ventricular filling pressure to optimal levels. In most patients the optimal level of PAWP (left ventricular filling pressure) ranges between 15 and 20 mmHg. Differences of opinion exist about the optimal level of left ventricular filling pressure in patients with acute myocardial infarction, because one study has shown maximum cardiac index at left ventricular end-diastolic pressures from 20 to 25 mmHg[110], and a second study has found maximum cardiac performance with pulmonary capillary wedge pressures between 14 and 18 mmHg[108]. These two studies may not be in con-

Table 13.4 Therapeutic subset classification in acute myocardial infarction

Subset	Systolic arterial pressure (mmHg)*	Left ventricle filling pressure (mmHg)*	Cardiac index (litre/min m²)*	Description	Therapy
1	<100	<10	<2.5	Hypovolaemic	Volume
2	100–150	>20	>2.5	Pulmonary congestion	Diuretics or nitrates
3	<100	10–20	>2.5	Peripheral vasodilation	None or vasopressors
4	<100	>20	<2.5	LV pump failure	Vasodilators
5	<80	>20	<2.0	Cardiogenic shock	Inotropic drugs/ Vasodilators/ Circulatory assist
6	<100	>25	<2.5	Mitral regurgitation VSD	Vasodilators → circulatory assist → surgery
7	<100	<15 (RVFP >12)	<2.5	Right ventricular infarct	Avoid diuretics. Volume if low LVFP

* These numbers are intended only as guidelines and not absolute haemodynamic parameters

flict because PAWP is usually lower than the simultaneously measured left ventricular end-diastolic pressure.

The choice of intravenous fluid to raise ventricular filling pressure is probably not critical. In most circumstances a rapid infusion, 100–300 ml of 5% dextrose in water, 0.45% saline, salt-poor albumin or dextran will increase filling pressure[111]. During this volume expansion the PAWP and cardiac output should be monitored closely. PAWP will increase with a concomitant increase in cardiac output. Fluid administration should be continued at an adjusted rate to maintain the left ventricular filling pressure in the range of 15–20 mmHg. If, despite an increase in left ventricular filling pressure, cardiac output fails to increase, coexistent left ventricular pump failure should be suspected. If PAWP increases rapidly to exceed 20 mmHg, and cardiac output does not increase significantly, fluid administration should be discontinued to avoid precipitating pulmonary oedema.

(2) Subset 2

Subset 2 represents a common group of patients with acute myocardial infarction who often have the symptom of dyspnoea. Haemodynamically they have a reasonable arterial pressure and cardiac index, but a high left ventricular filling pressure. Because this elevated filling pressure is the predominant haemodynamic abnormality, diuretics represent the therapy of choice. Diuretics such as frusemide reduce ventricular filling pressure by first increasing systemic venous capacitance, and then promoting a diuresis via the kidneys[112]. With successful diuresis and reduction of left ventricular filling pressure, dyspnoea should disappear. The PAWP should be carefully monitored during diuretic therapy to avoid lowering the filling pressure to hypovolaemic levels. Using basal pulmonary rales as a guide to left ventricular filling pressure can be misleading. Rales may take up to 48 hours to clear, despite a rapid reduction in filling pressure. Redistribution of blood flow to the upper lobes of the lungs on chest X-ray seems to correlate somewhat better than clinical rales with left ventricular filling pressures greater than 15 mmHg[113].

(3) Subset 3

Patients falling into subset 3 have peripheral vasodilation and, as a result, low systolic arterial pressure with a relatively normal cardiac index. This unusual situation results from a lack of the usual peripheral vasoconstriction, which attempts to maintain blood pressure, that is seen following acute myocardial infarction. With adequate cardiac output, despite low arterial pressure, specific therapy may not be needed. Vasoconstrictive drugs may be needed in those patients with extremely low pressure.

(4) Subset 4

Patients with moderate to severe left ventricular pump failure constitute subset 4. This common situation is manifested haemodynamically by a low arterial pressure, low cardiac index and an elevated left ventricular filling pressures (PAWP greater than 20 mmHg). In this situation, the major objectives of therapy are to reduce left ventricular filling pressure and to increase cardiac output, preferably without enhancing myocardial ischaemia. Vasodilator therapy can be extremely beneficial to these patients and can accomplish both therapeutic objectives. Many studies have been performed documenting the effectiveness of vasodilators in treating hypertensive, normotensive, acute and chronic heart failure[114-117]. Vasodilators, which are frequently referred to as afterload or impedance reducing agents, have their primary action in reducing resistance in the arteriolar and/or venous beds.

Sodium nitroprusside has vasodilator properties in both the arteriolar and venous circulation. Agents such as hydralazine are predominantly arteriolar dilators with very little venodilating properties. Nitrates, on the other hand, are predominantly venodilators. The predominant mechanism by which vasodilators increase cardiac output, in the setting of the left ventricular pump failure, is by reducing systemic arteriolar tone and systemic vascular resistance. Although cardiac performance is improved primarily by these peripheral vascular effects of vasodilators, other mechanisms exist. By decreasing both left ventricular diastolic pressure and volume, a reduction in myocardial oxygen demand may occur. Collateral flow to ischaemic myocardium may be enhanced by some vasodilators[118]. Left ventricular compliance may also be acutely increased by vasodilators[119]. The left ventricle will accommodate a larger volume at the same end-diastolic pressure during vasodilator administration. Because left ventricular end-diastolic volume is the important determinant of stroke volume, an increase in cardiac performance can occur at comparatively lower levels of filling pressure.

Several vasodilator agents have been used for the therapy of patients with pump failure complicating acute myocardial infarction. Intravenous sodium nitroprusside is the most useful vasodilator agent for use in treating the acute myocardial infarction patient with high left ventricular filling pressure and low cardiac output. Because of its arteriolar dilating effects a decrease in systemic vascular resistance will occur along with an increase in cardiac output. Because nitroprusside also has venodilating properties, a reduction in systemic and pulmonary venous pressures will occur, resulting in a decrease in the left ventricular filling pressure. An increase in cardiac output, along with a decrease in left ventricular filling pressure, indicates improved cardiac performance. These beneficial effects in cardiac performance should be expected only in those patients with high systemic vascular resistance and left ventricular filling pressures (subsets 4 and 5). No improvement, or a decrease in cardiac function, may occur in patients with normal or low ventricular filling pressures treated with a nitroprusside infusion. Proper selection of patients based on haemodynamics is mandatory. During an infusion of nitroprusside repeated haemodynamic measurements should be made to judge the response. In particular, arterial pressure, pulmonary capillary wedge pressure, cardiac output and systemic vascular resistance should be monitored. The therapeutic goal in vasodilator therapy of the failing left ventricle is to reduce pulmonary capillary wedge pressure and to increase cardiac output. A reduction in arterial pressure should not be used as the sole measure of the therapeutic effect of a vasodilator. Marked haemodynamic changes can occur despite little change in blood pressure.

(5) Subset 5

Subset 5 represents patients with cardiogenic shock. They are profoundly hypotensive, have a low cardiac index and high left ventricular filling pressure. A therapeutic approach for this difficult situation involves vasodilators, inotropic agents and often circulatory assist devices (intra-aortic balloon counterpulsation). Despite aggressive therapy the long-term prognosis for this group remains poor[120]. Presently, dopamine or dobutamine are the pressor amine agents of choice for inotropic stimulation in cardiogenic shock. Dopamine (3-hydroxytyramine) is a precursor of noradrenaline which stimulates both α- and β- receptors. Dopamine's activity appears to be dose dependent in most circumstances. Low doses have a direct renal vasodilating effect felt to be mediated through specific dopaminergic receptors. Dopamine stimulates the myocardium directly (β_2-receptors), and also indirectly through release of noradrenaline stores. At larger doses the predominant effect is α-constriction. Dopamine increases cardiac output and may decrease left ventricular filling pressure, implying improved cardiac performance, but the magnitude of this improvement appears to be dependent on initial cardiac function. In severe left ventricular pump failure there is less response. In patients with shock occurring as a complication of myocardial infarction, the improvement in cardiac output seen with dopamine is often due to an increase in heart rate and not to enhanced stroke volume[121]. Dopamine, like other inotropic agents used in the setting of myocardial infarction, may increase myocardial oxygen demand and enhance myocardial ischaemia.

Dobutamine, predominantly a β_1-receptor agonist, is the newest of the catecholamines[122]. It has weak α- and β_2-adrenergic activity[123]. It increases peripheral perfusion mainly through its effect on cardiac contractility without increasing afterload or excessive chronotropic effect. The complete haemodynamic and metabolic effects of this agent's use in cardiogenic shock have not yet been evaluated.

There are two special subsets of patients with complications of acute myocardial infarction which deserve special mention: right ventricular infarction and the mechanical lesions of acute mitral regurgitation or ventricular septal rupture.

Acute mitral regurgitation and ventricular septal rupture are both relatively uncommon complications of acute myocardial infarction. Both are usually catastrophic and heralded by the sudden appearance of a holosystolic murmur and subsequent severe left ventricular pump failure. The diagnosis of acute mitral regurgitation can be confirmed by the presence of large 'v' waves on the PAWP tracing. Abnormal systolic mitral valve motion may be noted on an M-mode echocardiogram, and it is often possible to visualize a ruptured chordae or papillary muscle with wide angle two-dimensional echocardiography. Similarly, the site of acute septal rupture may be visualized by two-dimensional echocardiography and abnormal septal motion appreciated. Because of the 'left to right' shunt through the ventricular septal rupture a step-up in oxygen saturation will be observed at the ventricular level when serial samples are taken from the right heart. The O_2 saturation in pulmonary arterial blood will be significantly higher than in right atrial blood.

The definitive treatment of acute mitral regurgitation and ventricular septal rupture is surgical. The timing of surgery must be individualized. If there is evidence of other organ system failure, the patient should be studied in the cardiac catheterization laboratory, and then taken to surgery. Vasodilator therapy is beneficial and improves forward cardiac output in these patients[124].

By decreasing forward systemic vascular resistance, vasodilators have been shown to increase cardiac output and decrease regurgitant volume in acute mitral regurgitation. Left to right shunting across the ruptured ventricular septum is, therefore, reduced. Intra-aortic balloon counterpulsation is often employed together with vasodilators (nitroprusside) to stabilize the patient through cardiac catheterization, and until surgery can be undertaken.

The final haemodynamic subset of importance to identify is right ventricular infarction. Right ventricular infarction is a common consequence of inferior or infero-posterior myocardial infarction. The diagnosis is suggested at the bedside by elevation of jugular venous pressure in the absence of clinical signs of left heart failure. Non-invasive studies such as M-mode or two-dimensional echocardiograms, or radionuclide cardiac imaging, can be almost diagnostic by demonstrating a dilated and hypocontractile right ventricle with a normal left ventricle[125]. Haemodynamic monitoring is helpful in assessing the severity of right ventricular dysfunction as well as for evaluating therapy. In acute right ventricular infarction the right ventricular filling pressure (right atrial pressure) is usually disproportionately elevated when compared to the left ventricular filling pressure. Occasionally equal diastolic pressures may be noted in all four chambers of the heart and differentiation of right ventricular infarction from tamponade can be difficult. The absence of a pericardial effusion on echocardiography and a dilated, instead of a compressed, right ventricle favours right ventricular infarction.

Hypotension and a low output state can be observed in right ventricular infarction and are related to the extent of the damage to both right and left ventricles. Occasionally, the right ventricular papillary muscles are involved, causing tricuspid valve regurgitation. Therapeutically, it is important to avoid diuretics in this syndrome, even though the right ventricular filling pressure (mean right atrial pressure) is elevated. Volume expansion is indicated to correct hypotension and low cardiac output. Severe right ventricular failure reduces the forward output of the right ventricle which is responsible for the venous return to the left ventricle. Volume expansion, even in the presence of high right ventricular filling pressure, may improve the forward output of the right ventricle, thus improving venous return to and output of the left ventricle. Venodilators, such as nitroprusside, should be used with caution and not administered to lower the elevated right ventricular filling pressure. The resulting systemic venous pooling of blood may precipitate hypotension and extension of infarct size.

(III) PRESERVATION OF THE ISCHAEMIC MYOCARDIUM

(1) Reduction of myocardial infarction size

The concept of myocardial infarct size limitation or the preservation of ischaemic myocardium is an extremely important one for all physicians caring for patients with acute myocardial infarction. All forms of therapy employed during the management of patients with myocardial infarction should be considered in the context of their effects on the ultimate extent of myocardial damage. As discussed earlier (Part I), the prompt treatment of arrhythmias is life saving. Prompt therapy also restores haemodynamic stability and, by correcting a rapid heart rate, helps prevent extension of infarct size. The use of inotropic agents in patients with acute myocardial infarction should be carefully considered. Drugs which increase contractility such as digitalis, isoprenaline (isoprotenerol) and dopamine all increase myocardial oxygen consumption. Therefore, in patients with coronary artery disease with limited coronary blood flow, myocardial ischaemia may be enhanced and myocardial injury extended. Despite their beneficial effect in raising blood pressure and cardiac output in patients with shock, these agents have been shown to produce deterioration in myocardial metabolism and increase the size of infarction[121,126-128]. It is therefore important to use inotropic agents only when an increase in contractility and augmentation of blood pressure are clinically needed.

The use of vasodilators to treat pump failure and their theoretical benefits to ischaemic myocardium have already been discussed. It must be pointed out that excessive reduction in the coronary perfusion pressure may increase existing myocardial ischaemia. Excessive decrease in diastolic blood pressure with vasodilators (< 60 mmHg) should be avoided to reduce the possibility of extensive myocardial injury.

(2) Experimental methods to estimate the size of a myocardial infarction

One of the major obstacles to the clinical investigation of the reduction of infarct size is an accurate method of infarct sizing. The lack of a precise sizing method that is clinically applicable has hindered all investigations into infarct size reduction. The current methods of sizing a myocardial infarction are electrocardiographic ST segment mapping, creatinine phosphokinase (CK) disappearance curves and, most recently, radionuclide scintigraphy. Considerable problems exist with each method. Limitations of precordial ST segment mapping include the phenomenon of spontaneous reduction in ST segment elevation in the early hours post infarction[129,130]. Additionally, ST segment elevation secondary to pericarditis may confuse analysis. Creatinine phosphokinase disappearance curves are determined from serial determination of serum CK levels over the first 24 hours of a myocardial infarction. By plotting the CK enzyme levels against time, the absolute amount of CK entering the circulation can be predicted from the area under the curve. Good correlations have been reported between the estimated total CK released and actual extent of myocardial infarction[131,132]. Serum CK level is a result not only of the rate of entry of CK into the blood, but also its rate of removal. Problems with continued myocardial necrosis and variable washout of CK from underperfused, infarcted areas affect the rate of entry into the blood. Variable clearance of CK by the reticuloendothelial system also affects the rate of removal.

As a result of these problems and others, several clinical studies have shown poor correlation between enzymatic and histologic estimates of infarct size[133-135]. Experimental studies with radionuclide scintigraphy employing technetium 99-m pyrophosphate indicate that it is a sensitive and relatively specific indicator of infarction. A reasonable correlation between the area of uptake of technetium 99-m pyrophosphate on a scan and the extent of histologic myocardial damage exists in preliminary studies[136,137]. Perhaps this technique alone or in combination with others will provide an accurate infarct sizing method.

(3) Experimental therapies to limit the extent of myocardial infarction

Briefly outlined, several experimental therapeutic approaches to reducing myocardial ischaemic injury are based on the following principles: decreasing myocardial oxygen demand, increasing oxygen supply, improving myocardial anaerobic metabolism, and protection from autolytic processes. Although beneficial effects have been demonstrated for all these agents in laboratory models and sometimes in human studies, the data is not conclusive enough at this time to recommend their routine clinical use.

(4) Decreasing myocardial oxygen demands

Propranolol, practolol and other β-adrenergic drugs reduce myocardial oxygen demand by reducing heart rate and myocardial contractility. Experimental studies employing CK curves and/or ST segment mapping to size myocardial infarction have shown a decrease in expected infarct size with β-adrenergic blockade[138-140]. The hazard of β-adrenergic blockade is that the reduction in myocardial contractility might induce pump failure. We are not routinely using β-adrenergic blocking drugs in all patients with acute myocardial infarction in hope of reducing infarct size, and we reserve their use for patients with angina, hypercontractility or rapid heart rates. Several randomized multicentre studies are now underway which may help to better define the role of propranolol for routine therapy of acute myocardial infarction.

(5) Increasing oxygen supply

There are several potential means to increase blood flow and oxygen delivery to ischaemic myocardium. An easy approach is to increase arterial oxygen tension, PaO_2. Several studies suggest a beneficial effect on infarct size and myocardial ischaemia by administration of 40–100% oxygen[141-143]. To increase myocardial perfusion directly, emergency myocardial revascularization has been employed but without consistent beneficial effect on long term prognosis[144-146]. The use of intra-aortic balloon counterpulsation to both increase perfusion pressure to improve collateral flow and to decrease oxygen demand by reducing preload and afterload has been studied[147-149]. As clinical studies at this time are too limited and serious complications do exist, this form of therapy cannot be recommended for routine prophylactic treatment of acute myocardial infarction.

(6) Improving metabolism and protection from autolytic process

Glucose–insulin–potassium (GIK) infusion, by decreasing the level of circulating free fatty acids, may theoretically reduce myocardial energy demands. Free fatty acids are frequently elevated early in acute infarction and have been shown to increase oxygen demand and enhance myocardial ischaemia. GIK infusion may also augment anaerobic metabolism by increasing ATP levels[150-152]. Clinical use of GIK has not, however, demonstrated a significant reduction in infarct size[153,154]. Glucocorticoids and hyaluronidase have been investigated as a means of reducing infarct size. The anti-inflammatory effects of glucocorticoids have been used to treat myocardial infarction. Theoretically, by stabilizing lysosomal membranes they may slow or prevent the release of hydrolytic enzymes and therefore prevent secondary damage to the myocardium[155-158]. However, available clinical studies fail to show a convincing beneficial effect[159-161]. The potential adverse effect of impaired healing and enhanced propensity to aneurysm formation or myocardial rupture has been suggested[162,163]. The enzyme hyaluronidase has been shown to decrease experimental infarct size[164,165]. Its exact mechanism of action is not known and only limited clinical studies have been done[166].

References

1. Meltzer, L. E. and Kitchell, J. B. (1966). The incidence of arrhythmias associated with acute myocardial infarction. *Prog. Cardiovasc. Dis.*, **9**, 50
2. Rothfeld, E. L., Bernstein, A., Crews, A. H. Jr., Parsonnet, V. and Zucker, I. R. (1965). Telemetric monitoring of arrhythmias in acute myocardial infarction. *Am. J. Cardiol.*, **15**, 38
3. Imperial, E. S., Carballo, R. and Zimmerman, H. A. (1960). Disturbances of rate, rhythm and conduction in acute myocardial infarction. A statistical study of 153 cases. *Am. J. Cardiol.*, **5**, 24
4. Julian, D. G., Valentine, P. A. and Miller, G. G. (1964). Disturbances of rate, rhythm and conduction in acute myocardial infarction. A prospective study of 100 consecutive unselected patients with the aid of electrocardiographic monitoring. *Am. J. Med.*, **37**, 915
5. Bashour, F. A., Jones, E. and Edmondson, R. (1967). Cardiac arrhythmias in acute myocardial infarction. II. Incidence of the common arrhythmias with special reference to ventricular tachycardia. *Dis. Chest*, **51**, 520
6. Brown, R. W., Hunt, D. and Sloman, J. G. (1969). The natural history of

atrioventricular conduction defects in myocardial infarction. *Am. Heart J.*, **78**, 460

7. Atkins, J. M., Leshin, S. J., Blomquist, C. G. and Mullins, C. B. (1973). Ventricular conduction blocks and sudden death in acute myocardial infarction. Potential indications for pacing. *N. Engl. J. Med.*, **288**, 281

8. Waugh, R. A., Wagner, G. S., Haney, T. L., Rosati, R. A. and Morris, J. J. Jr. (1973). Immediate and remote prognostic significance of fascicular block during acute myocardial infarction. *Circulation*, **47**, 765

9. Mullins, C. B. and Atkins, J. M. (1976). Prognoses and management of ventricular conduction blocks in acute myocardial infarction. *Mod. Concepts Cardiovasc. Dis.*, **45**, 129

10. Day, H. W. (1965). Effectiveness of an intensive coronary care area. *Am. J. Cardiol.*, **15**, 51

11. Killip, T. and Kimball, J. T. (1967). Treatment of myocardial infarction in a coronary care unit: a two year experience with 250 patients. *Am. J. Cardiol.*, **20**, 456

12. Goble, A. J., Sloman, G. and Robinson, J. S. (1966). Mortality reduction in a coronary care unit. *Br. Med. J.*, **1**, 1005

13. Rotman, M., Wagner, G. S. and Wallace, A. G. (1972). Bradyarrhythmias in acute myocardial infarction. *Circulation*, **45**, 703

14. Scott, M. E., Geddes, J. S., Patterson, G. C., Adgey, A. A. J. and Pantridge, J. F. (1967). Management of complete heart block complicating acute myocardial infarction. *Lancet*, **2**, 1382

15. Lown, B., Fakhor, A. M., Hood, W. B. Jr. and Thorn, G. W. (1967). The coronary care unit. *J. Am. Med. Assoc.*, **199**, 188

16. Day, W. (1968). Acute coronary care – a five year report. *Am. J. Cardiol.*, **21**, 252

17. Moss, A. J. and Akiyama, T. (1974). Prognostic significance of ventricular premature beats. *Cardiovasc. Clin.*, **6**, 273

18. Mogensen, L. (1971). A controlled trial of lidocaine prophylaxis in the prevention of ventricular tachyarrhythmias in acute myocardial infarction. *Acta Med. Scand.*, **513**, 1

19. Lawrie, M., Greenwood, T. W., Goddard, M., Harvey, A. C., Donald, K. W., Julian, D. G. and Oliver, M. F. (1967). A coronary care unit in the routine management of acute myocardial infarction. *Lancet*, **2**, 104

20. Dhurandhar, R. W., MacMillan, R. L. and Brown, W. B. (1971). Primary ventricular fibrillation complicating acute myocardial infarction. *Am. J. Cardiol.*, **27**, 347

21. deSoyza, N., Bissett, J. K., Kane, J. J., Murphy, M. L. and Doherty, J. E. (1974). Ectopic ventricular prematurity and its relationship to ventricular tachycardia in acute myocardial infarction in man. *Circulation*, **50**, 529

22. Lie, K. I., Wellens, H. J., Downar, E. and Durrer, D. (1975). Observations on patients with primary ventricular fibrillation complicating acute myocardial infarction. *Circulation*, **52**, 755

23. Wyman, M. G., Hammersmith, S. (1974). Comprehensive treatment plan for the prevention of primary ventricular fibrillation in acute myocardial infarction. *Am. J. Cardiol.*, **33**, 661

24. Lawrie, D. M., Higgins, M. R., Godman, M. J., Oliver, M. F., Julian, D. G.

and Donald, K. W. (1968). Ventricular fibrillation complicating acute myocardial infarction. *Lancet*, **2**, 523

25. deSoyza, N., Meacham, D., Murphy, M. L., Kane, J. L., Doherty, J. E. and Bissett, J. K. (1979). Evaluation of warning arrhythmias before paroxysmal ventricular tachycardia during acute myocardial infarction in man. *Circulation*, **60**, 814

26. Lie, K. I., Wellens, H. J., Van Capelle, F. J. and Durrer, D. (1974). Lidocaine in the prevention of primary ventricular fibrillation. A double-blind randomized study of 212 consecutive patients. *N. Engl. J. Med.*, **291**, 1324

27. Wyman, M. G., Lalka, D., Hammersmith, L., Cannom, D. S. and Goldreyer, B. N. (1978). Multiple bolus technique for lidocaine administration during the first hours of an acute myocardial infarction. *Am. J. Cardiol.*, **41**, 313

28. Benowitz, N. L. (1976). Clinical applications of the pharmacokinetics of lidocaine. In Brest, A. N. (ed.). *Cardiovascular Clinics*, p. 77. (Philadelphia: F. A. Davis)

29. Pewleur, H., Chaudron, J. M. and Reyns, P. (1977). Effects of disopyramide and aprindine on arrhythmias after acute myocardial infarction. *Eur. J. Cardiol.*, **5**, 397

30. Kidner, P. H. and Carmichael, D. J. S. (1978). Oral disopyramide in the prevention of ventricular arrhythmias following myocardial infarction in patients managed on the coronary care unit and open ward. *East Afr. Med. J.*, **55**, 403

31. Zainal, N., Jennings, G., Jones, B., Model, D., Turner, P., Besterman, E. M. M. and Kidner, P. H. (1976). Disopyramide in the treatment and prevention of arrhythmias following myocardial infarction. *J. Int. Med. Res.*, **4**, 71

32. Luomanmaki, K., Heikkila, J. and Hartel, G. (1975). Bretylium tosylate, adverse effects in acute myocardial infarction. *Arch. Intern. Med.*, **135**, 515

33. Day, H. W. and Bucaner, M. (1971). Use of bretylium tosylate in the management of acute myocardial infarction. *Am. J. Cardiol.*, **27**, 177

34. Grossman, J. I., Lubow, L. A., Frieden, J. and Rubin, I. L. (1968). Lidocaine in cardiac arrhythmias. *Arch. Intern. Med.*, **121**, 396

35. Bigger, J. T. Jr. and Heissenbuttel, R. H. (1969). The use of procainamide and lidocaine in the treatment of cardiac arrhythmias. *Prog. Cardiovasc. Dis.*, **11**, 515

36. Jewitt, D. E., Kishon, Y. and Thomas, M. (1968). Lignocaine in the management of arrhythmias after acute myocardial infarction. *Lancet*, **1**, 266

37. Kayden, H. J., Brodie, B. B. and Steele, J. M. (1957). Procaine amide – a review. *Circulation*, **15**, 118

38. Horowitz, L. N., Josephson, M. E., Farshidi, A., Spielman, S. R., Michelson, E. L. and Greenspan, A. M. (1978). Recurrent sustained ventricular tachycardia. III. Role of the electrophysiologic study in selection of antiarrhythmic regimens. *Circulation*, **58**, 986

39. Lang, T. W., Bernstein, H., Barbieri, F. F., Gold, H. and Corday, E. (1965). Digitalis toxicity. Treatment with diphenylhydantoin. *Arch. Intern. Med.*, **116**, 573

40. Bigger, J. T. Jr., Schmidt, D. H. and Kutt, H. (1968). Relationship between the plasma level of diphenylhydantoin sodium and its cardiac antiarrhythmic effects. *Circulation*, **38**, 363

41. Suzuki, T., Saitoh, Y. and Nishihara, K. (1970). Kinetics of diphenyl-hydantoin disposition in man. *Chem. Pharm. Bull.*, **18**, 405
42. Atkinson, A. J. Jr. and Davison, R. (1974). Diphenylhydantoin as an anti-arrhythmic drug. *Ann. Rev. Med.*, **25**, 99
43. Desai, J., Hirschfeld, D., Peters, R., Scheinman, M. and Gonzalez, R. (1978). Electromechanical dissociation associated with disopyramide. *Circulation*, **58** (Suppl. 2), II-178
44. Walsh, R. A. and Horwitz, L. D. (1979). Adverse hemodynamic effects of intravenous disopyramide compared to quinidine in conscious dogs. *Circulation*, **60**, 1053
45. Katz, R. L., Lord, C. O. and Eakins, K. E. (1967). Anesthetic-dopamine cardiac arrhythmias and their prevention by beta adrenergic blockade. *J. Pharmacol. Exp. Ther.*, **158**, 40
46. Kelliher, G. J. and Roberts, J. (1972). The effects of d(+) and d(−) practolol on ouabain-induced arrhythmia. *Eur. J. Pharmacol.*, **20**, 243
47. Balcon, R., Jewitt, D. E., Davis, J. P. H. and Oram, S. (1966). A controlled trial of propranolol in acute myocardial infarction. *Lancet*, **2**, 917
48. Bath, J. C. J. L., Blake, S., Bloom, R. A., Fleming, H. A., Franklin, A. J., Fulton, R. M., Jackson, E., Leckie, W. J. H., Melrose, A. G. and Turner, J. R. B. (1966). Propranolol in acute myocardial infarction. A multi-center trial. *Lancet*, **2**, 1435
49. Conolly, M. E., Kersting, F. and Dollery, C. T. (1976). The clinical pharma-cology of beta-adrenoceptor-blocking drugs. *Prog. Cardiovasc. Dis.*, **19**, 203
50. Terry, G., Vellani, C. W., Higgins, M. R. and Deig, A. (1970). Bretylium tosylate in treatment of refractory ventricular arrhythmias complicating myo-cardial infarction. *Br. Heart. J.*, **32**, 21
51. Bernstein, J. G. and Koch-Weser, J. (1972). Effectiveness of bretylium tosylate against refractory arrhythmias. *Circulation*, **45**, 1024
52. Cohen, H. C., Gozo, E. G. Jr., Langendorf, R., Kaplan, B. M., Chan, A., Pick, A. and Glick, G. (1973). Response of resistant ventricular tachycardia to bretylium: relation to site of ectopic focus and location of myocardial disease. *Circulation*, **47**, 331
53. Lown, B., Klein, M. D. and Hershberg, P. I. (1969). Coronary and pre-coronary care. *Am. J. Med.*, **46**, 705
54. Han, J., Millett, D., Chizzonitt, B. and Moe, G. K. (1966). Temporal dis-persion of recovery of excitability in atrium and ventricle as a function of heart rate. *Am. Heart. J.*, **71**, 481
55. Wellens, H. J. J., Bar, F. W., Gorgels, A. P. and Mucharaz, J. F. (1978). Electrical management of arrhythmias with emphasis on the tachycardias. *Am. J. Cardiol.*, **41**, 1025
56. Mason, J. W. and Winkle, R. A. (1978). Electrode-catheter arrhythmia induction in the selection and assessment of antiarrhythmic drug therapy, for recurrent ventricular tachycardia. *Circulation*, **58**, 971
57. Rothfeld, E. L., Zucker, I. R., Parsonnet, V. and Alinsonorin, C. A. (1968). Idioventricular rhythm in acute myocardial infarction. *Circulation*, **37**, 203
58. Schamroth, L. (1968). Idioventricular tachycardia. *J. Electrocardiol.*, **1**, 205
59. Rothfeld, E., Zucker, R., Leff, W. A. and Parsonnet, V. (1970). Idio-

ventricular rhythm in acute myocardial infarction: a reappraisal. *Circulation*, **42** (Suppl. 3), 193

60. Norris, R. M. and Mercer, C. J. (1974). Significance of idioventricular rhythms in acute myocardial infarction. *Prog. Cardiovasc. Dis.*, **16**, 455

61. Scheinman, M., Thorburn, D. and Abbott, J. A. (1975). Use of atropine in patients with acute myocardial infarction and sinus bradycardia. *Circulation*, **52**, 624

62. Adgey, A. A. J., Patton, J. N., Campbell, N. P. S. and Webb, S. W. (1979). Ventricular defibrillation: appropriate energy levels. *Circulation*, **60**, 219

63. Tacker, W. A., Jr., Galioto, F. M., Jr., Giuliani, E., Geddes, L. A. and McNamara, D. G. (1974). Energy dosage for human trans-chest electrical ventricular defibrillation. *N. Engl. J. Med.*, **290**, 214

64. Tacker, W. A., Jr., Geddes, L. A., Cabler, P. S. and Moore, A. G. (1974). Electrical threshold for defibrillation of canine ventricles following myocardial infarction. *Am. Heart J.*, **88**, 476

65. Geddes, L. A., Tacker, W. A., Jr., Rosborough, J. P., Moore, A. G. and Cabler, P. S. (1974). Electrical dose for ventricular defibrillation of large and small animals using precordial electrodes. *J. Clin. Invest.*, **53**, 310

66. Dahl, C. F., Ewy, G. A., Warner, E. D. and Thomas, E. D. (1974). Myocardial necrosis from direct current countershock. *Circulation*, **50**, 956

67. Peleska, B. (1965). Cardiac arrhythmias following condenser discharges led through an inductance: comparison with effects of pure condenser discharges. *Circ. Res.* **16**, 11

68. Gold, J. H., Schuder, J. C., Stoeckle, H., Granberg, T. A., Hamdani, S. Z. and Rychlewski, J. M. (1977). Transthoracic ventricular defibrillation in the 100 kg calf with unidirectional rectangular pulses. *Circulation*, **56**, 745

69. Campbell, N. P. S., Webb, S. W., Adgey, A. A. J. and Pantridge, J. F. (1977). Transthoracic ventricular defibrillation in adults. *Br. Med. J.*, **2**, 1379

70. Adgey, A. A. J., Campbell, N. P. S., Webb, S. W., Kennedy, A. L. and Pantridge, J. F. (1978). Transthoracic ventricular defibrillation in the adult. *Med. Instrum.*, **12**, 17

71. Lown, B., Crampton, R. S., DeSilva, R. A. and Gascho, J. (1978). The energy for ventricular defibrillation – too little or too much? *N. Engl. J. Med.*, **298**, 1252

72. Kerber, R. E. and Sarnat, W. (1979). Factors influencing the success of ventricular defibrillation in man. *Circulation*, **60**, 226

73. Holder, D. A., Sniderman, A. D., Fraser, G. and Fallen, E. L. (1977). Experience with bretylium tosylate by a hospital cardiac arrest team. *Circulation*, **55**, 541

74. Weberk, T., Janicki, J. S., Russell, R. O. and Rackley, C. E. (1978). Identification of high risk subsets of acute myocardial infarction. *Am. J. Cardiol.*, **41**, 197

75. Killip, T. and Gault, J. H. (1965). Mode of onset of atrial fibrillation in man. *Am. Heart J.*, **70**, 172

76. Hurwitz, M. and Eliot, R. S. (1964). Arrhythmias in acute myocardial infarction. *Dis. Chest*, **45**, 616

77. Lindsay, J. and Hurst, J. W. (1974). The clinical features of atrial flutter and their therapeutic implications. *Chest*, **66**, 114

78. Waldo, A. L., MacLean, W. A. H., Karp, R. B., Kouchoukos, N. T. and James, T. N. (1977). Entrainment and interruptions of atrial flutter with atrial pacing: studies in man following open heart surgery. *Circulation*, **56**, 737

79. Mounsey, P. (1967). Intensive coronary care: arrhythmias after acute myocardial infarction. *Am. J. Cardiol.*, **20**, 475

80. Hagemeijer, F. (1978). Verapamil in the management of supraventricular tachyarrhythmias occurring after a recent myocardial infarction. *Circulation*, **57**, 751

81. Pick, A., Langendorf, R. and Katz, L. N. (1961). A-V nodal tachycardia with block. *Circulation*, **24**, 12

82. Pick, A. and Dominquez, P. (1957). Nonparoxysmal A-V nodal tachycardia. *Circulation*, **16**, 1022

83. Chung, E. K. (1971). *Principles of Cardiac Arrhythmias*. (Baltimore: Williams and Wilkins)

84. Konecke, L. L. and Knoebel, S. B. (1972). Nonparoxysmal junctional tachycardia complicating acute myocardial infarction. *Circulation*, **45**, 367

85. James, T. N. (1961). *Anatomy of the Coronary Arteries*. (New York: Haeber Inc)

86. James, T. N. (1968). The coronary circulation and conduction system in acute myocardial infarction. *Prog. Cardiovasc. Dis.*, **10**, 410

87. Pick, A. (1963). A-V dissociation: a proposal for a comprehensive classification and consistent terminology. *Am. Heart J.*, **66**, 147

88. George, M. and Greenwood, T. W. (1967). Relation between bradycardia and the site of myocardial infarction. *Lancet*, **2**, 739

89. Adgey, A. A. J., Geodes, J. S., Mulholland, H. C., Keegan, D. A. J. and Pantridge, J. F. (1968). Incidence, significance, and management of early bradyarrhythmias complicating acute myocardial infarction. *Lancet*, **2**, 1097

90. James, T. N. (1961). Myocardial infarction and atrial arrhythmias. *Circulation*, **24**, 761

91. Hindman, M. C., Wagner, G. S., JaRo, M., Atkins, J. M., Scheinman, M. M., DeSanctis, R. W., Hutter, A. H., Yeatman, L., Rubenfire, M., Pujura, C., Rubin, M. and Morris, J. (1978). The clinical significance of bundle branch block complicating acute myocardial infarction. I. Clinical characteristics, hospital mortality, and one year followup. *Circulation*, **58**, 679

92. Langendorf, R. and Pick, A. (1968). Atrioventricular block, type II (Mobitz) – its nature and clinical significance. *Circulation*, **38**, 819

93. Rosenbaum, M. B., Elizari, M. V. and Lazzari, J. D. (1970). *The Hemiblocks*. p. 259. (Florida: Tampa Tracings)

94. Hecht, H., Kossman, C. E., Childers, R. W., Langendorf, R., Lev, M., Rosen, K. M., Pruitt, R. D., Truex, R. C., Utley, H. N. and Watt, T. B. (1973). Atrioventricular and intraventricular conduction: revised nomenclature and concepts. *Am. J. Cardiol.*, **31**, 232

95. Hindman, M. C., Wagner, G. S., JaRo, M., Atkins, J. M., Scheinman, M. M., DeSanctis, R. W., Hutter, A. H., Yeatman, L., Rubenfire, M., Pujura, C., Rubin, M. and Morris, J. J. (1978). The clinical significance of bundle branch block complicating acute myocardial infarction. II. Indications for temporary and permanent pacemaker insertion. *Circulation*, **58**, 689

96. Scanlon, P. J., Pryor, R., Blount, S. G., Jr. (1970). Right bundle branch block

associated with left superior or inferior intraventricular block: associated with acute myocardial infarction. *Circulation*, **42**, 1135

97. Lie, K. I., Liem, K. L., Schuilenberg, R. M., David, G. K. and Durrer, D. (1978). Early identification of patients developing late in-hospital ventricular fibrillation after discharge from the coronary care unit. *Am. J. Cardiol.*, **41**, 674

98. The Coronary Drug Project Research Group. (1973). Prognostic importance of premature beats following myocardial infarction: experience in the Coronary Drug Project. *J. Am. Med. Assoc.*, **223**, 1116

99. Ruberman, W., Weinblatt, E., Goldberg, J. D., Frank, C. W. and Shapiro, S. (1977). Ventricular premature beats and mortality after myocardial infarction. *N. Engl. J. Med.*, **297**, 750

100. Moss, A., DeCamilla, J., Davis, H. and Bayer, L. (1977). Clinical significance of ventricular ectopic beats in the early post-hospital phase of myocardial infarction. *Am. J. Cardiol.*, **39**, 635

101. Moss, A. J., Davis, H. T., DeCamilla, J. and Bayer, L. W. (1979). Ventricular ectopic beats and their relation to sudden and non-sudden cardiac death after myocardial infarction. *Circulation*, **60**, 998

102. Schulze, R. A., Jr., Strauss, H. W. and Pitt, B. (1977). Sudden death in the year following myocardial infarction. Relation to ventricular premature contractions in the late hospital phase and left ventricular ejection fraction. *Am. J. Med.*, **62**, 192

103. Swan, H. J. C., Ganz, W., Forrester, J., Marcus, H., Diamond, G. and Chonette, D. (1970). Catheterization of the heart in man with the use of flow directed balloon-tipped catheter. *N. Engl. J. Med.*, **283**, 447

104. Ganz, W., Donoso, R., Marcus, H. S., Forrester, J. S. and Swan, H. J. C. (1971). A new technique for measurement of cardiac output by thermodilution in man. *Am. J. Cardiol.*, **27**, 392

105. Forrester, J. S., Ganz, W., Diamond, G., McHugh, T., Chonette, D. and Swan, H. J. C. (1972). Thermodilution cardiac output determination with a single flow directed catheter. *Am. Heart J.*, **83**, 306

106. Chatterjee, K., Swan, H. J. C., Ganz, W., Gray, R., Loebel, H., Forrester, J. S. and Chonette, D. (1975). Use of balloon-tipped flotation electrode catheter for cardiac monitoring. *Am. J. Cardiol.*, **36**, 56

107. Forrester, J. S., Diamond, G., McHugh, T. J. and Swan, H. J. C. (1971). Filling pressures in the right and left sides of the heart in acute myocardial infarction. *N. Engl. J. Med.*, **285**, 190

108. Crexells, C., Chatterjee, K., Forrester, J. S., Dikshit, K. and Swan, H. J. C. (1973). Optimal level of left heart filling pressures in acute myocardial infarction. *N. Engl. J. Med.*, **289**, 1263

109. Forrester, J. S., Chatterjee, K. and Swan, H. J. C. (1976). Medical therapy of acute myocardial infarction by application of hemodynamic subsets. *N. Engl. J. Med.*, **295**, 1356 and 1404

110. Russell, R. O., Jr., Rackley, C. E., Pombo, J. *et al.* (1970). Effects of increasing left ventricular filling pressure in patients with acute myocardial infarction. *J. Clin. Invest.*, **49**, 1539

111. Chatterjee, K. (1977). Pump failure in acute myocardial infarction. Fluid and drug therapy. *Ann. Clin. Res.*, **9**, 124

112. Dikshit, K., Vyden, J. K., Forrester, J. S., Chatterjee, K., Prakash, R. and Swan, H. J. C. (1973). Renal and extrarenal hemodynamic effects of furosemide in congestive failure after acute myocardial infarction. *N. Engl. J. Med.*, **288**, 1087

113. McHugh, J. J., Forrester, J. S., Adler, L., Zion, D. and Swan, H. J. C. (1972). Pulmonary vascular congestion in acute myocardial infarction: Hemodynamic and radiologic correlations. *Ann. Intern. Med.*, **76**, 29

114. Judson, W. E., Hollander, W. and Wilkins, R. W. (1956). The effects of intravenous hydralazine on cardiovascular and renal function in patients with and without congestive heart failure. *Circulation*, **8**, 664

115. Franciosa, J. B., Guiha, N. M., Limas, C. J., Rodriguera, E. and Cohn, J. N. (1972). Improved left ventricular function during nitroprusside infusion in acute myocardial infarction. *Lancet*, **2**, 1650

116. Chatterjee, K., Parmley, W. W., Ganz, W. *et al.* (1973). Hemodynamic and metabolic responses to vasodilator therapy in acute myocardial infarction. *Circulation*, **48**, 1183

117. Chatterjee, K. and Parmley, W. W. (1977). The role of vasodilator therapy in heart failure. *Prog. Cardiovasc. Dis.*, **19**, 301

118. Mann, R., Cohn, P. F., Holman, B. L., Green, L. H., Markis, J. E. and Phillips, D. A. (1978). Effect of nitroprusside on regional myocardial blood flow in coronary artery disease. Results in 25 patients and comparison with nitroglycerin. *Circulation*, **57**, 732

119. Parmley, W. W., Chuck, L., Chatterjee, K., Swan, H. J. C., Klausner, S. C., Glantz, S. A. and Ratshin, R. (1976). Acute changes in the diastolic pressure volume relationship of the left ventricle. *Eur. J. Cardiol.*, **4**, (Suppl.), 105

120. Sanders, C. A., Buckley, M. J., Leinbach, R. C., Mundth, E. D. and Austen, W. G. (1972). Mechanical circulatory assistance. Current status and experience with combining circulatory assistance, emergency coronary angiography and acute myocardial revascularization. *Circulation*, **45**, 1292

121. Mueller, H. S., Evans, R. and Ayers, S. M. (1972). Effect of dopamine on hemodynamics and myocardial metabolism in shock following acute myocardial infarction in man. *Circulation*, **45**, 335

122. Sonnenblick, E. H., Frishman, W. H. and LeJemtel, T. H. (1979). Dobutamine: a new synthetic cardioactive sympathetic amine. *N. Engl. J. Med.*, **300**, 17

123. Robie, N. W., Nutter, D. O., Moody, C. and McNay, J. L. (1974). *In vivo* analysis of adrenergic receptor activity of dobutamine. *Circ. Res.*, **34**, 663

124. Chatterjee, K., Parmley, W. W., Swan, H. J. C., Berman, G., Forrester, J. and Marcus, H. S. (1973). Beneficial effects of vasodilator agents in severe mitral regurgitation due to dysfunction of subvalvar apparatus. *Circulation*, **48**, 684

125. Sharpe, N., Botvinick, E., Shames, D., Chatterjee, K., Massie, B., Schiller, N. and Parmley, W. (1976). Noninvasive diagnosis of right ventricular infarction: a common clinical entity. *Circulation*, **53** and, **54** (II), 76

126. Sonnenblick, E. H., William, J. F. Jr., Glick, G., Mason, D. T. and Braunwald, E. (1966). Studies on digitalis. XV. Effects of cardiac glycosides on myocardial force–velocity relations in nonfailing human heart. *Circulation*, **34**, 532

127. Bezdeck, W., Forrester, J., Chatterjee, K. *et al.* (1972). Myocardial metabolic effect of ouabain in acute myocardial infarction (AMI). *Circulation*, 45 and 46 (II), 113

128. Varonkov, Y., Sheh, W. E., Smirnov, V., Gukovsky, D. and Chaziv, E. (1977). Augmentation of serum CPK activity by digitalis in patients with acute myocardial infarction. *Circulation*, 55, 719

129. Madias, J. E., Venkatraman, K. and Hood, W. B. (1975). Precordial ST segment mapping. I. Clinical studies in the coronary care unit. *Circulation*, 52, 799

130. Haradarson, T., Henning, H., O'Rourke, R. A., Karlinger, J. S., Ryan, W. and Ross, J. Jr. (1978). Variability, reproducibility and applications of precordial ST segment mapping following acute myocardial infarction. *Circulation*, 57, 1096

131. Shell, W. E., Kjekshus, J. K. and Sobel, B. E. (1971). Quantitative assessment of the extent of myocardial infarction in the conscious dog by means of analysis of serial changes in serum creatine phosphokinase activity. *J. Clin. Invest.*, 50, 2614

132. Shell, W. E., Lavell, J. F., Covell, J. W. and Sobel, B. E. (1973). Early estimation of myocardial damage in conscious dogs and patients with evolving acute myocardial infarction. *J. Clin. Invest.*, 52, 2579

133. Ross, J., Jr. (1976). General discussion. *Circulation*, 53 (Suppl. 1), 111

134. Roe, C. R. and Starmer, C. F. (1975). A sensitive analysis of enzymatic estimation of infarct size. *Circulation*, 52, 1

135. Roe, C. R., Cobb, F. R. and Starmer, F. (1977). The relationship between enzymatic and histologic estimates of the extent of myocardial infarction in conscious dogs with permanent coronary occlusion. *Circulation*, 55, 438

136. Stokey, E. M., Buja, L. M., Lewis, S. E., Parkey, R. W., Bonte, F. J., Harris, R. A. and Willerson, J. T. (1976). Measurement of acute myocardial infarction in dogs with 99m Tc stannous pyrophosphate scintigrams. *J. Nucl. Med.*, 17, 1

137. Botvinick, E. H., Shames, D., Lappin, H., Tyberg, J. V., Townsend, R. and Parmley, W. W. (1975). Noninvasive quantitation of myocardial infarction with technetium 99m pyrophosphate. *Circulation*, 52, 909

138. Reimer, K. A., Rasmussen, M. M. and Jennings, R. B. (1976). On the nature of protection by propranolol against myocardial necrosis after temporary coronary occlusion in dogs. *Am. J. Cardiol.*, 37, 520

139. Pelides, L. J., Reid, D. W., Thomas, M. and Shillingford, J. P. (1972). Inhibition of beta blockade on the ST segment elevation after acute myocardial infarction. *Cardiovasc. Res.*, 6, 295

140. Peter, T., Norris, R. M., Clarke, E. D., Heng, M. K., Singh, B. N., Williams, B., Howell, D. R. and Ambler, P. K. (1978). Reduction of enzyme levels by propranolol after acute myocardial infarction. *Circulation*, 57, 1091

141. Ratliff, N. B., Hackel, P. V. and Mikat, E. (1969). Myocardial oxygen metabolism and myocardial blood flow in dogs with hemorrhagic shock. *Circ. Res.*, 45, 901

142. Maroko, P. R., Radvany, P., Braunwald, E. and Hale, S. L. (1975). Reduction of infarction size by oxygen inhalation following acute coronary occlusion. *Circulation*, 52, 360

143. Madias, J. E., Madias, N. E. and Hood, W. B. (1976). Precordial ST mapping.

I. Effects of oxygen inhalation on ischemic injury in patients with acute myocardial infarction. *Circulation*, **53**, 411

144. Smullens, S. N., Weiner, L., Kasparian, H., Brest, A. N., Bacharach, B., Noble, P. H. and Templeton, J. Y. Evaluation and surgical management of acute evolving myocardial infarction. *J. Thorac. Cardiovasc. Surg.*, **64**, 495

145. Dawson, J. T., Hall, R. J., Hallman, G. L. and Cooley, D. A. (1973). Mortality of coronary artery bypass after previous myocardial infarction. *Am. J. Cardiol.*, **31**, 128

146. Cheanvechai, C., Effler, D. B., Loop, F. D., Groves, L. K., Sheldon, W. C., Razavi, M. and Sones, F. M., Jr. (1973). Emergency myocardial revascularization. *Am. J. Cardiol.*, **32**, 901

147. Maroko, P. R., Davidson, D. M., Libby, P., DeLaria, G. A., Covell, J. W., Ross, J. Jr. and Braunwald, E. (1972). Effects of intraaortic balloon counterpulsation on the severity of myocardial ischemic injury following acute coronary occlusion. *Circulation,* **45**, 1150

148. Sugg, W. L., Webb, W. R. and Echer, R. R. (1969). Reduction of extent of myocardial infarction by counterpulsation. *Ann. Thorac. Surg.*, **7**, 310

149. Leinbach, R. C., Gold, H. K., Harper, R. W. *et al.* (1978). Early intraaortic balloon pumping for anterior myocardial infarction without shock. *Circulation*, **58**, 204

150. Mjos, O. D., Kjekshus, J. K. and Lekven, J. (1974). Importance of free fatty acids as a determinant of myocardial oxygen consumption and myocardial ischemic injury during norepinephrine infusion in dogs. *J. Clin. Invest.*, **53**, 1290

151. Opie, L. H., Bruyneal, K. and Owen, P. (1975). Effects of glucose, insulin and potassium infusion on tissue metabolic changes within first hour of myocardial infarction. *Circulation*, **52**, 49

152. Prather, J. W., Russell, R. O., Mantle, J. O., McDaniel, H. G. and Rackley, C. E. (1976). Metabolic consequences of glucose–insulin–potassium infusion in the treatment of acute myocardial infarction. *Am. J. Cardiol.*, **38**, 95

153. Norris, R. M., Heng, M. K., Singh, B. N. and Barrat-Boyes, E. (1975). The effect of glucose, insulin and potassium on hemodynamics and infarct size after myocardial infarction. *Circulation*, **52** (Suppl. 2), 107

154. Rogers, W. J., Segall, P. H., McDaniel, H. G., *et al.* (1979). Prospective randomized trial of glucose–insulin–potassium in acute myocardial infarction. *Am. J. Cardiol.*, **43**, 801

155. Spath, J. A., Lane, D. L. and Lefer, A. M. (1974). Protective action of methylprednisolone on the myocardium during experimental myocardial ischemia in the cat. *Circ. Res.*, **35**, 44

156. Vyden, J. K., Nagasawa, K., Rabinowitz, B. *et al.* (1974). Effect of methyprednisolone administration in acute myocardial infarction. *Am. J. Cardiol.*, **34**, 677

157. Hoffstein, S., Weissmann, G. and Fox, A. C. (1976). Lysosomes in acute myocardial infarction. Studies by means of cytochemistry and subcellar fractionation, with observations on the effects of methylprednisolone. *Circulation*, **53**, (Suppl. 1), 34

158. Welman, E., Selwyn, A. P. and Fox, M. B. (1979). Lysosomal and cytosolic

enzyme release in acute myocardial infarction: Effects of methylprednisone. *Circulation*, **59**, 730

159. Vogel, W. M., Zannoni, V. G., Abrams, G. D. and Lucchesi, B. R. (1977). Inability of methylprednisolone sodium succinate to decrease infarct size of preserved enzyme activity measured 24 hours after coronary occlusion in the dog. *Circulation*, **55**, 588

160. Morrison, J., Reduto, L., Pizzarello, R., Geller, K., Maley, T. and Gulotta, S. (1976). Modification of myocardial injury in man by corticosteroid administration. *Circulation*, **53** (Suppl. 1), 200

161. Peters, R. W., Norman, A., Parmley, W. W., Emilson, B. B., Scheinman, M. M. and Cheitlin, M. (1978). Effect of therapy with methylprednisolone on the size of myocardial infarcts in man. *Chest*, **73**, 483

162. Roberts, R., DeMello, V. and Sobel, B. E. (1976). Deleterious effects of methylprednisolone in patients with myocardial infarction. *Circulation*, **53** (Suppl. 1), 204

163. Bulkley, B. H. and Roberts, W. C. (1974). Steroid therapy during acute myocardial infarction. A cause of delayed healing and of ventricular aneurysm. *Am. J. Med.*, **56**, 244

164. Maroko, P. R. and Braunwald, E. (1973). Modification of myocardial infarct size after coronary occlusion. *Ann. Intern. Med.*, **79**, 720

165. Maclean, D., Fishbein, M. C., Maroko, P. R. and Braunwald, E. (1976). Hyaluronidase induced reduction in myocardial infarct size. Direct quantification of infarction following coronary artery occlusion in the rat. *Science*, **194**, 199

166. Maroko, P. R., Hillis, L. D., Muller, J. E., Tavazzi, L., Heyndrick, G. R. *et al.* (1977). Favorable effects of hyaluronidase on electrocardiographic evidence of necrosis in patients with acute myocardial infarction. *N. Engl. J. Med.*, **196**, 898

14
Acute Poisoning

NOEL WRIGHT

Acute poisoning now accounts for over 10% of all medical admissions and over 50% of medical admissions who are aged less than 45. Despite these very high rates the overall hospital mortality from poisoning remains less than 1% and the number of people dying from suicide continues to fall in Britain. The vast majority of cases in the adult population is self-induced and the mean age for the phenomenon is dropping slowly. Women outnumber men by a ratio of 1.5:1. Motivation for taking an overdose is often complex, including reasons such as a 'cry for help', manipulation of relatives, opting out and so forth, but almost all are not suicidal in intent. This is borne out by the difference in mean age of overdose patients admitted to hospital, which is around 25 years, whilst the mean age of subjects actually committing suicide is around the age of 50 years. Despite the absence of clear suicidal intent, all patients admitted to hospital should be assessed by a suitably trained person with a view to helping the patient and preventing repetition[1,2]. Accidental poisoning occurs commonly in toddlers and experimental self-poisoning in young adolescents. Though the total number of patients is great the majority are trivial from a physical point of view and do not require intensive care. Approximately 15% do require either intensive observation or active treatment and it is the management of this subgroup that forms the subject of this chapter. The contents are based on 3 years of experience in the Regional Poisoning Centre in Edinburgh followed by 6 years as director of this unit.

(I) DIAGNOSIS

Most cases present with a history of poisoning but a minority either fail to give the diagnosis or are sufficiently ill to make it impossible to obtain a history. Unfortunately it has been shown that even when a history is obtained from a patient, it is frequently misleading and up to 50% of patients either exaggerate or minimize the problem to some degree[3]. It is therefore always worthwhile, in a seriously poisoned patient, to seek confirmation of the diagnosis. Corroborative evidence both from the patient's relatives, from the GP or the pharmacist should be sought particularly in the seriously ill. Where possible, laboratory confirmation should be obtained of the drugs claimed to have been taken. In a recent survey one of the surprising findings was that over half the patients dying in hospital of self-poisoning did not have any premortem confirmation of the cause of the presenting illness[4].

Patients presenting in coma and no history of any kind are a relatively common problem, and though initial management does not often depend on which particular substance was taken it is wiser to identify the poison subsequently.

(II) INITIAL ASSESSMENT

As with all medical emergencies a detailed history and examination should be made and base lines established for level of consciousness, neurological status, cardiological status and respiratory status. A useful clinical grading of unconsciousness is:

Grade 0 fully conscious
Grade 1 drowsy but responsive to verbal commands
Grade 2 unconscious but responding to painful stimulus
Grade 3 unconscious but responding only to maximal painful stimulus
Grade 4 unconscious and not responding to pain in any way

The neurological status of the patient should be recorded, and the state of the pupils, the optic fundus, reflexes and plantars should all be noted. Respiratory function should be assessed; in particular the respiratory rate, the depth of breathing and the presence of both peripheral and central cyanosis should be noted. A Wright's spirometer may be used in the casualty department to give a rough guide as to the minute volume ventilation. Blood gases will, of course, confirm the presence of hypoventilation in borderline cases. Where there is any respiratory embarrassment the pharynx and larynx should be inspected, any foreign bodies removed, vomitus aspirated and an endotracheal tube inserted if the cough reflex is grossly depressed. Intermittent positive pressure ventilation should be instituted if there is hypoventilation. Where there is a diminished cough reflex, an oropharyngeal tube should be left in place. Circulatory status of the patient should also be assessed; pulse, blood pressure and peripheral perfusion should all be noted and the latter interpreted in the light of the patient's body temperature. The abdomen should also be examined. In deeply unconscious patients bowel sounds are frequently absent and in patients who have taken corrosives, perforation and intra-abdominal damage may give rise to changing physical signs.

(III) PRINCIPLES OF INTENSIVE THERAPY

These can be summarized as follows:

(1) Maintenance of vital functions.
(2) Prevention of further absorption.
(3) Identification of the poison.
(4) Acceleration of elimination of the poison.
(5) Symptomatic treatment.

The vast majority of cases of self-poisoning get better without active treatment; in fact the dramatic fall in mortality from barbiturate poisoning between the early and late 1950s was entirely due to the use of intermittent positive pressure ventilation (IPPV), together with other supportive treatment and the omission of stimulant drugs and other 'active' measures.

(I) Maintenance of vital functions

Intensive nursing care

Much of the success of supportive therapy is due to high standards of nursing care. Whilst the patient is unconscious, he should be turned hourly to relieve pressure on weight-bearing skin and passive movement should be instituted to avoid venous thrombosis and stiff muscles. Skin care should be performed and bullous lesions or superficial ulcers treated promptly to prevent infection. The patient should be nursed in a coma position, that is, on his side with his neck extended. If his cough reflex is depressed an oropharyngeal tube should be inserted and if a cough reflex is absent an endotracheal tube should be introduced. Dentures should be removed and respiratory toilet carried out at hourly intervals. When the patient begins to recover consciousness, bedside physiotherapy to the chest with encouragement to cough should also be performed. One of the major responsibilities of the nursing staff is to maintain accurate and regular observations of the patient's clinical condition. The pulse, blood pressure, respiratory rate, pupil size and response, central venous pressure and fluid balance should all be recorded.

Fluid and electrolyte balance

Patients who are deeply unconscious from hypnotic poisoning, or who have been vomiting frequently following ingestion of substances such as para-cetamol, may be mildly dehydrated. It is worthwhile restoring their extra-cellular fluid volume cautiously with one or two litres of dextrose/saline. Fluid balance should then be maintained with 2–3 litres of fluid per day. There is no need to use larger volumes unless a forced diuresis is indicated for elimination of the poison ingested. Urine output should be carefully monitored but unless the patient develops acute retention with a distended bladder the bladder should not be catheterized. An unconscious patient may be encouraged to pass urine by suprapubic pressure. If a bladder catheter is inserted then urine specimens should be sent regularly for bacterial culture.

Respiratory care

Patients who are deeply unconscious and who have an absent cough reflex require an endotracheal tube to be inserted and if there is hypoventilation, IPPV should be started. Plastic endotracheal tubes as opposed to rubber may be left in place for days without precipitating laryngeal irritation and inflammation (Chapter 7). However, there is a tendency for debris to accumulate at the tip of the tube and for obstruction to occur. It is therefore a reasonable precautionary measure to change the endotracheal tube at least once every 48 hours. After the tube has been inserted a chest X-ray should be obtained so that the position of its tip can be visualized; if it is near the carina the tube can be shortened. Though clinical examination will usually detect obstruction of a bronchus with consequent loss of aeration of the lung, this is not always the case. Ventilation should always be performed with adequately humidified air and bronchial toilet carried out at regular intervals.

Monitoring

Whilst a patient is in a ICU, daily urea, electrolytes and haemoglobin estimates should be carried out. As chest infection is one of the major com-plications of prolonged coma, daily chest X-rays should be obtained and bronchial secretion regularly cultured. Prophylactic antibiotics should not be used. Prolonged coma without superimposed infection may itself cause a raised white count and an elevation of temperature. Antibiotics should only be used when there are specific indications (Chapter 3).

(2) Prevention of further absorption

Once a substance has been ingested absorption may be reduced by gastric aspiration and lavage. The criteria for performing this procedure are clear:

(1) It should be performed only if a significant amount of toxic substances has been taken.

(2) It should be performed if the patient is seen within 4 hours of taking the drug or poison. Salicylates and tricyclic antidepressants are not emptied from the stomach into the small intestine as rapidly as other substances and the 4 hour rule does not apply. It is worthwhile carrying out a stomach washout up to 12 hours after a significant amount of aspirin has been ingested.

(3) Some claim that a stomach washout should not be performed if a corrosive substance has been taken. However, it is a question of balancing one risk against another. For example, paraquat is a strong corrosive but it is always worthwhile washing out the stomach when the patient is seen within 12 hours of ingesting this substance. A similar argument justifies the use of stomach washout with other corrosives. It must be borne in mind that there is a risk of perforation, particularly if significant amounts have been taken. The patients must be carefully observed after the procedure in order to detect evidence of peritonitis.

(4) If the patient does not have an adequate cough reflex an endotracheal tube should be inserted before the procedure is carried out.

(5) If kerosene or its derivatives, which cause a particularly destructive form of lipoid pneumonia, have been ingested a gastric lavage is best not performed.

When all poisoned patients who receive a stomach washout are considered, gastric lavage seems to be a remarkably safe if rather unaesthetic procedure. However, when only severely ill patients are considered the number that develop complications, such as aspiration pneumonia, arrhythmias during the procedure, epileptiform fits and perforation of the stomach, is remarkably high (up to 30% in one series)[4]. The procedure should only be performed in a seriously ill patient by someone who is experienced in the technique and where there are facilities for monitoring and treating complications that arise.

With these points in mind gastric lavage should be carried out with the patient lying on his left side and with his head tilted down. Vomitus will tend to run out of his mouth and not enter his lungs. A wide bore tube should be introduced into the mouth and the patient then persuaded to swallow so that it can be passed easily into the stomach. The contents of the stomach are then aspirated and a lavage carried out with 250 ml of warmed tap water. The contents of the stomach are aspirated after each aliquot has been introduced. The procedure should be continued until the returned fluid becomes clear of debris. The tube should then be removed with the patient still lying. If possible he should be persuaded to cough to clear the airways of any debris. A suction machine should be kept available and running throughout the procedure so that the lungs or mouth can be sucked out if any complications occur. It has been suggested that at the end of the procedure activated charcoal should be introduced in order to absorb any poison either left in the stomach or upper intestinal tract. The evidence that this improves prognosis is lacking, though this is the reason for the use of Fuller's earth in paraquat poisoning and oral desferrioxamine in iron poisoning, both of which have become generally accepted. If the patient is unconscious and has no cough reflex the procedure should only be performed after an endotracheal tube has been put in place. The stomach tube is replaced by a Ryle's tube and the stomach aspirated hourly.

(3) Identification of the poison

Whenever possible a sample of the offending substance should be obtained from the patient or from relatives accompanying him. A specimen of gastric aspirate should be kept and blood and urine samples obtained so that the laboratory is given every chance to identify the substance. Unidentified tablets are often a problem and if the casualty sister or pharmacist are unable to identify them the *Chemist and Druggist Directory* may be of help. In some parts of the country pharmacists have drug identification systems which may be of help.

(4) Acceleration of the elimination of poison

The only procedures that need be considered under this heading are forced acid and forced alkaline diuresis, haemo- and peritoneal dialysis and haemoperfusion. Diuresis procedures are of use if the active substance or an active metabolite is excreted in the urine in significant quantities. The increase in urine volume reduces the concentration difference between the tubular fluid and the interstitial fluid and minimizes back diffusion into the body. Alteration of urine pH may be used to render a weak acid or a weak base ionized and thus keep it in its least fat soluble form. In the case of weak acids, such as salicylates, urine should be made alkaline, whilst it should be made acidic for weak bases such as amphetamines.

A variety of different techniques have been advocated; perhaps the most popular for a diuresis is as follows:

(1)   sodium bicarbonate 1.26% or 1.4%, 500 ml,
(2)   5% dextrose, 1 litre,
(3)   normal saline, 500 ml, plus 20 mmol of potassium chloride.

This cocktail, totalling 2 litres of fluid, should be given in a fit young person once hourly during three successive hours thus totalling 6 litres. If the patient has any history of renal disease, heart disease, or is over the age of 45, the cocktail should be given at the rate of 1 litre per hour. Whilst the procedure is being carried out the patient should be carefully observed for any signs of fluid overload such as elevated jugular venous pressure, increased respiratory rate and basal crepitations, and the infusion stopped if these signs develop. The patient should also be reviewed by medical staff if a positive balance of more than 3.5 litres occurs.

Forced acid diuresis is rarely necessary but in those few cases an adequate regime to acidify the urine is as follows:

(1)   5% dextrose 500 ml plus 1.5 g ammonium chloride,
(2)   5% dextrose 500 ml,
(3)   normal saline 500 ml.

This should be given at the rate of 1 litre per hour and repeated four times over a 4 hour period. Electrolytes should be monitored throughout the procedure and the urine pH tested.

A mannitol diuresis is often complicated by electrolyte disturbances and should be avoided. Acetazolamide acts as a diuretic and induces alkalinization of the urine. It also causes a metabolic acidosis and has been shown to increase mortality in dogs poisoned with aspirin[6]; it should be avoided. Other diuretics such as frusemide may compete for tubular secretion of salicylic acid and reduce the efficacy of a diuresis. They should therefore be avoided unless there are signs of pulmonary congestion.

Haemodialysis, peritoneal dialysis and haemoperfusion have all been shown to increase the elimination of a number of substances. As with the forced diuresis, any procedure is only worth performing if a patient is seriously ill, if substantial improvement can be obtained and if significant amounts of active substance can be removed. For example, haemoperfusion will remove large amounts of both short acting and long acting barbiturates and may be worthwhile in patients who are Grade 4 unconscious and deteriorating. On the other hand tricyclic antidepressants are distributed throughout the body water and very substantially in fat depots. Though the drug may be absorbed on a charcoal column, such small amounts are eliminated by this means that the procedure is not worth carrying out[7].

Cases of poisoning which have benefited from these forms of therapy include phenobarbitone and other barbiturates, glutethimide, methaqualone, ethchlorvynol and meprobamate.

(5) Symptomatic treatment

Relief from unpleasant effects of poisoning should always be given where it is safe to do so. But in those cases where accurate assessment of patient progress is a major part of management, symptomatic treatment should not obscure this. Milk or antacids, for example, should be given to patients who have taken corrosives if they give relief.

Methaemaglobinaemia was common when phenacetin was freely available. Its presence is suggested by a slate grey colour of the extremities together with hyperventilation and respiratory distress in the absence of respiratory obstruction. Treatment consists of 10ml of 10% methylene blue given intravenously. The dye appears in the urine as a greenish pigment.

Cerebral oedema is a complication of severe hypnotic poisoning and also the inhalation of carbon monoxide. Standard treatment consists of 200ml of 20% mannitol given rapidly intravenously.

(IV) SPECIFIC POISONS

Substances have been selected for specific mention in this section on a basis of their commonness as clinical problems. They have been classified according to their major actions and then described according to the clinical problems associated with management.

(1) Barbiturates

Acute barbiturate poisoning remains the commonest single cause of death from suicide in this country. Despite improvements in patient care it remains also one of the commonest causes of death from self-poisoning after admission to hospital. It is interesting that this should be the case, as there has been a very considerable and significant fall in the total number of barbiturate poisoning incidents, presumably as a result of the curb on prescribing of these substances. Nowadays there is very little reason for their continued use as there are adequate alternatives.

Clinical features

Barbiturates have a major effect on the central nervous system where they cause depression of level of consciousness and depression of reflexes. They also have a depressant effect on the musculoskeletal system; in deep coma the limbs become flaccid, the pupils are usually equal but conjugate movement is lost and the light reflex may be depressed or absent; the corneal reflex is often absent. It is uncommon for the pupils to be unequal unless cerebral damage has occurred. Lateralizing signs are usually absent and their presence should strongly suggest co-existent brain damage. Barbiturates do not cause epileptiform fits and the only time that fits are seen is when there has been brain damage or alternatively during the recovery phase when acute withdrawal is being experienced by an addict.

Muscle tone is reduced in barbiturate overdosage and when this is severe and prolonged, peripheral vascular pooling takes place with resulting tissue hypoxia. Muscle damage ensues and this is borne out by high levels of a variety of serum enzyme activities, in particular serum creatinine phosphokinase; there is also elevation of serum fibrin degradation products, the erythrocyte sedimentation rate is increased and body temperature becomes elevated. These latter findings often do not occur until 24–72 hours after the overdose[8]. When the muscle damage is severe it is occasionally followed by muscle calcification.

Barbiturates cause depression of the cardiovascular system at a number of levels. Centrally there is a reduction in vasomotor tone; there is also a direct depressant effect on the smooth muscle of the peripheral arteriole and finally there is a depressant effect upon the myocardium. Decreased myocardial activity results in a poor cardiac output which tends to cause a high central venous pressure. The decreased peripheral vascular tone causes an increase in vascular capacity. The relative circulating volume is reduced resulting in a fall in central venous pressure. Thus, though there is a general depression of the cardiovascular system, the central venous pressure may be high or normal or even low.

Depression of the respiratory centre naturally enough causes hypoventilation. Hypoxaemia, hypercapnia and metabolic acidosis ensue. In one or two studies it has been noted that these features are out of proportion to the degree of hypoventilation and it has been suggested that barbiturates might have a direct effect upon the pulmonary vasculature, causing a capillary leak reminiscent of the 'shock lung' without preceding shock or hypoxia. An alternative explanation is ventilation/perfusion imbalance[9].

Barbiturates also have a depressant effect on the muscular activity of the gastrointestinal tract. In major overdosage it is not uncommon for a paralytic ileus to occur. Recovery of function with consequent mixing of the gastrointestinal contents and further absorption of barbiturates has been put forward as the reason for the swings in depths of consciousness which are sometimes seen in this form of overdosage.

Barbiturates and other hypnotics, together with tricyclic antidepressant drugs and even carbon monoxide, are all known to cause skin blisters. In barbiturate poisoning they appear in approximately 5% of cases and, thought more frequent in patients who have been deeply unconscious, they also occur in those who have suffered relatively trivial poisoning. Though they often, but not always, occur over pressure areas they are not necessarily related to trauma and it is thought that their occurrence is due to local hypoxia. As has already been indicated they are not specific for any particular kind of poisoning[10]. With the general depression of neurological function, hypothalamic control is also depressed. This is particularly important with respect to temperature and the local loss of muscle tone compounds this effect. Thus hypothermia is common both at home or in hospital when inadequate measures are taken to maintain body temperature.

Management

The mainstay of treatment of acute barbiturate poisoning is supportive treatment. If a patient gets into hospital without brain damage he should make a complete recovery. Initial assessment should be carried out in the Accident and Emergency Department where the necessary life-saving supportive treatment should be started. If a cough reflex is absent then an endotracheal tube should be put in place and if the minute volume is less than 4.0 l, IPPV should be started. The patient should be transferred quickly to an ICU where specialized nursing and monitoring is commenced. If the patient is Grade 2 unconscious or less he may go to a general ward but he must be carefully and regularly observed for indications of deepening coma. If this should occur he should be immediately admitted to an ICU and the dangers of respiratory depression and hypoxia avoided. If the systolic blood pressure is less than 80 mmHg in a patient less than 40 years of age, or 85 mmHg in a patient greater than 40 years, and in particular if there is poor peripheral perfusion as indicated by a low skin temperature of the extremities, poor capillary filling, and collapsed peripheral veins, then active treatment must be considered. In the first instance the body should be tilted so that the legs are higher than the head; this reduces peripheral pooling and increases venous return. Often this is sufficient; however, if no response is seen, then agents such as metaraminol, or alternatively, dopamine may be tried. Metaraminol should be given in small doses, for example 2.5 mg intramuscularly with the intention of raising the systolic pressure to approximately 100 mm Hg. This may be repeated once if there is an inadequate response. The use of metaraminol has been criticized because it may cause renal artery vasoconstriction and acute renal failure. However, with this particular dose regime there is little evidence that renal failure does occur. Dopamine has been used as an alternative to metaraminol. It is effective and possibly less nephrotoxic. The other approach to shock in barbiturate poisoning is the use of plasma expanders such as polygeline or dextran 70 or crystalloids, such as saline. Considerable amounts of fluid are frequently needed to raise the blood pressure and improve the peripheral circulation. Unfortunately, there is always the danger in those patients who have a jeopardized myocardium, that giving large amounts of fluid may precipitate pulmonary oedema. Central venous pressure monitoring should always be carried out when fluid expansion is undertaken; however, this does not always give warning of incipient pulmonary oedema. When the arterial pressure is low and the CVP is high, then there is a choice of either using an inotrope alone or risking a further infusion. This dilemma can be resolved by using a Swan–Ganz catheter to measure the PAWP (Chapter 7). When this measurement is normal or low a further infusion is safe; when raised, an inotrope should be used alone.

All patients who are in Grade 4 coma, whatever the minute volume ventilation, should have their blood gases estimated. Hypoxaemia and metabolic acidosis should be corrected. A chest X-ray should be performed as soon as possible after admission, firstly to ascertain whether the endotracheal tube is clear of the carina and secondly for evidence of aspiration pneumonia. If the latter has occurred then standard treatment is given which includes high doses of steroid together with prophylactic antibiotics*.

Hypothermia is quite common but does not required active treatment unless the core temperature has fallen below 32°C. When this is the case, active warming with an electric blanket placed over the patient should be instituted; the aim should be to gradually raise the temperature rather than to achieve a rapid change.

It can be seen by the above remarks that management is directed towards the symptoms rather than any specific drug level. Interindividual variation in sensitivity to barbiturates is great and it is not unknown for a patient to regain consciousness with a higher barbiturate level than that with which he was admitted. Short acting barbiturates are mainly metabolized and urinary excretion of active compound is small. There is no place for forced diuresis. With long acting barbiturates the situation is different, for example, barbitone is mainly excreted unchanged by the kidneys; 30% of an ingested dose of phenobarbitone appears unchanged in the urine. In cases of long acting barbiturate overdosage it has been customary to carry out a forced alkaline diuresis and there is no doubt that increased amounts of drugs can be eliminated by this procedure. However, it must be borne in mind that such seriously poisoned patients have depressed myocardiums and are prone to pulmonary oedema. These are the very patients in whom fluid overload is to be avoided. Recently[4] 15 cases of hospital deaths from hypnotic poisoning were studied. It was clear that the majority of deaths in those patients who

* Editor's note: Controversial! In the clinical situation, opinion is divided for and against 'blind' steroid and antibiotic.

were admitted without brain damage occurred following prolonged periods of coma which became complicated by respiratory infection. Phenobarbitone overdose patients are usually unconscious for prolonged periods. Thus 'aggressive' treatment with haemoperfusion may be indicated in this very small group of patients poisoned with long acting barbiturates who are deeply unconscious at the time of admission and who fail to improve over the succeeding 24 hours. Haemoperfusion through a charcoal column has been shown to be an effective technique[7,11-13]; it is also an easy technique. The problems of fluid shifts do not occur as they do in haemodialysis. A drawback is that an arteriovenous shunt may be required and this entails sacrifice of an artery. However, the superiority of haemoperfusion over aggressive conservative therapy, even in this highly selected group, is disputed[14].

Acute renal failure is an uncommon complication of barbiturate-induced hypotension and hypoxia. Presumably diminished renal perfusion occurs and acute tubular necrosis ensues. Management of this complication is the same as that for any case of acute renal failure. The prognosis is rather better than the average patient presenting with this condition.

(2) Glutethimide

Glutethimide is a relatively uncommonly used hypnotic marketed in Britain under the name of Doriden. The clinical picture of overdosage is very similar to that of barbiturates. A few patients develop papilloedema, unequal pupils and cerebral oedema. Treatment is similar to that of barbiturate poisoning, that is conservative in the vast majority of cases. Before the advent of haemoperfusion, haemodialysis had been tried and the merits of conservative management were debated[15,16]. However, haemoperfusion is efficient and vitiates all the problems of mixtures of fluids and fats in the haemodialysis machines. Mannitol (20%) 200ml intravenously of dexamethasone sodium phosphate is usually adequate for the treatment of cerebral oedema.

(3) Mandrax

This preparation, which is a combination of methaqualone (250 mg) and diphenhydramine (25 mg) used to be very popular as a hypnotic and then became popular as a drug of abuse. Because of this latter problem it has largely disappeared from the market. Overdosage results in prolonged coma together with hypertonia and hyper-reflexia[17]. Some claimed that the antihistamine acted as a mild respiratory stimulant and maintained ventilation rather better than occurred with the average hypnotic overdose. The antihistamine component theoretically would give rise to fits, increased reflexes and cardiac arrhythmias in overdosage. As with other hypnotics, blood levels are of relatively little use in assessment of a patient compared with thorough clinical examination and observation of his progress.

(4) Other hypnotics

Methyprylone (Noludar) is occasionally seen in overdosage and treatment is largely supportive[18]. Ethchlorvynol is not popular in this country but is elsewhere. It has an extremely long half-life and when taken in overdosage may cause extremely prolonged coma[19]. It is extracted on a charcoal column and haemoperfusion may well reduce the length of coma. Chloral hydrate, a relatively commonly used hypnotic, is seen surprisingly infrequently in overdosage. This may be because of its gastric irritant effect and relatively unpleasant taste. Overdosage causes coma and a clinical picture very similar to that of barbiturate poisoning though there have been recent reports of cardiac arrhythmias occurring in a few cases[20]. Chlormethiazole has recently become popular in the treatment of alcoholics and cases of overdosage have consequently occurred. The clinical picture is the same as for other hypnotic poisoning except for the occurrence of increased salivation[21]. Treatment is conservative.

(5) Tricyclic antidepressants

Compared with barbiturates tricyclic antidepressant drugs are a recent innovation. They are prescribed with increasing frequency to adults for depressive illness and to children for nocturnal enuresis. At present they account for approximately 12% of all adult admissions to hospital with poisoning and for a similar proportion of deaths from self-poisoning. There are a very large number of tricyclic preparations available on the market and now some quadracyclic compounds with a similar action are appearing. As yet there is no definite evidence that these different chemical structures produce a significantly different clinical picture in overdosage.

Clinical picture

The clinical picture in tricyclic antidepressant poisoning is dominated by central excitation and depression. They also have peripheral sympathomimetic activity. Thus the severely poisoned patient may, on admission, be deeply unconscious, but show increased reflexes and upward going plantar responses. Occasionally, despite depressed levels of consciousness, generalized epileptiform fits occur. Coma is usually not of very long duration unless one of the slow release preparations such as Lentizol has been ingested. Anticholinergic effects include widely dilated pupils, dry skin, retention of urine and paralytic ileus. Temperature regulation may be grossly impaired, partly because of the depressant effect on the central nervous system, and partly due to loss of peripheral organ activity such as sweating. Effects on the cardiovascular system are complex; sinus tachycardia is common and is of no particular significance. Prolongation of the QT interval on the e.c.g. appears to be dose related. A small proportion of patients, particularly the young, and possibly those with pre-existing heart disease, develop ventricular arrhythmias. These include multifocal ventricular tachycardia and ventricular fibrillation. Cardiac arrhythmias are said to occur long after recovery of consciousness and in some cases up to 5 days after the over-dosage[22]. Recovery from coma is often accompanied by hallucinations and disorientation; communication with the patient is also complicated by difficulty in understanding the drug-induced distorted speech.

Management

Tricyclic antidepressants are usually quickly absorbed from the small intestine. In overdosage there is a suggestion that gastric emptying is delayed and it may be worthwhile carrying out gastric aspiration and lavage up to 10 hours after a serious overdose. They are rapidly distributed throughout the body and because of their high lipid solubility pass into the fat cells. Only small amounts are present in the blood and 90% of that is protein bound. Elimination is via hepatic metabolism and in some cases active metabolites undergo enterohepatic recirculation. Only a very small proportion of active drug or metabolite appears in the urine.

Plasma drug concentrations appear to be related to the severity of symptoms but the assay is complex and time-consuming. It is not suitable for routine management of the patient. The drug can be easily detected in the urine. Management is therefore based on the patient's clinical state and is supportive. As with other drug overdoses respiratory status should be checked as soon as the patient is admitted. The patient should be placed on a cardiac monitor and in cases of serious poisoning should be maintained on the monitor for a least 48 hours and possibly 72 even though significant improvement in general clinical status may have occurred well before this time. If shock is not due to cardiac arrhythmias, it is usually short-lived. However, drugs such as metaraminol and dopamine should be avoided because part of the action of this group of drugs is due to sympathomimetic activity; it should be treated by plasma expansion, and should be monitored by central venous pressure measurements. Neurological excitation and epileptiform fits occur, especially during recovery from deep coma, and is best treated by diazepam. The most challenging complications of tricyclic antidepressant poisoning to treat are the cardiac arrhythmias. These appear to be partially dose related[23]. Sinus tachycardia is common and does not require any treatment. There is also prolongation of the QT interval and widening of the QRS complex. However, life-threatening ventricular arrhythmias also occur and are frequently resistant to standard methods of treatment. They are occasionally precipitated by generalized convulsions; presumably the accompanying hypoxia and metabolic acidosis have an arrhythmogenic effect. Immediate measures should be taken to correct any hypoxia or metabolic acidosis but if these measures fail then the author uses standard antidysrhythmic drugs, such as lignocaine or practolol. Others have used intravenous pyridostigmine to treat tachy-dysrhythmias, on the basis that these are due to the anticholinergic action of the tricyclic.

A little while ago physostigmine salicylate was proposed as an effective antidote to this form of poisoning[24]. It is a reversible cholinesterase inhibitor and unlike neostigmine, is capable of crossing the blood–brain barrier and thus reversing central cholinergic blockade. There is no doubt that patients who are given small doses rapidly regain consciousness. Unfortunately, complications such as severe bradycardia, excessive salivation and grand-mal fits also occur[25]. As this latter complication is particularly associated with life-threatening arrhythmias in tricyclic poisoning, its value is now questioned and it should certainly not be used unless the patient is in extremis. There is also some work on mice poisoned with tricyclic antidepressants which shows a greater mortality in those treated with physostigmine compared with those that were untreated[26]. Procedures such as forced diuresis, haemodialysis or haemoperfusion are all useless due to the low plasma levels and high volume of distribution of this group of drugs. Unlike hypnotic poisoning, death in tricyclic antidepressant intoxication frequently occurs within the first 48 hours and is often associated with cardiac arrhythmias. Death is not usually associated with the respiratory complications of prolonged coma.

(6) Salicylates

Salicylate poisoning accounts for approximately 10% of the adult patients admitted to hospital with self-poisoning. It also accounts for about 10% of all deaths from poisoning. There has been a slight reduction in total numbers over the past few years but this fall has occurred at the same time as the increase in patients admitted with paracetamol poisoning. Aspirin poisoning is also common in children but frequently has a significantly different clinical course.

Clinical features

Clinical presentation is very variable. Adult patients usually present to Casualty early, that is within 6 hours of taking the tablets. The vast majority are conscious, alert and orientated. They may be restless but confusion, drowsiness and coma are rare. A decreased level of consciousness is of particular significance, as these patients have the greatest morbidity[27]. Patients sometimes complain of restlessness, sweating and tinnitus and may be noted to be hyperventilating. However, especially in the early hours after ingestion of significant amounts of drug, there may be no signs or symptoms. Less common clinical features include hyperpyrexia, vomiting and severe dehydration.

Management

In all cases in which the diagnosis is suspected it should be confirmed by obtaining a serum salicylate concentration. As there is little correlation between severity of symptoms and the severity of poisoning, the seriousness of the situation can only be assessed by a drug level. Interpretation is helped if the time after ingestion is known. Absorption of aspirin, unlike paracetamol, continues over a considerable length of time and peak serum levels may be obtained up to 8 hours after ingestion. A level of 300mg/1 may be significant if the drug was taken 12 hours before the time of assay whereas such a level is almost within the therapeutic range 4–6 hours after ingestion. By and large, active treatment should be instituted if the drug level is over 500mg/1 up to 12 hours after ingestion and over 300mg after this time. The second necessary investigation in the assessment of a significantly poisoned patient is the acid–base status. Aspirin has a direct excitatory effect upon the respiratory centres in the brain stem, resulting in hyperventilation and a respiratory alkalosis. Salicylic acid is a weak acid with an uncoupling effect upon ATP; this tends to cause a metabolic acidosis. Blood gas analyses in an adult usually show a pH in the upper range of normal or above it, a low $PaCO_2$ and a normal PaO_2; the bicarbonate concentration tends to be below that predicted from the $PaCO_2$. In children, and a minority of adults, blood pH may be found to be low and these patients have a relatively poor prognosis. In acidotic or confused adults and all children, blood glucose should be assessed as hypoglycaemia is not uncommon.

Perhaps the most important principle to remember when treating salicylate poisoning is that, when indicated, active treatment should be started promptly. Death can occur early and with little warning. Gastric aspiration and lavage should be carried out on the strength of the history and instituted at any time up to 12 hours after ingestion. Gastrointestinal bleeding is uncommon despite the frequency with which the preparation causes haematemesis after therapeutic doses. The sheet anchor of treatment is a forced alkaline diuresis. This procedure enhances excretion of salicylate, corrects any hypovolaemia and ensures adequate blood glucose levels. A number of regimes have been suggested and that described on page 329 is adequate. This regime may cause the patient's blood pH to rise as high as 7.6 but there is no evidence that it has caused any harm whilst there is no doubt that it enhances excretion of salicylate[28]. It is not clear what is the best treatment for the combination of acidosis and decreased consciousness. The usual approach is to restore normal acid–base status by giving bicarbonate and then giving a standard diuresis. Care must be taken, as these patients are particularly prone to pulmonary oedema and may have primary capillary leak[29].

In severely poisoned patients who have renal failure or pulmonary oedema, it may be worthwhile using other methods to increase drug elimination. The most rapid and effective technique is haemoperfusion through a charcoal column but when this is not available, haemodialysis is also effective. Using these precise indications the technique will very rarely be necessary. It must always be borne in mind that the time taken to set up dialysis or perfusion is often as long as the time needed to complete a forced diuresis!

(7) Paracetamol

Paracetamol was first introduced in the late 1950s but sales did not become large until the middle 1960s. The first two cases of paracetamol poisoning were reported[30] in 1966, and since then there has been a gradual increase. To a certain extent it has supplanted aspirin and certainly these two substances have increased the proportion of non-prescribed drugs that are used as agents for self-poisoning. In therapeutic doses the drug is relatively effective as an analgesic with minor anti-inflammatory activity and is extremely non-toxic. This is not the case in overdosage.

Clinical features

As with aspirin poisoning, symptoms are not a reliable index of severity of poisoning. When the drug is taken in overdose the patient may vomit within the first 2–3 hours but rarely develop any other symptoms. Patients frequently appear at a hospital casualty department within a few hours of taking the overdose because they remained fully conscious and had second thoughts. Over the succeeding hours no specific symptoms develop, the patient may continue vomiting and develop epigastric pain. If a sufficiently large dose has been taken hepatic damage ensues; it reaches its peak, as

340

judged by liver function tests, between three and four days after ingestion. The more severe the poisoning the earlier these disturbances become apparent on biochemical testing. However, clinical signs of liver failure usually do not occur until 48 hours after ingestion even in the most severely poisoned cases.

Examination of the liver may reveal a tender enlarged organ during the first 3 days but this is not a reliable sign of liver damage. Jaundice may appear, but as hepatic damage is primarily hepatocellular it is only in severe cases that it is a major feature. In the very severe but non-fatal cases the hepatitic profile progresses to a cholestatic picture. Plasma levels of paracetamol usually reach their peak around 2 hours after ingestion and always by 4 hours. There is a clear relation between the plasma paracetamol levels corrected for time after ingestion and the occurrence and extent of liver damage. A level in excess of 200 mg/l at 4 hours after ingestion or 50 mg/l at 12 hours (Figure 14.1) are usually associated with liver damage if no treatment is given[31]. Levels less than this usually result in no liver damage or, at the worst, in minor changes. Previous ingestion of microsomal enzyme inducing drugs has a marginal effect in increasing the degree of liver damage[32]. The degree and extent of hepatic necrosis is relatively unpredictable in patients with alcoholic cirrhosis. There is a good relationship between the extent of liver damage and the plasma paracetamol half-life. Half-life following normal doses is approximately 2 hours, but following overdosage if it exceeds 4 hours then liver damage usually follows. If the half-life is in excess of 10 hours severe liver damage is certain and death a real possibility.

Management

Hepatic necrosis is not induced by paracetamol itself but by a toxic metabolite. This metabolite is formed by a P 450 dependent oxidative reaction. In the normal course of events the metabolite is scavenged by intracellular glutathione. In overdosage, glutathione stores are exhausted and the metabolite reacts with hepatic macromolecules finally resulting in cellular necrosis. Antidotal treatment has been directed towards either repleting intracellular glutathione or, alternatively, providing another suitable scavenging substance.

Despite paracetamol half-lives in severely poisoned patients being prolonged from as early as 4 hours after ingestion, it is possible to completely reverse hepatic necrosis with N-acetylcysteine, if it is given within 8 hours of ingestion. If the period between ingestion and treatment is between 8 and 12 hours hepatic necrosis may be reduced. Some authorities claim that treatment up to 15 hours may be useful but the evidence so far is unconvincing[33]. A variety of antidotes have been tried including cysteamine, penicillamine, dimercaprol and methionine[34]. The first substance to gain wide use was

341

cysteamine[35]. Though this is very effective it unfortunately causes considerable nausea and vomiting to the recipient. A more recently introduced antagonist is N-acetylcysteine, which is equally as effective as cysteamine and considerably less toxic[33]. It does not cause the serious gastrointestinal disturbances and in my own experience the side-effects are confined to restlessness with elevation of blood pressure. The dose regime is as follows:

150 mg/kg body weight over 15 minutes
50 mg/kg in 5% dextrose over 4 hours
100 mg/kg in 5% dextrose over 16 hours

As nausea and vomiting occur in over 50% of cases of paracetamol poisoning there is little justification for using oral preparations such as methionine when the patient is potentially seriously poisoned.

In those patients who present late, that is more than 12 hours after ingestion, antidotal treatment is not as effective. Various techniques may be used to predict those patients that will develop either severe hepatic damage or hepatic failure as opposed to minor changes. These include a paracetamol half-life greater than 10 hours, a prothrombin time more than three times normal and becoming progressively longer and the aminopyrine breath test[36]. Peak serum enzyme levels occur around the third day and if hepatic coma is to occur it usually appears between the third and fourth days after ingestion. Treatment in this situation remains speculative. It is customary for patients to be put on a liver failure regime. There is some evidence suggesting that dialysis and haemoperfusion in the period 12–18 hours after ingestion may be of help in borderline cases of very severe poisoning, but this is by no means proved. Finally, once hepatic failure has occurred treatment in no way differs from that of hepatic failure due to other causes.

(8) Opiate narcotics

Until recently poisoning with this group of drugs, which includes morphine, heroin, methadone, pethidine, dihydrocodeine, pentazocine and codeine, was usually either due to overdosage or misuse by addicts. However, over the last few years self-poisoning by the typical 'self-poisoning' patient with Distalgesic has occurred on a large scale. Distalgesic contains paracetamol and dextropropoxyphene and the latter has opiate-like actions.

Clinical features

Certain features distinguish opiate poisoning from that of hypnotics. Firstly though the patient may be unconscious, there is often a greater degree of respiratory depression than would be expected by the reduction in level of consciousness as compared with barbiturate overdosage. Pupils are often pinpoint though they remain equal and may be reactive. Hypotension is a common accompaniment. In addicts there is often evidence of repeated intravenous injections together with complications such as scars, abscesses and thrombosed veins. Another outstanding feature of Distalgesic poisoning is the synergism shown with alcohol. If an overdose of Distalgesic is taken at the same time as alcohol a proportion of patients develop rapid depression in level of consciousness and also disproportionate depression of respiration[37]. Patients appear to die with relatively low alcohol levels and relatively small overdoses with Distalgesic. Symptoms may appear very rapidly. It is not unknown for a fit young person to go from being fully conscious to Grade 4 unconscious in the space of 10 minutes.

Management

We now possess a specific and rapidly acting antagonist. This substance, naloxone, is chemically related to morphine; it reverses the respiratory depressant activity of opiates without having any respiratory stimulant activity of its own. It also reverses depression of consciousness and causes the pupils to dilate. Naloxone is a non-toxic substance and may be used as a therapeutic test in cases of coma where there is only a suspicion that opiates are involved. It sometimes causes an acute withdrawal syndrome in addicts and may cause laryngeal spasm in patients with severely depressed respiration. Naloxone has a relatively short half-life and its effects wear off in 15–30 minutes. It may be necessary to give repeated doses of the drug and because its mode of action is that of an antagonist, it may be necessary to give considerably more than the standard 2 mg dose. In the comatose patient full respiratory care should be instituted as well as giving the antidote. Failure to respond suggests that other substances have been taken or that severe brain damage has occurred.

(9) Phenothiazines

This group of drugs, which are often prescribed as major tranquillizers, were developed from the antihistamines. They are used in patients with psychotic illnesses and although an uncommon cause of self-poisoning, the death rate is high. They are rapidly absorbed from the gut and are widely distributed in the body, with consequent low blood levels. They tend to be excreted in the bile and then reabsorbed once again from the gut. Examples of drugs in this group include chlorpromazine, promazine, thioridazine, thiothixene and fluphenazine.

Clinical features

Patients are frequently drowsy or unconscious; neurological examination may show involuntary movements, but the reflexes are not usually increased to the same degree as is seen with tricyclic poisoning. The major features in the cardiovascular system are hypotension and tachycardia. Hypotension, which may be due to a combination of α-adrenergic blockage and central depressant action of the drug, may be severe and difficult to treat. The tachycardia is presumably partly a reflex response to the hypotension. Dysrhythmias may develop though they are not as common as with the tricyclic antidepressants. Profound hypothermia may be a major feature and is due to peripheral vasomotor collapse together with depression of the hypothalamus.

Management

Management is entirely supportive. The nature of the poisoning may be confirmed by toxicological examination of the urine but attempts to increase renal elimination of the drug, by forced diuresis or body clearance by dialysis and haemoperfusion, are entirely ineffective. The only feature that may require active intervention is drug-induced extrapyramidal dyskinesias including oculogyric crisis. Substances such as benztropine mesylate 2 mg intravenously may be given repeatedly if necessary. Cardiac arrhythmias have been treated with physostigmine[38].

(10) Amphetamine derivatives

Amphetamine sulphate, that is benzedrine, dexamphetamine sulphate (Dexedrine) and methylamphetamine are hardly ever prescribed nowadays for therapeutic reasons and cases of poisoning are usually associated with illicit use. When these substances are not obtainable, drugs such as fenfluramine and diethylpropion are used as substitutes. Whether or nor these latter two compounds have amphetamine-like actions in normal dosage, there is no doubt that in overdosage the clinical picture is identical.

Clinical features

The most obvious features are restlessness, tremor and irritability. In more severe cases there may be confusion, anxiety and aggressiveness; limb reflexes are often increased and pupils dilated. There is frequently pallor followed by flushing and tachycardia. Cardiac dysrhythmias have been reported, particularly in severe cases, and where death occurs this is frequently the cause. Gastrointestinal tract symptoms do occur but are more common on withdrawal of the drug from addicts.

Management

Usually the most urgent measure that is required is sedation; diazepam is probably the least toxic preparation but if this is insufficient, chlorpromazine is an alternative. Forced acid diuresis has been used[40] and it increases the renal excretion of amphetamine and fenfluramine. However, in the vast majority of cases it is not required.

(11) Paraquat

This substance has achieved immense popularity in the last decade or so as a herbicide. It has the property of killing vegetation but becoming inactive after contact with soil. Ground upon which paraquat has been sprayed may be sown days later. It is available to farmers and market gardeners in a 20% concentrated solution (Gramoxone, etc.) and is also available to the general public in the form of solid granules which contain 5% paraquat and diquat (Weedol, Pathclear). In the early 1960s the major cause of ingestion was accidental. The concentrate was frequently put into a container, such as a lemonade bottle, and then drunk by accident by another person. The makers mounted a very successful publicity campaign highlighting the toxic properties of paraquat, and discouraging its transfer to unmarked bottles. As a result accidental poisoning has diminished but deliberate poisoning has increased.

Clinical features

Paraquat is a strong corrosive and early clinical features are common to those of any corrosive substance. They consist of burns to the tongue, mouth and oesophagus. Frequently these are not apparent immediately after ingestion but appear 24–48 hours later. Large white necrotic areas develop which are often painless. There is repeated vomiting and occasionally superficial epithelium of the stomach or oesophagus is vomited up. In severe cases where an overwhelming amount of the substance has been ingested all organs are damaged. Hepatic and renal damage occurs and there may be encephalopathy, myocarditis and bleeding into the lungs. Death usually occurs within 72 hours. In less severe cases symptoms may be much less dramatic. The patient is usually nauseated, vomits, may develop renal failure and minor hepatic damage. Paraquat is actively taken up by

345

the lung and concentrated in the alveolar cells[47]. These cells proliferate and a diffusion block occurs resulting in hyperventilation, hypoxaemia and hypocapnia. It may take 2–3 weeks for the clinical features to develop and a death, distressing to the patient, staff and relatives, ensues. Some patients do not take sufficient paraquat to develop lung lesions but enough for it to be detected in both blood and urine. These patients may escape all toxic features and excrete the substance without any ill effects over a period of days after ingestion.

Treatment

On admission and solely on the basis of the history, the patient should have a gastric aspiration and lavage. Fuller's earth, 1 litre of 15% suspension with 200 ml of 20% mannitol, should be given in order to inactivate paraquat in the gut and induce purgation. It is a rather unappetising mixture and may need to be given by a nasogastric tube. If Weedol has been taken approximately 90% of patients survive, whereas if a concentrate has been ingested the mortality rate is 90%. Assessment of severity can now be made. A rapid qualitative test on the urine will indicate whether any paraquat is present in the body. A radioimmunoassay is available in specialist centres which allows assay of blood paraquat levels, which correlate with severity of poisoning[48]. A variety of treatments have been tried, ranging from steroids and cytotoxic drugs, L-propranolol, superoxide dismutase, haemoperfusion and haemodialysis. None of these regimes has been shown to alter the natural progression of the poisoning. At the moment there would not appear to be any useful treatment available once the substance has been absorbed. Though it is impossible to treat the lung lesion, all other complications should be treated energetically as they are all potentially reversible. Hepatic damage should be treated by routine measures. Renal failure should be managed as any other case of acute tubular necrosis. There are very few cases of paraquat poisoning on record in which a definite lung lesion has occurred where pulmonary oedema and aspiration of stomach contents into the lungs was absent and who have then survived. The lung lesion in the vast majority of cases is progressive and ultimately fatal. Until recently there˙was no method of assessing the severity of poisoning, so the various treatments regimes that have been tried may not have been adequately assessed and patients with significantly different degrees of poisoning inadvertently compared.

(12) Sodium chlorate

Sodium chlorate is an effective weedkiller and is generally available.

346

Clinical features

The patient initially develops nausea, vomiting, abdominal pain and diarrhoea. Severe intravascular haemolysis and haemoglobinaemia ensue later. Haemoglobinuria, together with direct action of sodium chlorate on the kidneys, results in acute tubular necrosis. Acute hepatic damage may also occur.

Treatment

Treatment is largely supportive; methylene blue, 100 ml of 10% solution may be given intravenously for methaemoglobinaemia. It has been claimed that dialysis removes significant amounts of the chlorate ion but it is not clear whether anything useful is achieved. Dialysis may also be necessary for treatment of the acute renal failure.

(13) Cholinesterase inhibitors

These may be subdivided into two groups, organophosphorus compounds, which include parathion, and carbamate insecticides. They act by irreversibly inhibiting cholinesterase. There is potentiation of post-ganglionic parasympathetic activity. Initial stimulation then block of skeletal muscle neurotransmission also occurs resulting in fasciculation and then paralysis. Stimulation followed by depression of the central nervous system results in coma and convulsions[49]. The organophosphorus insecticides form extremely stable links with acetylcholinesterase whilst carbamate insecticides, though combining with cholinesterase, undergo slow but spontaneous degradation and clinical symptoms do not persist for more than 6–8 hours.

Clinical features

Symptoms of gross parasympathomimetic overactivity including anorexia, vomiting, colicky abdominal pain and diarrhoea are characteristic. The patient is frequently restless with dilated pupils; unconsciousness and epileptiform fits may also occur. Later ventilation becomes depressed both because of paralysis of respiratory muscles and also depression of the respiratory centre. Pulse rate is often slow and hypotension together with shock may result.

Treatment

Pralidoxime is a specific antidote for this form of poisoning and causes breakdown of the organophosphorus/cholinesterase complex. It should only be used in organophosphorus insecticide poisoning. In the case of carbamate poisoning the half-life of the enzyme/toxin complex is relatively short lived. Treatment is otherwise symptomatic. Large quantities of atropine may be needed to correct the bradycardia; IPPV may also be required. Care should be taken with drug therapy because reduction in cholinesterase activity may potentiate their activity. This is particularly marked with opiates, antihistamines, phenothiazines and tricyclic antidepressants. Estimates of cholinesterase activity should be made as an index of progress and the patient should be kept at rest until it has reached 70% of normal.

(14) Cyanide

Industry is the commonest source of cyanide salts, which are used to clean or harden metal. It is also used in laboratories and occasionally this is the source of the poisoning agent. Cyanide reacts with cytochrome c thus inhibiting the last steps in cell oxidation; there is failure in utilization of oxygen despite adequate delivery.

Clinical features

Ingestion of large quantities, for example 1–2 g, results in congestion and irritation of the gastric mucosa. There is a rapid loss of consciousness together with convulsions and death usually follows within a few minutes. If rather less is taken, the patient complains of dizziness; he then becomes breathless, confused and finally shocked. This may progress to loss of consciousness and death. Serious complications usually occur within 4 hours of ingestion.

Treatment

Factories using cyanide often have emergency kits and the patient can be given amyl nitrite to inhale before leaving the site of the accident. In hospital the current treatment is oxygen and cobalt edetate (Kelocyanor). 600 mg should be given intravenously over 1 minute followed by a further 300 mg if the patient fails to improve. Cobalt has a greater affinity for cyanide radicals than ferric ions which are present in cytochrome c. This treatment may itself cause hypotension, tachycardia, vomiting and diarrhoea[50]. Since cobalt edetate can cause hypoglycaemia, dextrose should also be given. If these measures fail, 15 ml of a 3% solution of sodium nitrite should be given intravenously. This causes the formation of methaemoglobin which competes with cytochrome c for the cyanide radicals. This is followed by 25 ml of 50% sodium thiosulphate solution which forms sodium thiocyanide, a relatively non-toxic end product. Once again, therapy is often accompanied by nausea, vomiting and occasionally shock.

(15) Acids and alkalis

Acid and acid-like substances are mainly used for cleaning metals and other substances. They are also involved in industrial chemical processes. Alkalis are used in the manufacture of soaps and also as cleaning substances in the household. The main action of acid is to destroy cells by non-specific destructive activity whilst alkalis attack protein and fats thus producing large necrotic areas.

Clinical features

When swallowed they cause intense burning of the mouth, pharynx and stomach. This is usually accompanied by vomiting and diarrhoea. Damage may be severe enough to cause perforation of the oesophagus and stomach with ensuing peritonitis. Irritation of the epiglottis and larynx may cause acute epiglottitis and laryngitis leading to asphyxia. Absorption results in profound acid–base disturbance, shock and death. Frequently there are extensive burns around the mouth, buccal mucosa and tongue which can give rise to intense pain.

Treatment

There is some debate as to the value of gastric lavage; it has been suggested that the risks of causing perforation outweigh the possible advantages. However, this is by no means proven and in experienced hands a stomach washout may help. If perforation has not occurred, liberal fluids should be given in order to dilute the corrosive substances. Shock should be treated by standard methods and tracheostomy may be considered if severe pharyngeal oedema occurs. Treatment is supportive. All patients should be carefully followed up after the acute episode because oesophageal stricture is a common late complication.

(16) Phenolic compounds

Phenol and its derivatives are common constituents of antiseptics, disinfectants and preservation substances. They denature proteins and have a non-specific destructive effect upon cells and cell walls.

Clinical features

Acute poisoning is frequently accompanied by painless blanching or alternatively erythema around the mouth and chin. There is intense thirst, nausea, vomiting, diarrhoea and sweating. If poisoning is severe this may be followed by abdominal pain, disturbance of consciousness, convulsions and coma. Acute renal failure is a frequent complication and hepatic damage can also occur.

Treatment

Once again there is controversy about gastric lavage, but if this procedure is performed carefully it is probably worthwhile in cases seen shortly after ingestion. Management is largely supportive; methaemoglobinaemia should be treated with methylene blue, respiratory depression by mechanical ventilation (Chapter 7) and shock by standard methods (Chapter 5). Acute renal failure should be treated by peritoneal or haemodialysis as indicated by standard criteria.

(17) Carbon monoxide

Now that carbon monoxide is no longer present in household gas, the commonest sources are motor car exhaust fumes and incomplete combustion of natural gas[51]. Carbon monoxide has a 300 times greater affinity for haemoglobin than has oxygen; it binds with haemoglobin and prevents it being used for oxygen transport. Tissue hypoxia ensues. This form of poisoning has a high mortality and the removal of carbon monoxide from household supplies is probably the single most important cause of the recent fall in suicide rate.

Clinical features

Clinical features are almost entirely due to hypoxia. When a significant level of carboxyhaemoglobin is reached the subject hyperventilates, becomes confused and disorientated and may develop coma. Cerebral oedema consequent to hypoxia may cause papilloedema. Hypoxia also affects the myocardium causing e.c.g. changes and infarction. Permanent neurological damage and myocardial infarction frequently occur up to 96 hours after the poisoning episode, well after apparent recovery has occurred. Furthermore, a single episode of poisoning may cause a Parkinson-like syndrome many years after the event. No reliance should be placed on the bright cherry pink colour frequently quoted as a diagnostic aid in patients with carbon monoxide poisoning; this finding is infrequently seen in survivors.

Treatment

All cases should be considered to be potentially serious. Oxygen should be given as soon as possible. If poisoning is sufficiently severe to cause respiratory depression, then the patient should be intubated and given high concentrations of oxygen by intermittent positive pressure ventilation (Chapter 7).

(18) Miscellaneous drugs

Antihistamines

A wide variety of preparations in the group are available on the market. Their principal toxic action is due to anticholinergic activity. Patients may develop tachycardia, dilated pupils, hallucinations, restlessness, coma and convulsions[41]. Treatment is supportive. Nitrazepam should be given for epileptiform fits; physostigmine salicylate has been advocated to lessen the degree of coma, but as with tricyclic antidepressant drugs, it not infrequently precipitates grand mal epileptiform fits. Its use should therefore be avoided. Forced diuresis and dialysis are ineffective.

β-blocking drugs

The main effect of this group of drugs is bradycardia and depression of level of consciousness[42]. Standard treatment consists of gastric lavage, atropine for bradycardia and isoprenaline by infusion to sustain blood pressure; it may be necessary to give both these drugs in large doses to have any effect. Dopamine and dobutamine may be more effective alternatives to isoprenaline. Large doses of glucagon have been tried but the author has no evidence of the value of this drug in β-blocker overdosage.

Theophylline derivatives

This group of drugs, and particularly slow release aminophylline, if taken in overdosage, causes nausea, vomiting, abdominal discomfort and occasionally ileus. They also cause tachycardia and cardiac dysrhythmias. Treatment is largely supportive but in seriously poisoned patients, where there are high blood levels, charcoal haemoperfusion has been attempted. It is claimed that patients benefited from the procedure[43].

Monoamine oxidase inhibitors

Poisoning with this group of drugs has become relatively uncommon. In overdosage they cause agitation, hallucinations, tachycardia and hyperthermia. They have also been reported to cause both hypotension and hypertension. Treatment is largely supportive but sympathomimetic agents such as metaraminol, isoprenaline and dopamine should all be avoided when shock is being treated.

Sulfonyl ureas and insulin

The clinical features of poisoning with these two groups of substances are those due to hypoglycaemia. Treatment consists of adequate amounts of intravenous dextrose. When insulin is administered intramuscularly in unusually large amounts, hypoglycaemia continues over a prolonged period, presumably due to slow release from the site of injection. Treatment should be continued over this period and the patient carefully monitored when treatment is stopped. Phenformin in overdosage may in addition cause lactic acidosis.

Iron

Iron poisoning seems to be particularly common in young women and children, presumably reflecting the number of prescriptions given to pregnant mothers.

Often the patients are initially asymptomatic. A minority develop severe abdominal pain, nausea, vomiting and haematemesis consequent to an acute gastritis. Patients who are seriously poisoned develop hypovolaemia and shock between 6 and 12 hours after ingestion. 24 hours later metabolic acidosis, convulsion, coma and acute hepatic necrosis ensue. Symptoms and signs appear to be related to serum iron concentrations and it is very uncommon for serious complications to develop unless the peak serum iron has exceeded 2–3 times the maximum normal value. It should be remembered that iron is often slowly absorbed and single serum concentrations should be interpreted with caution[44].

Despite evidence of gastrointestinal irritation, gastric aspiration and lavage should be performed and 10 g of desferrioxamine which chelates iron, should be left in the stomach. Plasma iron levels should be obtained as soon as possible in order to confirm the history. If values over twice the upper limit of normal are obtained then 1–2 g of desferrioxamine should be given intramuscularly and the dose repeated 12 hourly. If the patient is shocked the antidote is given intravenously; the dose is 15 mg/kg each hour up to a total dose of 80 mg/kg in 24 hours. Treatment is otherwise supportive.

Ethanol

The most common type of ethanol poisoning is over-indulgence. Occasionally, and particularly in children, alcohol poisoning is caused by ingestion of solvents which may frequently contain other toxic substances. Ethanol causes central nervous system depression and its effect can be potentiated by sedative drugs.

The clinical features are well-known to most people but are potentially serious when there is depression of consciousness. Coma may be deep but is usually short lived. There is considerable risk of hypothermia and some subjects, particularly children, develop hypoglycaemia. This should be treated with intravenous dextrose.

Methanol

Methanol poisoning is most commonly seen in vagrants, but may on occasion be accidental.

Depression of level of consciousness, nausea and vomiting are the major clinical features but there is often a profound metabolic acidosis with acidotic (Kussmaul) respiration. Severely poisoned patients develop acute optic nerve papillitis resulting in loss of vision. Occasionally symptoms may be delayed for 12–18 hours.

Gastric lavage should be performed if the patient is seen within 4 hours of ingestion and supportive therapy should be instituted. The appearance of acidosis or a blood level in excess of 500 mg/l indicates serious poisoning. Sodium bicarbonate should be given to correct the acidosis. Ethanol competes with methanol for alcohol dehydrogenase and should be given to prevent the formation of formate. A loading dose of 0.6 mg/kg followed by an infusion of 66 mg $kg^{-1}h^{-1}$ has been recommended. Haemodialysis has also been advocated and there is no doubt that it does remove methanol very rapidly but there is no definite evidence that this therapy is any more effective than using ethanol. The two treatments have been used simultaneously[45,46].

(V) INFORMATION SERVICES

Information services on poisoning have existed for some years. In the United States, with its greater emphasis on individual responsibility, the information services are directly accessible to the public. They deal with ten times the number of calls from the same sized population as the more restrictive British services.

In Britain there is the National Poison Information Service which has a 'contact' in each capital of various principalities. The information is given only to medical or paramedical personnel and usually consists of annotated data retrieved from extensive files. Some regions, such as Newcastle and Leeds, have attempted to offer alternative information by arranging direct access to medical or paramedical staff who are trained in poisoning. Others, such as the West Midlands, offer clinical support.

Government Sponsored Poisons Information Services:

London	01-407 7600
Edinburgh	031-229 2477
Cardiff	0222-33101
Belfast	0232-40503

References

1. Kreitman, N. (1977). *Parasuicide*. (London: Wiley)
2. Editorial (1979). Policies on self poisoning. *Br. Med. J.*, **2**, 1091
3. Wright, N. (1980). An assessment of the unreliability of the history given by self poisoned patients. *Clin. Toxicol.*, **16**, 381
4. Wright, N. (1980). Common errors in the management of self poisoning. *J. R. Coll. Physicians London*.
5. Matthew, H. and Lawson, A.A.L. (1979). *Treatment of Common Acute Poisonings*. (Edinburgh: Churchill Livingstone)
6. Kaplan, S.A. and del Carmen, F.T. (1958). Experimental salicylate poisoning: Observations on the effects of carbonic anhydrase inhibitor and bicarbonate. *Paediatrics*, **21**, 762
7. Goulding, R. (1976). Experience with haemoperfusion in drug abuse. *Kidney Int.*, **10**, 338
8. Wright, N., Clarkson, A,R., Brown, S.S. and Foster, V. (1971). Effects of poisoning on serum enzyme activities, coagulation and fibrinolysis. *Br. Med. J.*, **3**, 347
9. Sutherland, G.R., Park, J. and Proudfoot, A.T. (1977). Ventilation and acid

base changes in deep coma due to barbiturate or tricyclic antidepressant poisoning. *Clin. Toxicol.,* **2**, 403

10. Arndt, K. A., Milne, M. C. and Parrish, J. A. (1973). Bullae, a cutaneous sign of a variety of neurological diseases. *J. Invest. Dermatol.,* **60**, 312
11. Barbour, B. H., Lasette, A. M. and Koffle, A. (1976). Fixed bed charcoal haemoperfusion for the treatment of drug overdose. *Kidney Int.,* **10**, 5
12. Vale, J. A., Rees, A. J., Widdop, B. and Goulding, R. (1975). Use of charcoal haemoperfusion in the management of severely poisoned patients. *Br. Med. J.,* **1**, 5
13. Rosenbaum, J. L., Kramer, M. S., Raja, R., Winsten, S. and Dalal, F. (1976). Haemoperfusion for acute drug intoxication. *Kidney Int.,* **10**, 5
14. Lorch, J. A. and Garella, S. (1979). Haemoperfusion to treat intoxication. *Ann. Intern. Med.,* **91**, 301
15. Chazen, J. A. and Cohen, J. (1969). Clinical spectrum of glutethimide poisoning. *J. Am. Med. Assoc.,* **208**, 837
16. Wright, N. and Roscoe, P. (1970). Acute glutethimide poisoning. *J. Am. Med. Assoc.,* **214**, 1704
17. Matthew, H., Proudfoot, A. T., Brown, S. S. and Smith, A. C. A. (1968). Mandrax poisoning, conservative management of 116 patients. *Br. Med. J.,* **2**, 101
18. Bailey, D. N. (1973). Methyprylon overdosage: interpretation of serum drug concentration. *Clin. Toxicol.,* **6**, 563
19. Gibson, P. F. and Wright, N. (1972). Ethchlorvynol in biological fluids: specificity of methods of assay. *J. Pharm. Sci.,* **61**, 169
20. Marshall, A. J. (1977). Cardiac arrhythmias caused by chloral hydrate. *Br. Med. J.,* **2**, 944
21. Illingworth, R. N. and Stewart, M. J. (1979). Severe poisoning with chlormethiazole. *Br. Med. J.,* **2**, 903
22. Masters, A. B. (1967). Delayed death in imipramine poisoning. *Br. Med. J.,* **3**, 866
23. Petit, J. M., Spiker, D. G., Rutwitch, J. F., Ziegler, V. E., Weiss, A. N. and Biggs, J. T. (1977). Tricyclic antidepressant plasma levels and adverse effects after overdose. *Clin. Pharm. Ther.,* **20**, 47
24. Slovis, T. L., Oh, J. E., Teitlebaum, D. T. and Lipscombe, W. (1971). Physostigmine therapy in acute tricyclic antidepressant poisoning. *Clin. Toxicol.,* **4**, 451
25. Newton, R. W. (1975). Physostigmine salicylate in the treatment of tricyclic antidepressant overdosage. *J. Am. Med. Assoc.,* **231**, 941
26. Vance, M. A., Ross, S. M., Millington, W. R. and Blumberg, J. B. (1977). Potentiation of tricyclic antidepressant toxicity by physostigmine in mice. *Clin. Toxicol.,* **11**, 413
27. Proudfoot, A. T. and Brown, S. S. (1969). Acidaemia and salicylate poisoning in adults. *Br. Med. J.,* **1**, 547
28. Lawson, A. A. H., Proudfoot, A.T., Brown, S. S., MacDonald, R. H., Fraser, G., Cameron, J. C. and Matthew, H. (1969). Forced diuresis in the treatment of acute salicylate poisoning in adults. *Q. J. Med.,* **38**, 31
29. Hormaechea, E., Carlson, R. W., Rogoue, H., Uphold, J., Henning, R. J. and Weil, M. H. (1979). Hypovolaemia, pulmonary oedema and protein changes in

severe salicylate poisoning. *Am. J. Med.,* **66**, 1046
30. Davidson, D.G.D. and Eastham, W.N. (1966). Acute liver necrosis following overdose of paracetamol. *Br. Med. J.,* **2**, 497
31. Prescott, L.F., Wright, N., Roscoe, P. and Brown, S.S. (1971). Plasma–paracetamol half life and hepatic necrosis in patients with paracetamol overdosage. *Lancet,* **1**, 519
32. Wright, N. and Prescott, L.F. (1973). Potentiation of previous drug therapy of hepatoxicity following paracetamol overdosage. *Scott. Med. J.,* **18**, 56
33. Prescott, L.F., Illingworth, R.N., Critchley, J.A.J.H., Stewart, M.J., Adam, R.D. and Proudfoot, A.T. (1979). Intravenous N-acetylcysteine: the treatment of choice for paracetamol poisoning. *Br. Med. J.,* **2**, 1097
34. Prescott, L.F., Park, J., Sutherland, G.R., Smith, I.J. and Proudfoot, A.T. (1976). Cysteamine, methionine and penicillamine in the treatment of paracetamol poisoning. *Lancet,* **2**, 109
35. Hughes, R.D., Gazzard, B.G., Hamid, M.A., Trewby, P.N., Murray-Lyon, I.M., Davis, M., Williams, R. and Bennett, J.R. (1977). Controlled trial of cysteamine and dimercaprol after paracetamol overdose. *Br. Med. J.,* **2**, 1395
36. Saunders, J.B., Wright, N. and Lewis, K.O. (1980). Predicting the outcome of paracetamol poisoning. *Br. Med. J.,* **1**, 279
37. Carson, D.J.L. and Carson, E.D. (1977). Fatal dextropropoxyphene poisoning in Northern Ireland. *Lancet,* **1**, 894
38. Weisdorf, D., Kramer, J., Goldberg, A. and Klawans, H.L. (1978). Physostigmine for cardiac and neurologic manifestations of phenothiazine poisoning. *Clin. Pharm. Ther.,* **24**, 663
39. Veltri, J.C. and Temple, A.R. (1975). Fenfluramine poisoning. *J. Paediatr.,* **87**, 119
40. Riley, I., Corson, J., Haiden, J. and Oswald, I. (1969). Fenfluramine overdosage. *Lancet,* **2**, 1162
41. Cowen, P.J. (1979). Toxic psychosis with antihistamines reversed by physostigmine. *Postgrad. Med. J.,* **55**, 556
42. Kahn, A. and Muscar-Baron, J.M. (1977). Fatal oxprenolol poisoning. *Br. Med. J.,* **1**, 552
43. Lawyer, C., Aitchison, J., Sutton, J. and Bennett, W. (1978). Treatment of Theophylline neurotoxicity with resin haemoperfusion. *Ann. Intern. Med.,* **88**, 516
44. Eriksson, F., Johansson, S.V., Mellstedt, H. and Strandberd, O. (1974). Iron intoxication in two adult patients. *Acta Med. Scand.,* **196**, 231
45. Genda, A., Gault, H., Churchill, D. and Hollomby, D. (1978). Haemodialysis for methanol intoxication. *Am. J. Med.,* **64**, 749
46. McCoy, H., Cipolle, R.J., Ehlers, S.M., Sawchuk, R.J. and Zaske, D.E. (1979). Severe methanol poisoning. *Am. J. Med.,* **67**, 804
47. Rose, M.S., Smith, L.L. and Wyatt, I. (1974). Active uptake of paraquat by the lung. *Nature, (London),* **252**, 314
48. Proudfoot, A.T., Stewart, M.S., Levitt, T. and Widdop, B. (1979). Paraquat poisoning: significance of plasma paraquat concentrations. *Lancet,* **2**, 330
49. Smith, D.M. (1971). Organophosphorus poisoning from emergency use of a handsprayer. *Practitioner,* **218**, 877
50. Bryson, D.D. (1978). Cyanide poisoning. *Lancet,* **1**, 92
51. Venables, G.S. (1977). Carbon monoxide: a forgotten poison. *Lancet,* **2**, 461

15
Guillain-Barré syndrome

HENNING SUND KRISTENSEN

The Guillain-Barré type of polyneuritis has several other names, among which are post-infectious polyneuropathy and inflammatory polyradiculo-neuropathy. Sometimes the names Landry and Strohl are also attached to the syndrome. The former reported ten cases in 1859 and the latter was a co-author of Guillain and Barré who in 1916 described the clinical picture and characteristic findings in the spinal fluid. The Guillain-Barré syndrome has the following symptoms:

(1) An acute onset over 3 weeks.

(2) Lower motor neuron involvement with symmetrical ascending paresis, sometimes progressing to severe or even total paralysis.

(3) Muscle pain can be severe; the muscles are tender and this must influence the nursing care. In comparison paraesthesiae and especially sensory loss are minimal.

(4) Elevated protein but no pleocytosis in the spinal fluid.

(5) Recovery of normal or almost normal muscular strength in most of the survivors.

There is no cerebral involvement or signs of acute infection, but about one half of the patients report preceding mild respiratory or gastrointestinal symptoms. Other preceding and probably provoking factors described are

357

Mycoplasma pneumoniae infection, vaccination or operations. Symptoms arising from the autonomic nervous system present a problem and may contribute to the significant death rate. The disease is uncommon and often not recognized at the onset. Some patients are initially considered as hysterical. The disease is life-threatening when the muscles controlling respiration and swallowing are severely affected. On the other hand the chance of full recovery is good if the patient can be carried through the life-threatening period. Therefore the disease has always represented a definite challenge to intensive care units.

Tank and cuirass respirators were introduced into the Blegdam Hospital in the late 1930s, chiefly for the treatment of respiratory failure due to poliomyelitis, which was very common at that time. Patients with respiratory failure due to other diseases were also admitted, so that during the last 40 years the Blegdam Hospital received most of the severe cases of polyneuritis from Greater Copenhagen. The following account is a continuation of the study from this department by Ravn[1], who reported on experiences up to 1964.

(I) ASSESSMENT

The routine monitoring of severe cases of polyneuritis has included, whenever possible, the determination of the vital capacity by a simple gasometer connected to the patient by a valve and a mouthpiece. When respiratory failure was imminent the vital capacity was tested several times a day and the blood pressure, pulse and respiratory rates were determined hourly.

Deglutition was tested by examining the pharynx. When secretions started to accumulate and suction was required to clear the pharynx, a naso-gastric tube was passed and the patient was not allowed to take anything by mouth. When doubt existed as to deglutition, the patient was asked to swallow a mouthful of water. Impaired deglutition was indicated by a tense manoeuvre of swallowing, sometimes broken down into two or more steps and maybe followed by cough as a sign of fluid entering the airway. In cases where the respiratory muscles were not too weak, a permanent head-down position offered a good protection from aspiration in cases of impaired deglutition. However, few patients would tolerate this regimen. It is extremely important to watch for the signs usually preceding under-ventilation. Such signs are fatigue, irritability, slight disorientation, impaired sleep, increased blood pressure and tachycardia. X-rays of the chest were necessary to supplement auscultation. In properly monitored patients, examination of the arterial blood gas tensions should play a minor role at this stage of the disease, since IPPV should be started in time to prevent the development of abnormal arterial gas tensions.

Patients with the Guillain–Barré syndrome should be carefully looked after by experienced personnel and should be transferred to the ICU in the following situations: (1) paresis of the respiratory muscles with a vital capacity of about 1.5 litres or less in normal adults, even when deglutition is normal and there are no pulmonary complications, (2) impaired deglutition or lung complications irrespective of the vital capacity.

(II) INTENSIVE THERAPY

(1) Respiratory care

Great effort was made to prevent lung complications and to treat them when they appeared. The position of the patient was changed at least every second hour and especially in the more severely paralysed patient. The position was varied between right and left side and supine position. As far as possible, a drainage position was used in the cases where it was thought valuable, but often it had to be modified and the periods of drainage shortened according to the tolerance of the patient. Accumulation of secretions in the airways was looked for by auscultation and by placing the hands on the thorax when the patient tried to breathe deeply or during lung physiotherapy. In patients with weak respiratory muscles, secretions may be 'silent' for long periods and yet can suddenly cause alarming symptoms.

(2) Intermittent positive pressure ventilation (IPPV)

Indications for artificial ventilation

The most common indication for IPPV was progressive paralysis of the respiratory muscles to the point of exhaustion. In such patients the arterial blood gases were normal. At the time when artificial ventilation was started the vital capacity was between 0.5 and 1.0 litres in normal adults. In other patients pulmonary complications contributed to the decision to start IPPV. Such complications can arise because of pre-existing bronchitis but are probably more often due to aspiration caused by impaired deglutition. In this group the vital capacity is higher at the start of IPPV than in the previous group. In the patients who require IPPV, about two thirds have impaired deglutition. In about a quarter of the patients ventilatory failure is present at the start of IPPV. The hypoventilation was either proved by examination of the arterial gases or was obvious from the clinical evaluation. In a few patients the ventilatory failure is acute and usually described as respiratory arrest.

Programme for IPPV

Patients are intubated under general anaesthesia at the time when IPPV is considered necessary. Should a muscle relaxant be used, suxamethonium is contraindicated and a non-polarizing agent is substituted. During our early years, tracheostomy was performed immediately following intubation, but later the operation has been postponed to normal working hours, usually the next day. During the period between the start of IPPV and tracheostomy, the patients were nasotracheally intubated and often sedated by the addition of nitrous oxide to the gas mixture, delivered from the ventilator. A tracheostomy was carried out at the level of the second or third tracheal ring and a cuffed tube inserted. From 1964 to 1978 the Lundia ventilator was used exclusively. This is an extremely simple machine, delivering a pre-set volume at a pre-set rate. In 1978 the Lundia was replaced by the Servo ventilator which is more up to date in design and just as reliable.

The regimen described for the pre-respirator period was continued after tracheostomy. Because the Lundia ventilator has no sighing mechanism, deep manual ventilation was performed for short periods together with suctioning of the airways. This procedure was carried out at regular intervals of 2–4 hours. Suction was performed with sterile catheters handled with a clean disposable glove. Chest physiotherapy was given routinely and intensified when atelectasis occurred. Bronchoscopy as a therapeutic measure was not performed and positive end-expiratory pressure was applied in only two cases.

Weaning from the respirator was usually without any problem. It was never attempted before the patient was able to breathe comfortably on his own. The patients were told, which was true, that we had never seen a patient with a Guillain–Barré syndrome who failed to regain spontaneous respiration and it was of no importance whether the return to spontaneous respiration took place during this week or the next. In a few cases it was necessary to push the patients a bit, but kindly, remembering that it is never justified or appropriate to try to force a patient to breathe spontaneously. Once spontaneous respiration was regained the cuff tracheal tube was replaced by a smaller tube without cuff or by a silver cannula. This tube or cannula was occluded for longer and longer periods according to the improvement in respiratory muscle function. The tube was finally removed when the tube could be closed all the time and the patient was able to clean his airway without suction. The average duration of artificial ventilation and of tracheostomy was 40 and 52 days respectively.

Antibiotic therapy was guided by microscopy of tracheal secretion and the results of culture and sensitivity test.

360

(3) Nutrition and fluid therapy

As previously mentioned, two thirds of the patients who needed IPPV had impaired swallowing. In these patients a nasogastric tube was passed at the time of tracheostomy. Most of the remaining patients also required a naso-gastric tube in order to maintain a sufficient intake of fluid and food. The food given via the tube was a simple one consisting of a daily amount for adults of 2 litres of milk, 1 litre of water, 150 g of sugar, 5 g of sodium chloride, and vitamins. In cases of gastric retention or intolerance, other types of food were tried but were often not tolerated any better. In patients with gastric retention of longer duration intravenous nutrition was given. Urinary catheters were necessary in almost all cases, often for periods of several weeks.

(4) Physiotherapy

Much effort was made to position the patient comfortably in the bed and to avoid contractures. Sometimes the patient suffered from severe restlessness or pain in his muscles, especially in the period of returning muscle power. Such patients were treated with hot packs in the same way as the polio patients in the 1950s. Frequent changes of position sometimes relieved the discomfort but often mild analgesic drugs had to be given.

(5) Psychological problems and their management

A paresis of a degree which necessitates IPPV is, of course, a severe strain on the psychological resources of everyone. The ability to speak is usually lost completely because of the cuff tube and/or impairment of the muscles of the mouth, pharynx and larynx. Even the facial and ocular muscles can be paralysed so that the patient is unable to express himself and to show what he likes or dislikes. The vision is often blurred. In four of the author's cases there was complete paralysis of the voluntary musculature, leaving the patients totally unresponsive for periods varying from a few days to several weeks. In this situation the nursing staff and the doctors may tend to forget that the patients are real, living and conscious human beings, but it is extremely important that they do not. In order to focus on this problem and thereby to ensure that the patient was treated in an acceptable way at all stages, interviews were held with patients after their recovery. It was obvious from these interviews that the patients lose interest in what is going on in the world – if they had any such interest previously! Instead they concentrate on their immediate personal situation. They want to be repeatedly informed on their progress and they want detailed explanations in advance of the procedures carried out. The persons best fitted to inform the patient are those actually nursing them at the bedside. The nursing staff should therefore be sufficiently informed to pass on the appropriate information to the patient. It is important that when the patient is moved in the bed he is turned by flat hands and enough of them to avoid causing pain in tender muscles. Also it must be remembered that suction of the airways has to be done as quickly and effectively as possible. The patient feels it extremely helpful to be taken care of by nurses with experience in all the problems associated with the situation.

As to entertainment, most patients prefer soft music. They do not want to listen to records of operas or classical novels, even if they are fond of both. After recovery they told us that time did not pass slowly, even at the climax of the disease. From time to time mild anxiolytic drugs may be given. Diazepam is such a drug and also sometimes relieves muscle pain. It is no surprise that many patients lose confidence that they will ever recover. In this situation former patients who had recovered from the disease were asked to come and tell the patients about their own experiences. This contact with previous patients has often proved more effective in maintaining the morale of the patient than anything else. It should be added that this policy, especially the interviews, also seemed to support the understanding and confidence of the nursing staff.

(6) Steroid treatment

This unit does not use a steroid to treat the Guillain–Barré syndrome and a controlled trial did not show any benefit[2]. These drugs have been used in cases requiring IPPV but did not reduce the duration of ventilator treatment[3]. The potential dangers of using a steroid during IPPV are very real, masking the signs of secondary bacterial infection and inducing immuno-incompetence (Chapter 2). There is one clear-cut indication for a steroid, relapsing polyneuritis[4], which is in a variant of the Guillain–Barré syndrome. When, following weaning from the respirator, the paralysis starts all over again, prednisolone, 60 mg a day is given until the disease remits. The dose is then reduced progressively.

(III) COMPLICATIONS

Our long experience in Copenhagen has indicated that most of the complications of the Guillain–Barré syndrome are preventable. This applies both during spontaneous respiration and IPPV.

(1) Circulatory

In patients observed in general wards, ventilatory failure can go unnoticed and lead to hypoxic cardiac arrest. The author has observed three such cases with one death. During IPPV, cardiac arrest, pathological variations in the heart rate and hypertension have been attributed to autonomic neuropathy[3,6]. In this unit only one case of cardiac arrest was seen during artificial ventilation of 53 patients. It occurred in a 70-year-old man with arteriosclerotic heart disease during preparation for tracheostomy. The patient survived without sequelae. Otherwise no significant circulatory trouble likely to be due to autonomic neuropathy was seen. Thromboembolism is an important complication of the paralytic state (Chapters 4, 12, 16) and pulmonary embolism killed three of the patients in the writer's total series of 125 cases. The incidence of thromboembolism may, in the future, be reduced by the routine use of low dosage heparin.

(2) Pulmonary

The most frequent complication was the accumulation of secretions in the airways often due to aspiration of saliva, food or vomit. In a few cases lung symptoms in patients with impaired function of the respiratory muscles could be handled without tracheostomy and respirator treatment. Retained secretions are an important indication to start IPPV. Atelectasis can occur during IPPV and then require even more chest physiotherapy. Bacterial infection can result in consolidation (pneumonia) and is usually due to gram-negative rods or staphylococci. The author has seen one case of pulmonary abscess but this healed spontaneously. Pulmonary infection can prolong IPPV or kill the patient; none of the author's patients died from this cause.

Tracheal stenosis occasionally complicates IPPV (Chapter 7) and occurred in three of the author's patients without finally hindering removal of the tube or cannula. Bacteraemia can arise from the lung, urinary tract or intravenous cannulae. This problem is described in detail in Chapter 3.

(IV) RESULTS

Since the Guillain–Barré syndrome does not kill directly, then all the patients should recover! Consequently, death is due to pre-existing disease – as is the case with chest injuries, tetanus, botulism, poisoning, or to complications, most of which are preventable. In the patient breathing spontaneously, hypoxic cardiac arrest or aspiration syndrome can occur unless the criteria for intensive care are enforced or IPPV is delayed because assessment is wrongly based on the blood gas findings; both are readily preventable. Thromboembolism can cause death at any time from the paralysis to the convalescent stages. In the writer's series, one death occurred because the patient disconnected himself from the ventilator. Bacterial infection is an important cause of morbidity and mortality; this topic is detailed in Chapter 3. The death rate during intensive care differs much in the series published (see Table 15.1). With good ICU facilities death rates of about 5-10% may be anticipated nowadays. Of the patients who recover with the aid of IPPV, a majority do so completely, a minority (one in four in the author's series) have disabilities due to residual paresis, usually in the legs.

Table 15.1   Results of IPPV used to treat Guillain-Barré syndrome

		Patients			
Reference	Period	Total	Survived	Died during artificial ventilation	Died after artificial ventilation
1	1949–52	9	1	8	
1	1953–63	33	22	11	
author	1964–78	53	51	3	1
3	1953–66	35	31	4	2
8	1967–74	32	30	2	
9	1967–76	41	33	8	
10	1968–75	45	25	20	(infants and children)

References

1.   Ravn, H. (1967). The Landry-Guillain-Barré syndrome. *Acta Neurol. Scand.*, **43**, (Suppl. 30)
2.   Hughes, R. A. C., Newsom-Davis, J. M., Perkin, G. D. and Pierce, J. M. (1978). Controlled trial of Prednisolone in acute polyneuropathy. *Lancet,* **2**, 750
3.   Hewer, R. L., Hilton, P. J., Smith, A. C. and Spalding, J. M. K. (1968). Acute polyneuritis requiring artificial ventilation. *Q. J. Med.*, **37**, 479
4.   Joong, S. (1978). Subacute demyelinating polyneuropathy responding to corticosteroid treatment. *Arch. Neurol.*, **35**, 509
5.   Henschel, E. O. (1977). The Guillain-Barré syndrome, a personal experience. *Anaesthesiology*, **47**, 228
6.   Edmonds, M. E. and Sturruck, R. D. (1979). Autonomic neuropathy in the Guillain-Barré syndrome. *Br. Med. J.,* **2**, 668
7.   Frison, J. C., Sanchez, L., Garnach, A., Bohil, J., Olivero, R. and Miguel, C. (1980). Heart rate variations in the Guillain-Barré syndrome. *Br. Med. J.,* **281**, 649

8. O'Donohue, W. J., Jr., Baker, J. P., Bell, G. M., Muren, O., Parker, C. L. and Patterson, J. L. Jr. (1976). Respiratory failure in neuromuscular disease. *J. Am. Med. Assoc.*, **235**, 733
9. Dowling, P. C., Menonna, J. P. and Cook, S. D. (1977). Guillain-Barré syndrome in Greater New York-New Jersey. *J. Am. Med. Assoc.*, **238**, 317
10. Garcia, S. F., Cordero, J., Olivos, P., Mogilevich, S., Dattoli, P., Sánchez, E., Inostroza, E., Zamorano, J., Espina, E., Boettcher, M., del Valle, G. and Carrillo, L. (1977). Sindrome de Guillain-Barré y Strohl, Forma Landry. Manejo con respirador mecánico. *Rev. Chil. Pediatr.*, **48**, 10

16
Tetanus

ROBERT EDMONDSON, MARY COOKE AND MICHAEL FLOWERS

Selected cases of tetanus require intensive care to survive. It is an irony that the disease is rare in those countries with intensive care units. The intensive care of the tetanus patient exemplifies all the essentials of this service: defined criteria for admission, nurses with appropriate knowledge and skills (Chapter 19), readily available medical expertise, reliable equipment, and, lastly, the appropriate attitudes. This chapter is based on extensive experience of a regional tetanus unit established at Leeds General Infirmary in 1954.

(I) PATHOPHYSIOLOGY

Tetanus has been well-described and recognized since antiquity. It is still an important cause of mortality world-wide and it was considered by Bytchenko[1] to be responsible for 50 000 deaths a year. The disease is common in underdeveloped countries where neonatal and uterine tetanus is seen, and tetanus occurs as a result of going barefoot. Drug addiction also predisposes to the disease. However, the overall incidence of tetanus in a population is now clearly related to the degree of immunity in that population, and the effectiveness of prophylactic immunization is well documented[2]. In Western countries tetanus is now a rare disease; for example only 17 cases were reported in England and Wales in 1977. The disease was shown to be transmissible in 1883, but it was not until the introduction of improved anaerobic techniques by McIntosh and Fildes in 1916, that the way was open to the study of the causative organism.

(1) Clostridium tetani

The properties of this organism are reviewed by Willis[3]. *Clostridium tetani* is a spore-bearing gram-positive bacillus. It is found in cultivated soil and in the gut of man and animals, particularly herbivores. The organism has a characteristic drumstick appearance due to the terminal spore. Although strict anaerobiosis is required for the isolation of *Cl. tetani*, there are no particular technical difficulties in isolating this organism as there are with some other strict anaerobes.

The cultural appearance of the organism is characteristic; it spreads over the medium with a fine delicate swarming growth. Concentrated agar media and antitoxin may be used to suppress swarming. Inhibition of swarming by tetanus antitoxin is specific and is therefore of diagnostic value. The organism may be fully identified by its biochemical properties, being non-proteolytic and non-saccharolytic. It, however, produces indole and a diffuse opacity in milk agar and has a number of volatile metabolic products which may be identified by gas liquid chromatography. The most important characteristic of *Cl. tetani* is the production of a potent exotoxin. This will be discussed later.

(2) Diagnosis

The diagnosis of tetanus is made clinically; the isolation of the organism from cases of the disease is not always possible and indeed *Cl. tetani* may be isolated from the wounds of patients with no symptoms of the disease. It is particularly difficult to demonstrate the characteristic drumstick organism by gram-staining of a smear from an infected wound and it has been suggested that the use of a fluorescent labelled antibody technique may be of value[4]. If an excised wound is to be examined, the tissue can be inoculated into cooked meat broth and onto blood agar plates which are incubated anaerobically. Swabs from infected wounds are examined in the same way.

(3) Prophylaxis

Only a brief summary of this interesting subject is given here. The subject

367

has been reviewed by Furste and others[5-7]. The importance of surgical treatment of wounds and of antibiotic administration, particularly of penicillin,
cannot be overstressed. However, the most important aspect is to produce
active or passive immunity. Generally, active immunization by tetanus
toxoid is the method of choice. All infants should be immunized by giving
the 'triple antigen' and immunity should be boosted in all individuals at
risk, or when a wound is sustained. There are few contraindications to
tetanus toxoid, which is so effective that tetanus could be eliminated in
developed countries. Active immunization does not confer immediate
immunity to the non-immune patient and those who require such protection
should be given combined active and passive immunization. Human antitetanus immunoglobulin is now preferable to equine antitoxin[8].

(4) Tetanus toxin

The most important characteristic of *Cl. tetani* is its ability to produce
exotoxin. However, non-toxigenic strains of the organism are not unusual.
The mouse is the animal employed to demonstrate toxin production by *Cl.
tetani*, two animals being used for each test. One animal is protected by the
subcutaneous injection of 0.5 ml of antitoxin one hour before injection with
the virulent organism. Signs of tetanus develop in the unprotected animal:
these are the development of stiffness in the injected leg, then the tail and a
gradual spread to involve the whole of the body. The slightest stimulus produces a generalized spasm in the animal. These dramatic symptoms and
those of the disease in man are entirely due to the production of a single
toxin, the neurotoxin or tetanospasmin. *Cl. tetani* also produces a haemo-
lysin, tetanolysin, but this is not involved in the production of the
symptoms of the disease.

The neurotoxin is of great interest. It is one of the most potent toxins
known, exceeded only by botulinus toxin and it has a highly specific action
on the nervous system. However, little is known of the chemical groups
which are responsible for its toxicity. It is a protein with a high molecular
weight; this prevents its elimination through the kidneys and results in a
long half-life in the blood. Time is therefore available for its penetration
into neural tissue. Much interest has centred on the mechanism by which
tetanus toxin reaches the central nervous system. It is now generally
accepted that this is via the regional motor nerve trunks and it is interesting
that this route is similar to that described for the rabies virus. The question
arises as to whether the route is via the axon or within the perineuronal
clefts. This problem has been studied using ^{125}I-labelled toxin and histoauto-
radiography[9], and it has been shown that the toxin enters the axons of peripheral nerves and reaches the spinal cord by transport within the axon. This
occurs not only in motor neurons but also in sensory and autonomic fibres.

Investigations of this type are also valuable in studying the distribution of toxin in the spinal cord. In local tetanus, radioactivity is concentrated in the ventral ipsilateral segment of the cord; it precedes the onset of symptoms and persists for long periods[10]. Only a few motor neurons are involved. Habermann and Wellhöner[10] believe that generalized tetanus is, from a pharmacokinetic point of view, similar to local tetanus. In both situations the toxin first has to enter the peripheral nerves before following the path described. The persistence of toxin in the central nervous system is also of importance. Toxin is avidly fixed by ganglioside, the degree of fixation being related to the number and position of sialic acid residues. The action of tetanus toxin in the central nervous system is to block inhibitory spinal reflex mechanisms and this produces the characteristic symptoms of the disease. However, in the clinical disease it is well established that sympathetic overactivity also occurs. Episodes of tachycardia and hypertension are seen and there are increased concentrations of catecholamines in the blood and urine. In experiments on the sympathetic outflow in the renal nerve of the cat, inhibition in the spinal cord was reduced. There is also evidence that some peripheral synapses are susceptible to tetanus, but this is probably not of great importance in the human disease.

(II) DIAGNOSIS

Because of its rarity in Western countries many doctors have never seen a case of tetanus. This, together with the fact that the initial diagnosis is purely clinical, can lead to mistaken diagnosis. Once seen, the clinical features of tetanus are very characteristic, but it is important to be aware of variations in the pattern of presentation and the conditions that can mimic the disease.

(1) Presenting features

The colloquial name of 'lockjaw' is very accurate because trismus and dysphagia are the initial feature of most cases. The muscular hypertonicity then spreads to the neck, back, abdomen and limbs. When the disease is severe, muscular spasms of increasing frequency and duration are superimposed on this hypertonicity, resulting in crush fractures of the vertebrae and death from respiratory failure and exhaustion (Figure 16.1). Spasm of the facial muscles results in the classical risus sardonicus (Figure 16.2) and even when the symptom is stiffness of the neck, back or abdomen, trismus is almost always present on examination.

Two variations of the classical presentation are occasionally seen and may cause diagnostic difficulty. In 'cephalic tetanus' a wound around the

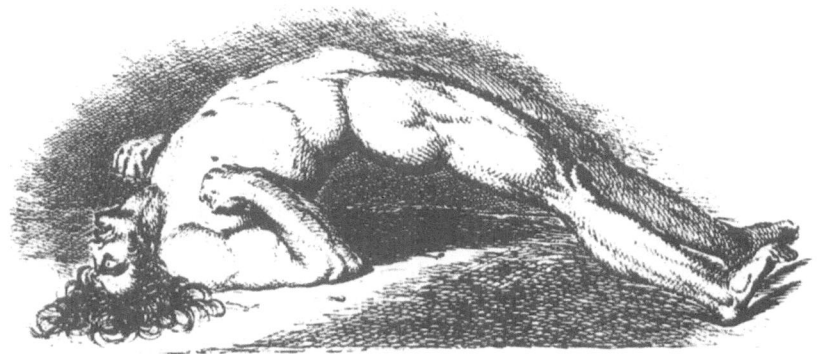

Figure 16.1 A soldier wounded at the Battle of Corunna in 1809. Taken from *Anatomy and Philosophy of Expression* by Sir Charles Bell, KH

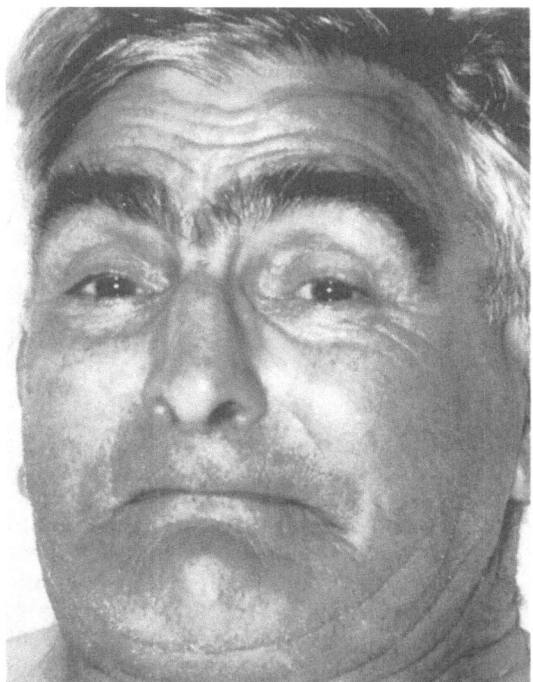

Figure 16.2 Trismus and risus sardonicus

head and neck may cause cranial nerve palsies, usually a unilateral facial palsy and sometimes weakness of the extra-ocular muscles, resulting in diplopia. In local tetanus there is hypertonicity of the muscles adjoining the wound, especially when the latter is sited in a limb. Both these variations usually progress to generalized tetanus and Figure 16.3 shows a patient with trismus, risus sardonicus and a left facial weakness following scalp and facial wounds, The presenting feature in 100 cases seen at Leeds are shown in Table 16.1.

Table 16.1 Presenting feature in 100 cases seen at Leeds from 1961 to 1977

Trismus and dysphagia	75
Neck and back rigidity	14
Cephalic tetanus	6
Local tetanus	3
Abdominal 'pain'	2

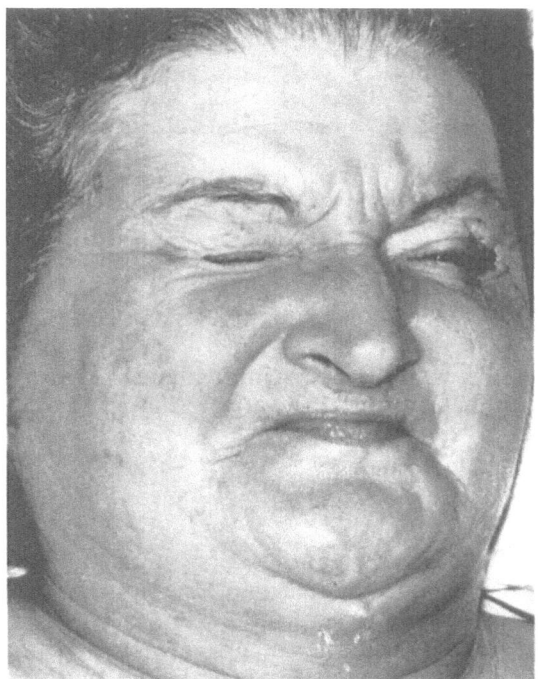

Figure 16.3 Cephalic tetanus. Trismus and left facial palsy

371

The incubation period

This is the interval between wounding and the onset of the first symptom of tetanus. In severe cases the incubation period tends to be short but a long interval is no guarantee of a mild attack (Figure 16.4).

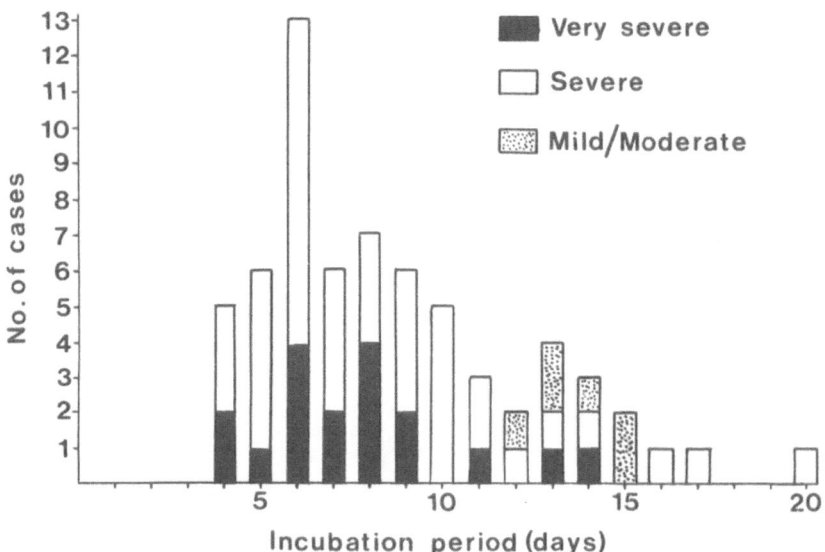

Figure 16.4   Incubation periods of tetanus

Period of onset

This is the interval between the first symptom and the first spasm and this also correlates with the severity of the attack (Figure 16.5).

The wound

A wound likely to be the source of infection is found in only about 60% of cases, so absence of such a wound certainly does not exclude the diagnosis. Tetanus occasionally follows surgery and infection of areas of broken skin such as varicose ulcers, epitheliomas and pressure sores. Neonatal tetanus is virtually unknown except in countries where the practice of applying dung to the umbilical cord is still commonplace.

372

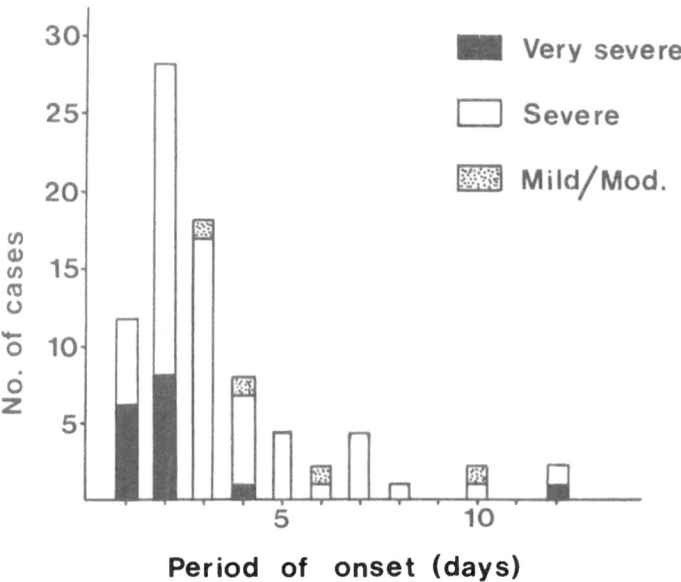

Figure 16.5 Period of onset

Immunization

Previous confirmed immunization with a full course of tetanus toxoid will virtually exclude the diagnosis and if the patient has not been immunized but received antitetanus serum at the time of wounding then tetanus is unlikely.

Differential diagnosis

Local pathology such as tonsillitis, dental abscesses or tempero-mandibular joint problems cause trismus, but are usually fairly obvious and there is no hypertonicity of other muscles. Hysteria can produce trismus and spasm of other muscles and must be excluded. Our tetanus unit once received a patient, tracheotomized and paralysed with curare, whose spasms proved to be hysterical in origin. Dystonic reactions to phenothiazine drugs, particularly metoclopramide (Maxolon) and Fentazin can present a most bizarre clinical picture with generalized muscular rigidity, but the facial contortion is unlike tetanus and the mouth is often open and the tongue protruding (Figure 16.6). The condition responds dramatically to an anti-

373

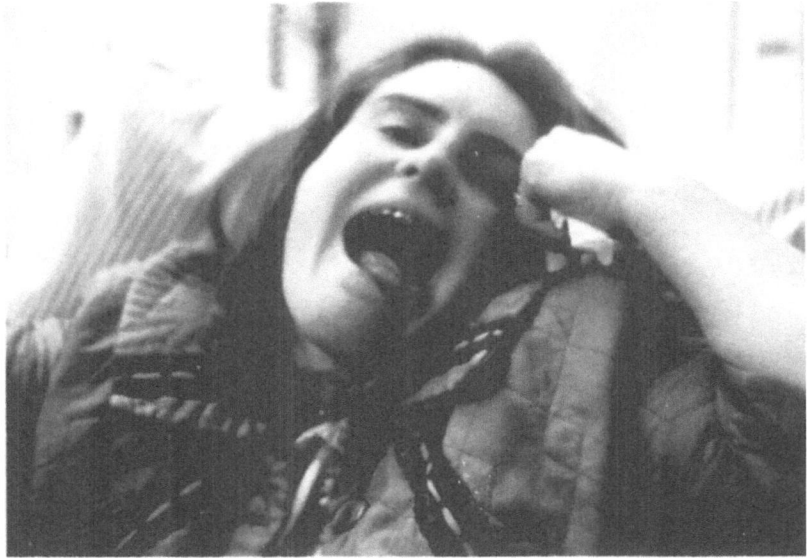

Figure 16.6 Dystonic reaction to Maxolon

parkinsonian drug such as benztropine. If the diagnosis is in doubt, time will quickly resolve the issue. The patient should be admitted to the ICU for observation and assessment as described below.

(III) GRADING THE SEVERITY

Tetanus varies in severity from a mild disease when the patient is hardly troubled by trismus and muscle stiffness, to a disease which ends in a terrifying and agonizing death within 48 hours of its onset. In the early stages both the time course and the ultimate severity of the disease are difficult to predict. The incubation period and time of onset do correlate with the severity but are not sufficiently reliable to influence management.

The first principle in the management of early tetanus is to prepare for a rapid deterioration in the patient's condition. The patient should therefore be admitted to an ICU for assessment where facilities for rapid intubation, paralysis and ventilation are immediately available. A secure i.v. line is established, thiopentone, atropine and suxamethonium drawn up in syringes ready and an appropriate endotracheal tube prepared. A trained ICU nurse must be present all the time and an anaesthetist (or other person capable of skilled and rapid intubation) available within seconds. Similar

374

precautions must be taken if the patient is to be transported either between or within hospitals. At this stage of assessment, and having ensured his safety, the patient should then be disturbed as little as possible. Injections should be kept to a minimum, a urinary catheter is not usually necessary and the passage of a nasogastric tube is positively contraindicated since it may provoke laryngeal spasm. Nothing should be given orally as this can also provoke laryngeal spasm and would increase the risk of regurgitation and pulmonary aspiration of gastric contents during a spasm.

We grade the severity of tetanus according to the method devised in this unit by Ablett[11]. The grading is useful in that each category is treated by a different regime.

Grade I–mild

Mild to moderate trismus and general spasticity. Little or no dysphagia. No respiratory embarrassment.

Grade II–moderate

Moderate trismus and general spasticity. Some dysphagia and respiratory embarrassment. Fleeting spasms.

Grade III (a)–severe

Severe trismus and general spasticity. Severe and prolonged spasms, both on stimulation and spontaneous.

Grade III (b)–very severe

Severe plus autonomic dysfunction, particularly sympathetic overactivity.

It is important to stress that any one patient may or may not progress rapidly through the grades of severity: a patient judged as mild on admission may remain so or may progress so rapidly that paralysis is required within hours. The onset of the autonomic disturbance of the very severe category is not usually seen until 2–4 days after the patient has required paralysis and lasts some 7–10 days before settling slowly. Patients presenting as local or cephalic tetanus are likely to progress to generalized tetanus and should receive the same care and assessment.

Using this grading we found that, of 100 patients admitted to the Leeds General Infirmary Intensive Care Unit between 1961 and 1977, the distribution of severity was: very severe 21, severe 69, moderate 3, mild 7.

Other workers found a different incidence of severity, e.g. Busuttil[12], using a similar method of classification, found that, of 194 cases in the Maltese Islands 51% were mild, 12% moderate and 37% severe. Garnier[13], reporting on a series of 230 cases in Haiti, found a similar distribution of severity. There are several possible explanations for these discrepancies.

(1) In the United Kingdom only the more severe cases are referred from district hospitals to regional tetanus units such as Leeds. This may account for some of the discrepancy.

(2) The severity of tetanus may vary in different locations.

(3) Centres with intensive care facilities may be more inclined to designate spasms and respiratory embarrassment as severe and life threatening than hospitals in underdeveloped countries dealing with vast numbers of cases with limited resources. There may be some truth in this explanation. Nevertheless, in spite of our policy of early establishment of an artificial airway, we have, on several occasions, been caught out by sudden and unexpected spasms severe enough to threaten the patient's life.

(1) Time course of the disease

Although there is considerable variation in the incubation period and period of onset, the duration of the established illness is fairly uniform whatever the grade of severity. The signs become progressively more severe during the first week, reach a plateau during the second week and wane in the third week. Some stiffness may persist for a further 2–3 weeks.

(IV) SPECIFIC TREATMENT

Treatment may be conveniently divided into two sections – specific measures to eliminate and neutralize tetanus toxin, which should be performed as soon as the diagnosis is made, and supportive treatment which varies according to the grade of severity.

(1) Wound excision

A wound can be identified as the likely source of tetanus in about 60% of cases, although often of apparently minor nature (Figure 16.7). However, when explored there is usually a deep seated focus of infected and necrotic tissue surrounding a foreign body, such as a splinter, thorn, piece of gravel or dirt. The wound is excised widely, all contaminated tissue is removed and sent for microscopical examination and culture. When several wounds are suspect, each must be explored. Occasionally amputation of an affected digit is required. The wound is left open and packed with gauze soaked in hydrogen peroxide or paraffin gauze impregnated with an antibacterial agent. After 5 days the wound can be closed by direct suture, split skin grafting or left to granulate. Although wound excision is an obviously logical and necessary measure, those patients in our series without a wound did not run a noticeably more severe course. Surgery which would produce permanent disability is probably not justifiable. For example, partial amputation of a finger is justified, but a thumb should be preserved if at all possible. There is no case for major amputation or other mutilating surgery. Local infiltration of antitetanus serum (ATS) around the wound has been employed and will do no harm, but is probably unnecessary if an appropriate systemic dose is given.

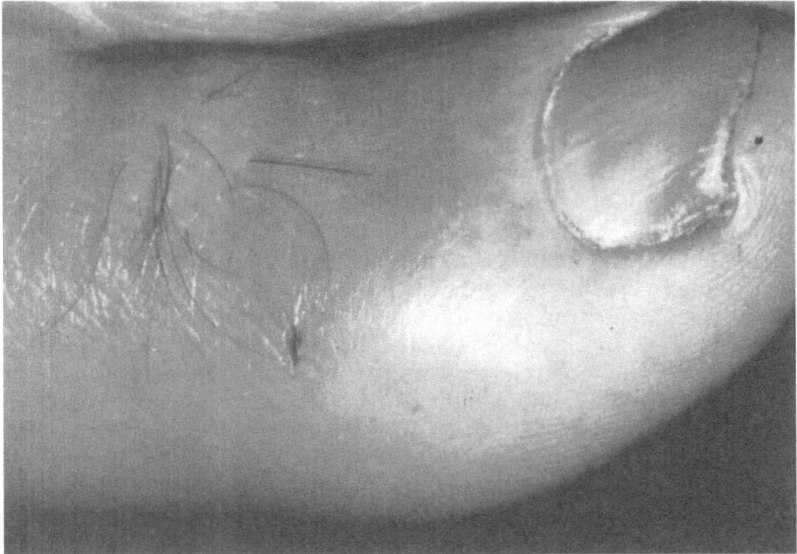

Figure 16.7   This wound, caused by a garden fork, was fatal

(2) Antibiotics and antitetanus serum

Cl. Tetani remains sensitive to penicillin so that a course of 1 mega unit of benzyl penicillin should be given i.m. 6 hourly for 1 week and then stopped.

377

Other antibiotics should only be given if specifically indicated for inter-current infection.

Antitetanus serum is a more controversial area of treatment, although a safe and rational policy has become easier to devise since the introduction in recent years of commercially available human ATS preparations. Clinical trials of ATS, given in varying doses and by differing routes of administration, are difficult in Western centres because of the relatively small numbers of cases seen. Reliance must therefore be placed on experimental findings together with the results of trials in the underdeveloped countries involving very large numbers of cases.

The first question to be asked is 'has ATS any therapeutic value'? The answer appears to be 'yes', although the influence is not dramatic. A careful clinical trial in Nigeria[14] showed that patients given 200 000 units of horse ATS fared better than those given none. A subsequent trial in Bombay[15] showed that 10 000 units was as effective as the larger doses and a survey of cases treated in the USA suggested that as little as 500 units could be equally effective[16].

The therapeutic effect of antitoxin is to neutralize toxin passing from the wound into the circulation and antitoxin has no power to reverse the action of toxin which is already producing a clinical effect[17]. Recently there has been a revised interest in Sherrington's work on antitoxin given intrathecally by the lumbar or cisternal route. Antitoxin given in this way might neutralize toxin which has already reached the CNS or is ascending the peripheral nerves. Sanders[18], working in a unit without intensive care facilities, reported a remarkably low death rate of 7% after the use of 200 units of horse ATS given intrathecally. The benefit of this route of administration was not, however, confirmed by Vakil[19] in Bombay who used 250 units of human ATS injected into the cisterna magna. If this route is used the nature and concentration of any preservative in the preparation must be carefully ascertained, because it could be toxic to the CNS. Burroughs Wellcome state that their human antitoxin (humotet) is formulated for intramuscular use only, and cannot be recommended for other routes, one of the reasons being the 0.01% thiomersal used as a preservative. When given i.m., however, there can be a delay of up to 48 hours in reaching peak blood levels[20] and the i.v. route is therefore preferable. It has been suggested[21,22] that, although many preparations are not recommended for intravenous use, they can probably be given safely by slow i.v. infusion. One dose of antitoxin provides adequate blood levels for about 4 weeks, especially if human antitoxin is used, because there is no risk of early immune elimination. This covers the period of the illness.

At Leeds our ATS policy is unadventurous but safe. We give one i.m. dose of 30 IU/kg humotet because we are not yet convinced that the alleged benefits of other routes outweigh the risks. Much work, both laboratory and clinical is, however, continuing in this field and will be followed by those involved in treating tetanus. Since an attack of tetanus does not confer immunity the first dose of a tetanus toxoid course should be given at the same time as the antitoxin, but in a different injection site.

(V) SUPPORTIVE TREATMENT

Having given the specific treatment, the aim of supportive treatment is to keep the patient alive and reasonably comfortable until natural remission occurs in 2–4 weeks. Provided that no complications develop, full recovery without residual neurological complications is to be expected[23]. Each of the three grades of tetanus is managed by a different regime.

(1) Grade I (mild tetanus)

These patients, who have no dysphagia or respiratory embarrassment present little problem. Diazepam will help to relieve the symptoms of trismus and spasticity. Once it is established, by a few days observation that the disease is not progressing beyond grade I, the patient may be allowed a light diet, i.v. therapy is discontinued, diazepam is given orally and the patient nursed on an ordinary ward. Although the disease is mild the time course appears to be as long as the severe disease with symptoms persisting for several weeks.

(2) Grade II (moderate tetanus)

The distinguishing features of this group are dysphagia, dyspnoea and minor spasms. They are at risk of developing laryngeal spasm, especially during passage of a nasogastric tube or if salivation is excessive. Lung expansion is restricted and coughing is ineffective due to spasticity of the respiratory muscles. They are therefore at risk of repeated minor hypoxic incidents, compounded by absorption collapse and infection due to retained secretions. Liberal use of sedatives, such as diazepam, relieves some of these problems but the depression of consciousness adds others. Tracheostomy removes the danger of upper airway obstruction due to laryngeal spasm or depression of consciousness; it allows the chest to be kept clear by suction and physiotherapy and renders safe the passage of a nasogastric tube. Having safeguarded the airway by tracheostomy, diazepam can then be given in large doses together with pethidine, which has less constipating effect than morphine. The patient continues to breathe spontaneously.

(3) Grade IIIa (severe tetanus)

When spasticity becomes more severe and spasms cause marked opistho-tonos and apnoea for more than 15–20 seconds, then muscle relaxants and IPPV are essential. This decision requires fine judgement, for even in the best intensive care unit, prolonged paralysis produces complications. However, undue delay in starting IPPV can lead to repeated severe hypoxic insults, exhaustion and even crush fractures of the vertebrae.

Neuromuscular blockade

The choice of drug is not too important. We use d-tubocurarine when there is a tendency to tachycardia and hypertension and pancuronium when the patient shows bradycardia and hypotension. During the first 2 weeks an average dosage of 15–20 mg d-tubocurarine hourly is given intravenously. This dosage completely abolishes spasticity, but spasms can be seen coming through as 'twitches' which, with experience, can be distinguished from the 'twitches' of a semi-paralysed patient trying to communicate with his attendants. Towards the end of the hour the patient has regained sufficient muscular power to communicate with his nurse, either by protruding his tongue or faintly squeezing her hand. This communication is valuable to the morale of both patient and attendants; it is of particular value in the early diagnosis of intra-abdominal complications and allows assessment of sedation and analgesia. After 2 weeks the relaxant can be given at pro-gressively longer intervals and usually stopped after 3 weeks. The duration

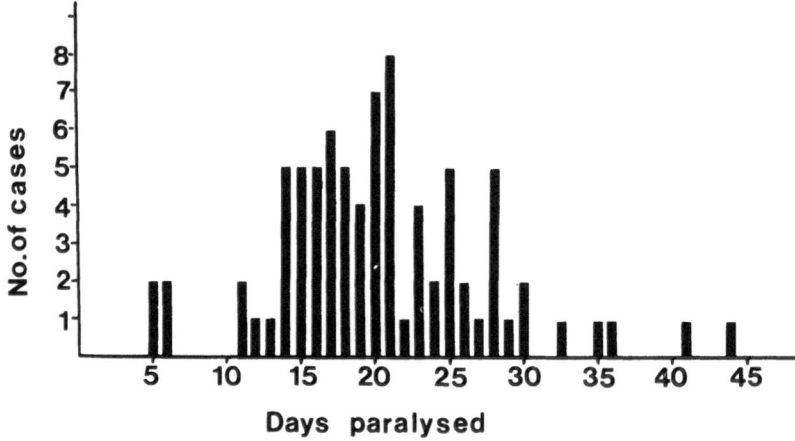

Figure 16.8 Duration of relaxant therapy

of the relaxant therapy in the Leeds series[23] is shown in Figure 16.8. Those paralysed for short periods were less severe, requiring relaxants only at the peak of their illnesses. Those paralysed for longer periods had usually developed complications which delayed their weaning. In two cases paralysis was mistakenly continued, the residual stiffness being due to drug-induced Parkinson's disease in one case and cerebral damage in another. Towards the end of the illness the relaxant drugs can be given intra-muscularly if an i.v. line is no longer necessary. Suxamethonium may be given in the early stages of tetanus but is contraindicated in the later stages because cardiac arrest has followed its use in the recovery phase.

Sedative drugs

Tetanus does not impair consciousness. Sedative and analgesic drugs should therefore be given, firstly to make the patient mentally and physically as comfortable as possible, and secondly to 'damp down' autonomic dys-function, especially the sympathetic overactivity. Diazepam has replaced the 'lytic cocktail' (pethidine, promethazine and chlorpromazine) as the drug of choice. Diazepam sedates, reduces anxiety, produces desirable amnesia and its muscle relaxant properties enable dosage of neuromuscular blockers to be reduced. It can be given i.v., i.m. or orally. Since diazepam is irritant by the i.v. or i.m. route and is well absorbed orally, this is the route of choice when the gastrointestinal tract is functioning. Dosage must be tailored to the patient's needs, because the individual requirements vary widely. The aim should be to keep the patient heavily sedated but rousable. This is especially important during the first 2 weeks or when there is evidence of sympathetic overactivity. During this period the average dosage for adults is 10 mg orally 4–6 hourly, with i.v. supplements if necessary. Generous analgesia should also be given to prevent pain from the tracheostomy and excised wound. Pethidine is perhaps preferable to morphia as it has less constipating effect and a dose of 50 mg i.m. 4–6 hourly alternating with diazepam is given for the first 2 weeks. Short painful or unpleasant procedures such as chest physiotherapy, wound dressings, enemata and rectal washouts are covered by nitrous oxide. After 2 weeks sedative drugs are progressively reduced and a hypnotic may be usefully given to try and restore the patient's sleep cycle.

(4) Grade IIIb (very severe tetanus)

Patients with very severe tetanus develop a characteristic syndrome of sus-tained but labile hypertension, tachycardia, dysrhythmias, peripheral vasoconstriction, profuse sweating and salivation, pyrexia and gastrointestinal stasis. This syndrome was studied by Kerr and workers in Oxford[24] and was seen in about 20% of the Leeds series. It developed 1–4 days after starting neuromuscular blockade and lasted 7–10 days. It is postulated that the syndrome is due to tetanus toxin acting on the sympathetic nervous system. The effects are comparable to those on the somatic motor neurones, with acute 'spasms' or overactivity imposed on a raised basal level of sympathetic activity. Similarly the autonomic spasms can be either spontaneous or precipitated by stimulation of the patient. The hypothesis is supported by finding that raised plasma and urinary catecholamine levels coincided with clinical signs[24,25]. A contrasting cardiovascular problem of hypotension and bradycardia is occasionally seen. This was investigated by Corbett et al.[26], who concluded that the hypotension was due to impaired neural cardiovascular control, rather than myocardial failure due to prolonged sympathetic stimulation (although this can occur and is probably the basis of the so called 'toxic myocarditis' of tetanus). This syndrome of hypotension and bradycardia can occur spontaneously but more particularly following tracheal suction and can progress to cardiac arrest[23,26]. If any hypoxia occurs during this procedure, this will enhance vagal reflexes arising from stimulation of the airway and interruption of ventilation[27].

The patient with very severe tetanus therefore presents the following therapeutic challenges:

(1) Control of fluctuating hypertension, tachycardia and cardiac dysrhythmias.

(2) Control of occasional episodes of hypotension and bradycardia.

(3) Replacement of massive fluid and electrolyte losses due to profuse sweating and salivation and sometimes large gastric aspirates.

(4) Provision of parenteral nutrition where there is complete gastrointestinal stasis.

However, before attributing these symptoms, particularly the cardiovascular changes, to the disease itself, a careful search must be made for more mundane causes. For example collapse of a lobe of the lung, retained bronchial secretions or a pneumothorax can cause hypoventilation with resulting hypertension, tachycardia, sweating and dysrhythmias.

The sympathetic overactivity may or may not kill the patient and it is therefore difficult to decide when therapy is essential. There are two lines of therapy – sedation or β-blockers – used alone or together. Heavy sedation undoubtedly 'damps down' the disturbances. Diazepam can be used in very large doses and is less toxic than older drugs such as chlorpromazine. Analgesia and further sedation is provided by regular dosage of opiate. The overactivity is abolished completely by anaesthesia but the agents are too toxic for long term use. Nitrous oxide would be the ideal agent if it were not for its effects on the bone marrow.

The second and logical approach to the problem is the use of specific adrenergic blockage. β-blockers have proved particularly useful in the control of tachycardia and dysrhythmias. Prys-Roberts et al.[28] used propranolol when there was persistent tachycardia of more than 120/min and the patient had a normal temperature and blood gas tensions. They used 0.2 mg i.v. increments until dysrhythmias were suppressed and the heart rate fell to 100/min. Propranolol 10 mg 6 or 8 hourly was given via nasogastric tube for maintenance. If hypertension was still a problem they gave bethanidine. More recently, Dundee[29] has successfully used the combined α- and β-blocking agent, labetalol, to produce cardiovascular stability, but because of the fluctuant nature of the sympathetic overactivity this can result in episodes of severe hypotension. β-blockers can precipitate acute cardiac failure in patients dependent on sympathetic myocardial drive, and leave the vagal element of complex reflexes, such as those arising from tracheal stimulation, unopposed. In the Leeds series two young and previously fit patients given 10 mg of propranolol 6 hourly via nasogastric tube developed sudden bradycardia and cardiac arrest during tracheal suction. Buchanan[30] reports the death of a seven-year-old child with tetanus who developed acute pulmonary oedema after propranolol.

Our present policy, therefore, is to use a basic regime of heavy sedation, covering episodes of acute overactivity, with additional i.v. sedation or the administration of N_2O. If these fail, small increments of a β-blocker are given intravenously and the oral route is avoided because of irregular absorption.

(5) Treatment of hypotension and bradycardia

The problems of acute hypotension and bradycardia, especially following tracheal suction, have been described and the importance of avoiding hypoxia must be emphasized. Hypotension without obvious cause usually responds to raising the foot of the bed, raising the arterial carbon dioxide tension and minor painful stimuli described by Corbett[26]. Should these measures fail, then the patient's fluid balance and drug regime should be carefully reassessed.

(6) Maintaining fluid balance and nutrition

These problems are not peculiar to tetanus and can be dealt with along standard lines (Chapter 1). It should be emphasized, however, that large losses from salivation and sweating are difficult to quantify and the total daily fluid requirements during the acute phase may be 6–8 litres. Fluid overload must, however, be avoided and peripheral oedema is not uncommonly seen in the second week. This oedema is probably multi-factorial in origin: prolonged immobility, IPPV, falling serum albumin levels and perhaps a degree of cardiac failure may all contribute. The oedema responds readily to a diuretic such as frusemide.

Most patients can be fed by nasogastric tube. There is usually a period of gastrointestinal stasis in the very severe cases with a silent but not distended abdomen. However, as most patients are well nourished before their illness, parenteral nutrition is not usually necessary unless the stasis persists for more than a week. Occasionally frank paralytic ileus is seen and the naso-gastric tube should be aspirated regularly to prevent acute gastric dilation. Constipation is usual and aperients, enemata and rectal washouts are fre-quently required. This problem is not to be taken lightly, because in the Leeds series constipation resulted in intestinal obstruction in one case and stercoral perforation of the caecum in another.

(7) Other aspects of management

Pyrexia

Most severe cases have a low grade pyrexia during their illness. If temperatures higher than 38.5 – 39 °C occur it may be caused by autonomic dysfunction or be due to intercurrent infection and it is very important to distinguish between the two, because attributing the pyrexia to autonomic dysfunction can result in a fatal delay in identifying and treating infection.

Anaemia

Most patients show a slow but steady fall in haemoglobin levels so that transfusion of 2 units of blood is required at approximately weekly inter-vals. If a more rapid fall occurs, gastrointestinal bleeding is the most likely cause.

Deep venous thrombosis

This is an ever present threat to a patient paralysed for this length of time. General measures such as frequent passive limb movements, calf massage and maintenance of normal hydration are important. In Leeds we gave low doses of heparin (5000 units s.c. 8 or 12 hourly) to the last 12 patients.

Jenkins and Keep[31] reported fatal pulmonary embolism in a tetanus patient on this regime and recommended full anticoagulation.

The recovery phase

Residual stiffness, especially in the calf muscles, may persist for several weeks and active physiotherapy is essential to prevent a contracture and ensure full mobilization. In the Leeds series, residual cranial nerve palsies were seen in all those presenting with cephalic tetanus and occasionally in others. Recovery occurred in 2–3 weeks in all except one patient, whose bulbar palsy was so severe that motor neurone disease was suspected. Nevertheless he made a complete recovery over 6 months. Disorientation, emotional lability, and depression during recovery are common but usually clear spontaneously in 1–2 weeks.

(VI) RESULTS

Apart from the specific therapy already dealt with, the treatment of severe tetanus is an exercise in the prolonged care of the paralysed patient and the treatment of complications which arise during this period of 3–4 weeks. The problems are only too familar to those involved in intensive care. The mortality in the Leeds series was 10% and the causes of death are shown in Table 16.2. Early resort to tracheostomy and paralysis in severe tetanus prevents deaths directly attributable to the disease, but a price is paid in complications of the treatment regime. Most of the complications in Table

Table 16.2 Causes of death in the Leeds series

Sex	Age	Severity of tetanus	Cause of death
M	87	severe	tension pneumothorax
M	24	very severe	unexpected cardiac arrest
F	66	very severe	unexpected cardiac arrest
M	71	very severe	haemorrhage from acute gastric erosions
M	57	severe	bronchopneumonia
M	57	severe	bronchopneumonia
F	68	severe	staphylococcal pneumonia
F	5	very severe	anaphylactic reaction to horse ATS
F	55	severe	pulmonary embolism
M	14	very severe	cerebral damage, probably due to cerebral venous infarction

16.2 are avoidable, but as many patients are elderly and have pre-existing cardiorespiratory disease, there must continue to be a significant mortality rate using this method of treatment. Mortality rates in other series vary widely from 7% to over 60% and results from intensive care units in Western countries, where experience of the disease is limited, are sometimes not as good as those obtained by conservative regimes in countries such as India, where vast numbers of cases are treated; this fund of experience should not be dismissed lightly. However, there can be no doubt that neuromuscular blockade and intensive care are essential to save the more severe case of tetanus. The disease is one of the most challenging and rewarding that intensive care staff are called upon to treat. If the patient can be kept alive and free of major complications, complete restoration of health will ensue with a normal life expectancy: this can be said of few other diseases seen in the intensive care unit.

References

1. Bytchenko, B. (1966). Geographical distribution of tetanus in the world, 1951–60: a review of the problem. *Bull. WHO.*, **34**, 71
2. Boyd, J. S. K. (1946). Tetanus in the African and European theatres of war, 1939–1945. *Lancet*, **1**, 113
3. Willis, A. T. (1977). *Anaerobic Bacteriology.*, Ch. 4 (London: Butterworths)
4. Batty, I. and Walker, P. D. (1967). In *International Symposium of Immunological Methods of Biological Standardization.* Vol. 4, p. 73. (Royamont, 1965)
5. Furste, W. (1974). Four keys to 100% success in tetanus prophylaxis. *Am. J. Surg.*, **128**, 616
6. Smith, J. W. G., Laurence, D. R. and Evans, D. G. (1975). Prevention of tetanus in the wounded. *Br. Med. J.*, **3**, 453
7. Fraser, D. W. (1976). Preventing tetanus in patients with wounds. *Ann. Intern. Med.*, **84**, 95
8. Editorial. Human antitoxin for tetanus prophylaxis (1974). *Lancet*, **1**, 51
9. Erdmann, G., Wiegand, H. and Wellhoner, H. H. (1975). Intra-axonal and extra-axonal transport of ^{125}I-tetanus toxin in early local tetanus. *Arch. Pharmacol.*, **290**, 357
10. Habermann, E. and Wellhoner, H. H. (1974). Advances in tetanus research. *Klin. Wochenschr.*, **52**, 255
11. Ablett, J. J. L. (1967). In Ellis, M. (ed.). *Symposium on Tetanus in Great Britain*, Leeds United Hospitals
12. Busuttil, A., Pace, J. B. and Muscat, J. A. (1974). Traditional treatment of 194 cases of tetanus. *Br. J. Surg.*, **61**, 731
13. Garnier, M. J. (1975). Tetanus in patients three years of age and up. A personal series of 230 consecutive patients. *Am. J. Surg.*, **129**, 459
14. Brown, A., Mohamed, S. D., Montgomery, R. D., Armitage, P. and Laurence, D. R. (1960). Value of a large dose of antitoxin in clinical tetanus. *Lancet*, **2**, 227

15. Vakil, B. J., Talpule, T. H., Armitage, P. and Laurence, D. R. (1968). A comparison of the value of 200 000 IU of tetanus antitoxin (horse) with 10 000 IU in the treatment of tetanus. *Clin. Pharmacol. Ther.*, **9**, 465

16. Blake, P. A., Feldman, R. A., Buchanan, T. M., Brooks, G. F. and Bennett, J. V. (1976). Serologic therapy of tetanus in the United States, 1965-1971. *J. Am. Med. Assoc.*, **235**, 42

17. Adams, E. B., Laurence, D. R., and Smith, J. W. G. (1969). *Tetanus*. (Oxford: Oxford University Press)

18. Sanders, R. K. M., Martyn, B., Joseph, R. and Peacock, M. L. (1977). Intrathecal antitetanus serum (horse) in the treatment of tetanus. *Lancet*, **1**, 974

19. Vakil, B. J., Armitage, P. and Laurence, D. R. (1975). Foundation meriux trial of intrathecal ATS. In *Proceedings of the International Conference of Tetanus*. p. 423. (Daker Senegal)

20. Turner, T. B., Velasco-Joven, E. A. and Prudovsky, S. (1958). Studies on the prophylaxis and treatment of tetanus. *Bull. Johns Hopkins Hosp.*, **102**, 71

21. Reed, W. D. *et al.* (1973). Infusion of hepatitis-B antibody in antigen-positive active chronic hepatitis. *Lancet*, **2**, 1347

22. Schwander, D. and Wigmann, A. (1973). *Schweiz Med. Wochenschr.*, **103**, 1184

23. Edmondson, R. S. and Flowers, M. W. (1979). Intensive care in tetanus management, complications and mortality in 100 cases. *Br. Med. J.*, **1**, 1401

24. Kerr, J. H. *et al.* (1968). Involvement of the sympathetic nervous system in tetanus. Studies on 82 cases. *Lancet*, **2**, 236

25. Benedict, C. R. and Kerr, J. H. (1977). Assessment of sympathetic overactivity in tetanus. *Br. Med. J.*, **2**, 806

26. Corbett, J. L., Spalding, J. M. K. and Harris, P. J. (1973). Hypotension in tetanus. *Br. Med. J.*, **2**, 423

27. De Burgh Daly, M., Angell-James, J. E. and Elsner, R. (1979). Role of carotid-body chemoreceptors and their reflex interactions in bradycardia and cardiac arrest. *Lancet*, **1**, 764

28. Prys-Roberts, C. *et al.* (1969). Treatment of sympathetic overactivity in tetanus. *Lancet*, **1**, 542

29. Dundee, J. W. and Morrow, W. F. K. (1979). Labetalol in severe tetanus. *Br. Med. J.*, **1**, 1121

30. Buchanan, N., Smit, L., Cane, R. D. and De Andrade, M. (1978). Sympathetic overactivity in tetanus fatality associated with propranolol. *Br. Med. J.*, **2**, 254

31. Jenkins, J. and Keep, P. (1976). Fatal embolism despite low-dose heparin. *Lancet*, **1**, 541

17
Botulism

PETER BALL AND ROWLAND HOPKINSON

Botulism is a rapidly progressive neuroparalytic disease which follows the ingestion of toxin produced by the vegetative forms of *Clostridium botulinum*. This organism is an anaerobic gram-positive spore-bearing bacillus, which is widely distributed in soil and organic aquatic sediments throughout the world. Seven types of *Cl. botulinum* (groups A–G) have been recognized, of which types A, B and E are usually associated with the production of disease in humans.

The intensive care unit, which concentrates the skills required for ventilatory assistance (IPPV), circulatory support, physiotherapy and parenteral feeding, has a vital role in the management of patients with severe paralytic botulism. The ICU will also have available the technology required to monitor the use of neuromuscular blockade antagonists used in treatment.

(I) EPIDEMIOLOGY

The spores of *Cl. botulinum* are released when environmental conditions are unfavourable to the vegetative forms of the organism. They are highly resistant to heat and other external influences and may survive for long periods in their natural habitat. Under favourable anaerobic conditions, these spores germinate and during vegetative multiplication a toxin is produced. This may occur naturally. For example, saprophytic growth of type C strains in decaying vegetation occurred in the Great Lakes of the USA. The toxin was ingested by wildfowl, causing large outbreaks of the disease.

The chain of events leading to the human disease usually involves an intermediate foodstuff which has become contaminated with spores and has been subject to anaerobic conditions favourable to toxin production. Fresh food has never caused botulism, and, except in infants (see below), ingestion of spores in the absence of preformed toxin does not cause disease. Occasional cases have followed contamination of traumatic wounds by *Cl. botulinum*[1].

Food-borne botulism usually follows the faulty preservation of food, either at home or commercially, but may also occur when food is allowed to decompose and is then eaten raw. Cooking immediately prior to eating renders food safe, as the toxin is inactivated by temperatures above 70°C in a matter of minutes. However, when food is inadequately preserved, surviving spores are able to produce toxin and the resultant product if uncooked, is potentially lethal.

In the United Sates, three quarters of all cases are due to the faulty home preservation of food[2]. Garden vegetables, in particular peppers and beans, are usually implicated. The practice of home bottling and canning is widespread in the United States and does much to explain the high incidence of the disease (ten outbreaks per year) compared with that in the United Kingdom (seven outbreaks in 50 years) where home processing is uncommon. The custom of eating decomposing fresh fish contaminated by type E strains has led to a considerable number of deaths in the Japanese and Eskimos.

An unusual form of food-borne disease, infant botulism, has recently been described following colonization of the gut by vegetative *Cl. botulinum*[3]. In one case the source appeared to be honey and in subsequent investigations spores were found in about 10% of samples tested. No other cases have been attributed to this source, which would be harmless to older subjects.

(II) PATHOGENESIS AND CLINICAL PRESENTATION

The features of botulism following ingestion of toxin-containing food vary little with either the source or with the type of *Cl. botulinum* involved. Ingested toxin is rapidly absorbed from the digestive tract and reaches nervous tissues via the circulation. It then becomes irreversibly fixed to unmyelinated motor neurofibrils proximal to the myoneural junction (MNJ). This produces paralysis by reducing the release of acetylcholine.

The paralysis is, therefore, unaffected by cholinesterase inhibitors. All cholinergic motor endings, including those of the parasympathetic, are equally affected. Sympathetic endings were thought to be immune, but animal studies and the evidence from recent human cases[4] have demonstrated sympathetic dysfunction.

Electromyographic studies show the MJN abnormality, characterized by a marked reduction in number and amplitude of evoked and spontaneous end-plate potentials[5]. Repetitive stimulation produces a potentiative effect similar to those observed in the Eaton–Lambert syndrome but shows fluctuations over periods of time[6]. In infant botulism the e.m.g. demonstrates 'brief, small, abundant, motor-unit action potentials' which are considered to be characteristic[3].

The delay between ingestion of toxin and onset of clinical symptoms is seldom greater than 48 hours. When large amounts of toxin, particularly of type E, have been ingested, symptoms can appear within 12 hours. The prodromal features are nausea, vomiting, dizziness and faintness, reminiscent of food poisoning due to staphylococcal and clostridial enterotoxins; thereafter, all similarity with such diseases ends. Diarrhoea is exceptional and the major clinical manifestations of botulism are neurological. The effect of the toxin is exclusively on motor nerves and sensation and consciousness are unimpaired. Cranial nerve disturbance usually precedes systemic paralysis by some hours. Paralysis of extrinsic and intrinsic ocular muscles leads to ptosis, loss of eye movements and sluggish, dilated pupils. These eye signs are typical but not invariable and pupillary reaction can be normal[6]. The bulbar cranial nerves are next involved, resulting in dysarthria and dysphagia, followed by progressive systemic paralysis and ventilatory failure. In the untreated case death then ensues.

This fully developed picture is seen in only a few patients. Others will have ingested a smaller quantity of toxin which results in a much milder illness. This is exemplified by a recent outbreak in the United States which followed the ingestion of a sauce made from home-canned peppers. 59 people became ill, of whom 53 were hospitalized. In 14 no neurological signs developed and of nine who developed respiratory paralysis only three required IPPV. This report described an association between oculomotor nerve dysfunction and severe respiratory paralysis[7]. However, when large quantities of toxin are ingested, severe paralysis is invariable.

In mild cases and those surviving IPPV gradual recovery takes place. The period of recovery is dependent on the extent of paralysis and is variable. Some severely paralysed patients recover spontaneous ventilation within a few weeks, but others may require IPPV for up to three months. Recovery is related to the proliferative arborization of the motor end-plate, resulting in new synaptic links between neurone and muscle.

The features of infant botulism include failure of suckling and swallowing, pooling of oral secretions, cranial nerve deficit, generalized 'floppy' hypotonia and, in some cases, sudden apnoea[3]. Most infants affected have recovered spontaneously, but recent evidence from the United States has suggested an association with the 'sudden infant death syndrome'[8]. About 80 cases of infant botulism have now been described in the United States and one case has now been reported in the United Kingdom.

(III) LABORATORY DIAGNOSIS

Definitive diagnosis requires identification of specific *Cl. botulinum* toxin in clinical specimens. In adults and older children, the serum usually contains detectable quantities of toxin for some days (unless antitoxin has been given: see below). Vomit and faeces may contain toxin, and, occasionally, spores and vegetative bacilli, but specimens are less valuable for laboratory examination. In infant botulism the reverse is true; serum is unlikely to yield toxin, but faeces usually contain both toxin and the organism for several weeks.

Toxin is identified by the production of a characteristic paralysis in mice following intraperitoneal inoculation of either serum or faecal extracts. Protection is demonstrated by inoculating mice with material pre-treated with type-specific monovalent antitoxin. This both proves the diagnosis and identifies the type involved.

Attempts should also be made to identify toxin and spores in the food, which should be sealed in a suitable container and retained for examination. The food source should be handled with care as inoculation of toxin into the skin of a handler can cause the disease.

The hospital bacteriologist should be informed immediately of all suspected cases, so that appropriate specimens may be obtained for diagnosis. It should be noted that *Cl. botulinum* is a category B1 pathogen and, therefore, most laboratories will have to forward specimens to the Central Public Health Laboratory for analysis. This procedure and the time required for protection studies will delay the definitive diagnosis for a variable period. Treatment is therefore started on clinical suspicion alone.

(IV) MANAGEMENT

The management of an outbreak of botulism includes the treatment of the disease and the investigation. In all cases of food-borne disease the Medical Officer for Environmental Health should be informed of the circumstances. Where relevant the place and the date of purchase of food, brand and product names and batch numbers of implicated commercial food will be needed as such foodstuffs may require to be withdrawn urgently from retail sale.

The treatment of individual cases requires the administration of polyvalent antitoxin, and may include the use of neuromuscular blockade antagonists and intensive care in severely affected patients requiring cardio-respiratory support. Many of the clinical problems posed by botulism are common to other neuroparalytic diseases such as poliomyelitis or polyneuritis, or conditions such as tetanus which may require prolonged IPPV. In botulism, respiratory failure, bulbar palsy and autonomic disturbance are of particular note, but the disease poses two additional problems. Firstly, the paralysis is of rapid onset and progression and, secondly, foodborne botulism may claim a number of victims simultaneously.

(1) Intensive supportive therapy

On admission the patient will be in progressive ventilatory failure, the severity of which will be determined by the amount and type of toxin ingested and the time since ingestion. Initial intervention will, in many instances, depend on a rapid clinical assessment of the degree of hypoventilation and the adequacy of the airway. Blood gas analysis, peak flow measurements and spirometry are useful baseline parameters, but should not delay intubation and ventilation if the condition of the patient so dictates.

Intubation should be preceded by pre-oxygenation via face mask and breathing bag. Aspiration of gastric contents should be guarded against by the application of cricoid pressure and the provision of suction apparatus. The endotracheal tubes employed should be implant-tested and have high-volume, low-pressure cuffs to reduce tracheal damage. Tubes fitted with regulators preventing cuff pressure in excess of 25 mmHg are recommended, but if these are unavailable then the cuff pressure should be set to obtain the minimum leak.

Intubation is performed by using a low dose of a rapidly acting anaesthetic agent assisted by suxamethonium. Thereafter muscle relaxants and respiratory depressants should be avoided as they may invalidate assessment and the effects of antitoxin and blockade antagonist therapy. However, it should be remembered that botulism does not impair consciousness or sensation and that, despite verbal explanation and reassurance of the patient, sedation and analgesia may be required, using tranquillizing doses of benzodiazepines.

Saline depletion and dehydration following vomiting are likely, and an intravenous line and central venous line should be inserted. An indwelling arterial line will facilitate the frequent blood gas analyses required during IPPV. Arterial cannulation also permits nursing and physiotherapy procedures and assessment of the Valsalva manoeuvre and postural change[4]. The arterial cannulation site should be changed frequently to minimize the risk of infection or thrombosis. Blood gas analysis should be complimented by simultaneous measurements of the inspired oxygen fraction, preferably by an oxygen analyser. Initially, blood gas and inspired gas analysis will be necessary 4 hourly and, subsequently, following changes in gas flows.

Respiratory paralysis, once established, may take weeks or months to recover. Therefore, as soon as the need for long-term ventilation is established, an elective tracheostomy should be performed. We prefer Lanz tracheostomy tubes. Chest physiotherapy with postural drainage is essential to clear secretions. Regular bronchoscopy was also required in the Birmingham patients. Physiotherapy should be integrated with bagging and suction by the nursing staff. The autonomic dysfunction may lead to marked swings of blood pressure during such sessions.

The choice of ventilator will be influenced by availability, but management may be facilitated by the use of a machine which adjusts to changes in pulmonary compliance (e.g. Servovent). Ventilation should be commenced with a tidal volume of 12.5 ml/kg and at a minute volume adjusted to obtain normocapnia and normal pH. Additional humidification, with apparatus such as Fischer–Paykel heated water bath units, is essential. Servo-controlled monitoring of the airway temperature is an advantage. The technique of intermittent mandatory ventilation (IMV)[9] was used in the four Birmingham patients. This method allows the mechanically ventilated patient to breathe spontaneously between each mandated inspiration. This confers a number of benefits. In contrast with other systems, IMV avoids prolonged hypocapnia which can itself reduce cardiac output and cerebral blood flow, and increase oxygen consumption. The reduction in mean intrathoracic pressure during spontaneous inspiration will enhance venous return and cardiac output. IMV also prevents the respiratory incoordination which often follows prolonged IPPV. Patients quickly learn to inspire between mandated cycles and even when spontaneous and mandated breaths coincide, the resulting rise in intrathoracic pressure appears of little consequence and may be regarded as the equivalent of a sigh. IMV also permits the measurement of spontaneous tidal and minute volumes. In our experience the IMV circuits of the Brompton–Manley, Bennett MA1 and Seimens–Elema 900 ventilators functioned satisfactorily. When necessary PEEP is applied to counteract hypoxaemia (Chapter 7).

(2) Autonomic dysfunction

As previously implied, serious cardiovascular consequences may follow the autonomic blockade of botulism. Cardiac denervation can lead to severe bradycardia which is unresponsive to atropine[4]. Marked hypotension may also result. This, together with a loss of other vasomotor reflexes suggests that the blockade is both sympathetic and parasympathetic. Hypotension may require the use of an inotropic agent, such as dopamine or dobutamine, which should be administered via a central venous catheter (Chapter 5).

Intestinal ileus may occur and nasogastric suction should then be instituted. It is recommended that phenoxymethyl penicillin (500 mg, 6 hourly, for the first 36 hours) should be given via the nasogastric tube to eliminate any vegetative *Cl. botulinum* in the gut. In food-borne botulism, at least in the adult, the value of this therapy is unproven. The nasogastric tube may also be used to administer prophylactic antacids when the pH of the gastric contents falls below 3.0. Stress ulcers, which caused significant bleeding in one of our patients, should be treated with intravenous cimetidine*.

Acute urinary retention is to be expected and a bladder catheter should be inserted. Secondary cystitis may be avoided by the use of bladder lavage twice daily with a solution of chlorhexidine or noxythiolin.

(3) Nutrition

Although return of intestinal motility during recovery will allow tube feeding, parenteral nutrition is likely to be required initially. A silicone central venous catheter introduced via the internal jugular or subclavian route may be used for this purpose. However, if prolonged intravenous nutrition is envisaged, the extended subcutaneous tunnel technique should be used as an added precaution against infection.

(4) Infection

Routine cultures of catheters, the tracheostomy, sputum and wounds should be undertaken. The results should be interpreted in relation to the clinical and laboratory signs and with the knowledge that all the sites mentioned become colonized by bacteria. Prophylactic antibiotics must be avoided.

Fever is most likely to indicate chest infection, urinary infection or bacteraemia and demands full examination, chest X-ray and relevant cultures. It should be noted that cultures of gram-negative bacteria from tracheostomy sites and tracheal aspirates are usually due to colonists. In our experience pneumonia is most likely to be due to pneumococci or staphylococci and is only rarely gram-negative. The incidence of gram-negative infection increases, however, if antibiotics have been given. Where the cause of fever is undetermined and the patient's condition is worsening, a

* Editor's note: alkali is more effective; see page 148.

combination of benzyl penicillin and gentamicin should be prescribed pending the results of bacteriological cultures.

(5) Antitoxin therapy

Botulism toxins reach the nervous system via the circulation and whilst in the blood are amenable to neutralization by type-specific antitoxin. Following fixation to nervous tissue, these toxins are no longer neutralizable. Hence, to be of value, antitoxin must be administered urgently, often before bacteriological confirmation of the diagnosis. However, although the onset of neurological signs implies neuronal fixation, toxin may continue to circulate for a week or more thereafter[10]. Therefore, antitoxin should still be given even when considerable time has elapsed.

There is no doubt about the efficacy of type E antitoxin. One study demonstrated a mortality of only 3.5% of treated patients compared with 30% in untreated subjects[11]. However, the response to types A and B antitoxin is less well-documented although type A antitoxin is effective in experimentally intoxicated monkeys[12]. Antitoxins are specific to the individual toxins and unless the toxin type is known, polyvalent antitoxins must be used. The antitoxin available in the United Kingdom (Lister Institute) has trivalent activity against types A, B and E (the usual human serotypes) and is equine in origin. It contains a standardized activity of 1000 IU anti-A, 700 IU anti-B and 100 IU anti-E per ml. As might be expected with equine antitoxins, reactions may occur. In a recent study[13], an overall reaction rate of 21% was noted, immediate hypersensitivity reactions being encountered in 10% and serum sickness in 7%. It is therefore, advisable to administer a test dose of 0.2 ml of antitoxin subcutaneously 20–30 minutes before the main dose of 80 ml of trivalent Lister antitoxin, which is given intravenously. This dose may require to be repeated 4–6 hourly until symptoms either cease to appear or subside. Supplies of Lister antitoxin are available on a regional and subregional basis in the United Kingdom and their location will be known to hospital pharmacists and Directors of Public Health Laboratories.

(6) Neuromuscular blockade antagonists

In 1949, Burgen, Dickens and Zatman[14] demonstrated the neuromuscular blocking action of *Cl. botulinum* toxin in an isolated rat diaphragm preparation and showed that nerve conduction and muscular response to direct stimulation were normal; the block was thus localized to the MNJ. It was further shown that, although the motor end-plates remained normally sensitive to acetylcholine, the output of acetylcholine following motor nerve stimulation was greatly reduced. This was thought to be due to failure of transmission in the pre-terminal motor fibril, as acetylcholine synthesis was unaffected by toxin.

These findings and the resultant electrical abnormalities resemble those of the Easton–Lambert syndrome[6] in which guanidine hydrochloride has been shown to act as a neuromuscular blockade antagonist. Guanidine, which enhances acetylcholine release[15] and a similar antagonist, germine monoacetate, have subsequently been used with some success in botulism[6,16-18]. Treatment with guanidine produces rapid reversal of e.m.g. abnormalities and sustained improvement in ocular and peripheral muscle paralysis. Doses of 10–20 mg kg^{-1} day^{-1}, by mouth, are effective in mild to moderate paralysis, but guanidine has proved ineffective in more severe cases[19] even in dosage of 45 mg kg^{-1} day^{-1} and has much less effect on paralysed respiratory muscle[5]. The poor response of severely paralysed patients, who usually require IPPV, limits the therapeutic usefulness of guanidine. Guanidine may also cause gastrointestinal mucosal irritation leading to abdominal discomfort, nausea and vomiting, and possible gastrointestinal bleeding. In higher doses paraesthesias and muscle fasciculation have occurred[19]. Studies with germine monoacetate in rabbits suggested that it might be of value in botulism[20] but in a human case it showed no advantage when combined with guanidine[18].

Recent work *in vitro*[5] has demonstrated that the reduction in motor end-plate potential in botulism is due to decrease in evoked quantal release of acetylcholine, in turn related to a reduction in the sensitivity of the acetylcholine release mechanism to calcium. A rise in intracellular calcium concentration, whether caused by tetanic nerve stimulation, a calcium ionophore or by prolongation of the nerve action potential by tetraethylammonium, was shown to result in increased acetylcholine release. Further studies[21] showed that guanidine had a similar effect and might act by interfering with intracellular calcium binding, thereby prolonging and enhancing the effects of calcium ions entering the terminal during the motor action potential. Subsequent studies in rat muscle *in vitro* showed that guanidine had this effect only in the presence of an ambient calcium concentration of 3–4 mmol/l. However, another agent, 4-aminopyridine (4-AP) was shown to be effective at physiological calcium concentrations and to be at least 20 times more active than guanidine[22]. Further, in animal studies, 4-AP was able to completely, if only transiently, reverse paralysis induced in rats by type A toxin.

Following this evidence and reports of the successful use of 4-AP in the Eaton–Lambert syndrome[23,24] studies in cases of botulism showed that intravenous dosage of 0.35–0.5 mg/kg of 4-AP produced significant increases in amplitude of evoked motor action potentials over periods of 45–60 minutes[4]. These effects were increased by the simultaneous administration of neostigmine and were potentiated and prolonged following a second dose of 4-AP. Clinically, single doses of this order produced dramatic improvement in ocular and peripheral muscle power, a rise of around 20 mmHg in systolic blood pressure and the return of bowel sounds. However, no appreciable increase in respiratory muscle power, as measured by spontaneous tidal volume, was observed and increased dosage of 4-AP (1.5 mg/kg by intravenous infusion over 4 hours) resulted in grand mal convulsions without further benefit.

(VI) PROGNOSIS

The outcome of intoxication with botulism toxin will depend chiefly on the amount of toxin ingested, the delay in giving specific antitoxin and, in those requiring intensive care, individual factors such as previous cardiorespiratory status. The mortality in the United States in the last decade has fallen to under 30%, comparing favourably with that earlier in the century (greater than 60%) and presumably reflecting ease of access to and availability of intensive care facilities. In all surviving cases complete recovery may be expected but this can take a year or more[6].

(VI) CONCLUSION

Botulism follows the ingestion, or rarely inoculation, of specific toxins formed by an anaerobic spore-bearing saprophyte, *Cl. botulinum*. The major symptoms are of those of general and respiratory paralysis caused by the neuromuscular blocking action of the toxins, which act by reducing the release of acetylcholine into the synaptic cleft of the myoneural junction. The mainstays of treatment are antitoxin, which will neutralize circulating toxin, and intensive supportive therapy. Guanidine hydrochloride and 4-aminopyridine, neuromuscular blockade antagonists which enhance acetylcholine release, may be of value in mild or moderate paralysis but not in severe respiratory paralysis. In severe cases a considerable mortality is to be expected, but the survivors can expect the paralysis to recover over a period of months.

References

1. Merson, M. H. and Dowell, V. R. (1973). Epidemiologic, clinical and laboratory aspects of wound botulism. *N. Engl. J. Med.*, **289**, 1005
2. Horwitz, M. A., Hughes, J. M., Merson, M. H. and Gangarosa, E. J. (1977). Food-borne botulism in the United States, 1970–1975. *J. Infect. Dis.*, **136**, 153
3. Arnon, S. S., Midura, T. F., Clay, S. A., Wood, R. M. and Chin, J. (1977). Infant botulism: epidemiological, clinical and laboratory aspects. *J. Am. Med. Assoc.*, **237**, 1946
4. Ball, A. P., Hopkinson, R. B., Farrell, I. D., Hutchison, J. G. P., Paul, R., Watson, R. D. S., Page, A. J. F., Parker, R. G. F., Edwards, C. W., Snow, M., Scott, D. K., Leone-Ganado, A. and Hastings, A. (1979). Human botulism caused by *Clostridium botulinum* type E: The Birmingham outbreak. *Q. J. Med.*, **48**, 473
5. Cull-Candy, S. G., Lundh, H. and Thesleff, S. (1976). Effects of botulinum toxin on neuromuscular transmission in the rat. *J. Physiol.*, **260**, 177
6. Cherington, M. (1974). Botulism: ten year experience. *Arch. Neurol.*, **30**, 432
7. Terranova, W., Palumbo, J. N. and Breman, J. G. (1979). Ocular findings in botulism type B. *J. Am. Med. Assoc.*, **241**, 475
8. Arnon, S. S., Midura, T. F., Damus, K., Wood, R. M. and Chin, J. (1978). Intestinal infection and toxin production by *Clostridium botulinum* as one cause of the sudden infant death syndrome. *Lancet*, **1**, 1273
9. Lawler, P. G. P. and Nunn, J. F. (1977). Intermittent mandatory ventilation. *Anaesthesia*, **32**, 138
10. Koenig, M. G., Drutz, D. J., Mushlin, A. I., Schaffner, W. and Rogers, D. E. (1967). Type B botulism in man. *Am. J. Med.*, **42**, 208
11. Dolman, C. E. and Iida, H. (1963). Type E botulism: its epidemiology prevention and specific treatment. *Can. J. Public Health*, **54**, 293
12. Oberst, F. W., Crook, J., Cresthull, P. and House, M. J. (1968). Evaluation of botulinum antitoxin, supportive therapy, and artificial respiration in monkeys with experimental botulism. *Clin. Pharmacol. Ther.*, **9**. 209
13. Merson, M. H., Hughes, J. M., Dowell, V. R., Taylor, A., Barker, W. H. and Gangorosa, E. J. (1974). Current trends in botulism in the United States. *J. Am. Med. Assoc.*, **229**, 1305
14. Burgen, A. S. V., Dickens, F. and Zatman, L. J. (1949). The action of botulinum toxin on the neuromuscular junction. *J. Physiol.*, **109**, 10
15. Otsuka, M. and Endo, M. (1960). Effect of guanidine on neuromuscular transmission. *J. Pharmacol. Exp. Ther.*, **128**, 273
16. Cherington, M. and Ryan, D. W. (1968). Botulism and guanidine. *N. Engl. J. Med.*, **278**, 933
17. Cherington, M. and Ryan, D. W. (1970). Treatment of botulism with guanidine: early neurophysiological studies. *N. Engl. J. Med.*, **282**, 195
18. Cherington, M., and Schultz, D. (1977) Effect of guanidine, germine and steroids in a case of botulism. *Clin. Toxicol.*, **11**, 19
19. Faich, G. A., Graebner, R. W. and Sato, S. (1971). Failure of guanidine therapy in botulism A. *N. Engl. J. Med.*, **285**, 773

20. Cherington, M., Soyer, A. and Greenberg, H. (1972). Effect of guanidine and germine on the neuromuscular block of botulism. *Curr. Ther. Res. Clin. Exp.*, **14**, 91

21. Lundh, H., Cull-Candy, S. G., Leander, S. and Thesleff, S. (1976). Restoration of transmitter release in botulinum-poisoned skeletal muscle. *Brain Res.*, **110**, 194

22. Lundh, H., Leander, S. and Thesleff, S. (1977). Antagonism of the paralysis produced by botulinum toxin in the rat. *J. Neurol. Sci.*, **32**, 29

23. Lundh, H., Nilsson, O. and Rosen, I. (1977). 4-aminopyridine – a new drug tested in the treatment of Eaton–Lambert syndrome. *J. Neurol. Neurosurg. Psychiatry.*, **40**, 1109

24. Agoston, S., van Weerden, T., Westra, P. and Broekert, A. (1978). Effects of 4-aminopyridine in Eaton–Lambert syndrome. *Br. J. Anaesth.*, **50**, 383

18
The recovery room

JOHN FARMAN

The recovery room is a ward adjacent to the operating theatres where patients recover from the immediate effects of their operations and their anaesthetics. Its function is to ensure the safe recovery of all patients. The idea is by no means new. Nightingale[1] wrote that 'it is not uncommon, in small country hospitals, to have a recess or small room leading from the operating theatre, in which patients remain until they recover'. Nevertheless there are many hospitals in which some, or even all, operating theatres have ˒no recovery room. Patients recovering from anaesthesia and surgery are still taken on hazardous journeys back to their wards in lifts, along corridors and even through the open air[2].

Although the ideal arrangement for the majority of patients would be the provision of a well-equipped recovery room adjacent to every operating theatre, it would be unrealistic to expect this in every case. What is essential is that any patient recovering from an anaesthetic should be under the care of a competent nurse, who has been trained for the job and who has certain basic items of equipment at her disposal. For this reason it is preferable to think in terms of the Recovery Nursing Service, rather than simply the recovery room, however well-equipped. A recovery room without its own nursing staff is little better than the arrangements criticized above. On the other hand it is entirely feasible to provide an efficient service in every hospital, even where the theatres are widely dispersed[3].

The justification for a proper recovery nursing service is provided by the wide range of disturbing and often life threatening complications which occur in the early postoperative period. Many of these are inevitable consequences of general anaesthesia, some are occasional complications, while others arise from the operation rather than from the anaesthetic. While a single complication is unlikely to cause death, multiple complications are by no means rare. A sequence of complications, such as respiratory obstruction leading to cyanosis and then to cardiac arrest, is particularly feared by all doctors and nurses looking after these patients.

Responsibility for the safety of the patient during the phase of recovery from anaesthesia and surgery lies primarily with the anaesthetist and the surgeon. This point has been well made by Wylie[4] in a discussion of deaths associated with anaesthesia: 'An example of commonly delegated responsibility is in the immediate postoperative and postanaesthetic period when a nurse is left to care for the patient. Recovery areas in operating theatre suites have saved many lives that might otherwise have been lost in open wards, yet the delegation of responsibility to a nurse in a recovery area does not absolve the anaesthetist from a continuing interest in his patient.' On the other hand, responsibility for providing an adequate nursing service lies with the employing health authority. The individual doctor has a duty to point out the need and to request that sufficient trained nurses be employed. Recently courts both in the United Kingdom and abroad have decided that accidents occurring to patients in the recovery period were the responsibility of the hospital rather than of the individual anaesthetist[5-7]. As Andrewes[3] has pointed out, to have special recovery nurses 'may well be an added expense, but to have anything less than this may prove to be very, very expensive indeed'.

(I) ORGANIZATION OF THE RECOVERY SERVICE

(1) Equipment and drugs

This can be considered under three headings[8]. Firstly, there are those basic items which should actually be within reach of the recovery nurse whenever a patient is receiving care. Secondly, there are items which may be needed in an emergency and which should always be available. Lastly, there are drugs and equipment which are occasionally needed and which it may therefore be convenient to have in the recovery area. Basic equipment for the recovering patient consists of an oxygen source, flowmeter and mask, oral airway, tipping bed or trolley (with cot sides), self-inflating bag and face mask, suction source with catheter and pharyngeal ends and a sphygmomanometer. Means of summoning help must also be available and the lighting must be good. The range of equipment for emergency use is larger and is similar to that found in other parts of the hospital. The usual resuscitation equipment must always be present (for endotracheal intubation and for intravenous infusion), as must syringes, needles and the usual selection of drugs (e.g. atropine, neostigmine, naloxone, an analeptic, an opioid, an anti-emetic, a sedative, a vasopressor, sodium bicarbonate). The third category of equipment is of intensive care type. It is convenient to keep such items in a recovery room serving a number of theatres, but problems of cost and siting arise when recovery areas are scattered. Much time will be wasted in an emergency fetching things from a central storage location. An e.c.g. monitor, ventilator, defibrillator, infusion pump, chest drainage set or brochoscope may be required. Similarly a stock of intravenous fluids, giving sets, blood warmers and filters will be needed. Depending on which surgical specialities are involved, patients may also need a wide variety of drugs in addition to those mentioned above. These will include antibiotics, frusemide, insulin, a range of inotropic agents, mannitol, hydrocortisone, salbutamol, an antihistamine, cimetidine, relaxants, 50% glucose and an anticonvulsant.

(2) Recovery on the ward

Hospitals constructed in the early days of anaesthesia usually had their operating theatres adjacent to the surgical wards. This allowed rapid transfer of the unconscious postoperative patient back to the ward. On operation days the cases would be grouped near to Sister's desk. Resuscitation equipment was kept ready and the nurses were taught how to look after the recovering patient. This arrangement is still found in older hospitals. It is capable of working well, and provided that the ward is really adjacent to the theatre, that the nurses receive appropriate training and that up-to-date equipment is available, it is safe and satisfactory. Indeed, it is likely to be safer to take a patient to such a well-equipped ward than to a remote recovery room, particularly if a lift journey is involved. An alternative approach, described by Andrewes[3], is the employment of a team of recovery nurses, headed by a nursing officer (senior nurse), who attend all recovery areas in the hospital whenever operations are to be performed. The nurses find the same facilities in all these areas, whether in a purpose-built recovery room, a theatre lobby or part of a ward. A very high standard of training and skill can be achieved with this system.

(3) The recovery room

The ideal physical arrangement for patients having the great majority of operations is to pass directly from the operating theatre to a nearby recovery room. This should be immediately accessible to the medical staff working in the theatres and so for these reasons should be within the theatre clean area. This concept is embodied in the DHSS Hospital Building Note[9]. However, where more than one group of theatres is served or when a recovery room is a later addition to the theatre suite, this may not be possible. In general, experience has shown that room is needed for one and a half patients per theatre[9,10]. The actual number will depend upon the type of surgery performed[8]. For example, a rapid series of minor procedures may fill as many as three beds per theatre. Again, an isolated theatre may need a larger proportion of beds compared with a multi-theatre suite in which the large recovery room can more easily cope with a rush of cases. The recovery room is often combined with a patient reception area, sharing ancillary rooms. The reception area functions as a buffer store, allowing patients to be assembled for final preparation and preventing delays to the theatre schedule. The recovery room may also fulfil this function, holding patients until it is convenient to return them to the ward.

In general, patients are wheeled to the theatre suite in their own beds. They are then lifted on to the operating table (or on to a detachable table top), usually in the anaesthetic room. The patient is placed back on to his bed at the end of the operation, prior to entering the recovery room. In older hospitals doors and corridors may be too narrow for beds, so patients are collected from the wards on trolleys. These trolleys can be tilted head downwards, have drop sides and can carry an oxygen cylinder and foot-operated suction apparatus[11]. The patients remain on the trolleys until their return to the ward.

(4) Postoperative intensive care unit

In highly specialized fields of surgery, such as neurosurgery and cardiac surgery, it is customary to have special intensive care units to which patients are transferred immediately after operation. Such a unit is geared to the appropriate surgical speciality, taking only their cases. Other features of these units are the 24 hour service and relatively long patient stay.

Administratively, this type of unit does not blend easily with the general recovery nursing service. The main object of such units is to continue the intensive care received during the operation into the postoperative period. Recovery of consciousness and spontaneous respiraton may well be secondary, and it is common to continue IPPV and the use of sedative drugs for many hours after admission. Such specialized units deal with a limited range of problems, permitting management to follow a routine course. Indeed in units of this type, therapeutic requirements may be so predictable that they can be automated. Examples are blood transfusion after cardiac surgery[12] and infusion of mannitol in head injury patients[13].

(5) Relationship of recovery room to general intensive care unit

This has been the subject of some consideration. Practice varies even between hospitals which have well-provided recovery rooms, but usually only a small proportion of patients will pass from the recovery room to the ICU. In the author's hospital these account for no more than 2% of cases. Eltringham[15] found that only 33 cases out of 10013 (0.33%) went to the ICU. Patients going to the ICU are those with severe intercurrent disease (for example chronic lung disease), those who have undergone major operations and those in whom serious complications have developed. Where there is no proper recovery room, then there will be a greater need to send such patients to the ICU. However, most recovery rooms can cope with short-term intensive care (for example, the patient with suxamethonium apnoea who needs ventilating for an hour). Hedstrand and Holmdahl[16] have considered the requirements of different types of hospital. They estimated that 20% of patients recovering from general anaesthesia can return to the ward immediately. The remainder should go to a recovery room, with the option of proceeding to an ICU if necessary. However, where the recovery room is on the way out of the theatres, all patients will pass through. It is in any case preferable to decide whether to send the patient to the ICU only after a period of observation in the recovery room. There are circumstances under which the functions of the recovery room and ICU may be combined in a single unit. This may be because there is no ICU[10,17] or, in the case of a small hospital, because there is little justification for a separate ICU. Stead[18] has described such a combined unit in a 291 bed hospital: in one year there were 2835 theatre cases and 40 patients needing intensive care. However, in spite of obvious similarities in the work of these two types of unit, there are also differences. The average length of stay is 1–2 hours in the recovery room, but 1–2 days in the ICU. The recovery room works hardest in the daytime but the ICU has to work round the clock. Lastly, it has been observed that the nurses who like recovery work may dislike intensive care and vice versa. Where units are combined or share facilities, a separate nursing area should be kept available for intensive care, for both administrative and microbiological reasons.

(6) Recovery staffing

The aim is to have a nurse looking after every patient throughout the immediate period of recovery. Andrewes[3] has emphasized the great importance of having one nurse to one patient at all times. Fisher[6] described a patient developing respiratory obstruction leading to permanent brain damage when a nurse was in sole charge of four recovering patients. It follows that the grouping of recovery facilities in a central unit will not reduce the number of bedside nurses needed, although it will assist the provision of off-duty rotas and meal breaks. At times of peak load the ideal ratio will not be achieved unless there is relative under-employment at other times. These periods are needed for routine equipment care and administrative procedures. By the use of flexible working hours and by the employment of part-time staff these inequalities can be largely eliminated. The recovery nurses should be under the command of a senior nurse who teaches and supervises them. He or she will usually be subordinate to the senior theatre nurse, although where there is a service covering the whole hospital the post should be more senior (e.g. Nursing Officer in the United Kingdom)[3]. It is essential that the recovery nurses receive training in their work. Training must be locally organized[3] in the absence of any agreed national standards. Recovery nursing should be regarded as a specialty like other similar branches of nursing. EEC nurse training requirements for student nurses now include one week in the recovery service. Their training is also the responsibility of the senior nurse. It is regrettable that there is, at any rate in the United Kingdom, no course of training (recognized by the Joint Board of Clinical Nursing Studies) for those who supervise and teach recovery nursing, although some JBCNS theatre courses include recovery work[19]. Suitable courses are urgently needed[20].

It is important that a member of the medical staff plays an administrative role in the recovery room. Although this role can be filled by a surgeon or intensivist, it seems more appropriate to the work of the anaesthetist, who in any case spends a large part of his time in the theatre suite. Together with the senior nurse, decisions are made about the correct equipment, facilities and procedures. Usually there are no medical staff specifically attached to the recovery service, which in an emergency will call on the patient's own anaesthetist or surgeon, or else summon the hospital resuscitation team. In general, individual surgeons and anaesthetists will continue to carry responsibility for their patients during the recovery period.

It is impossible to consider staffing without taking into account the pattern of demand. The service caters mainly for patients recovering from elective procedures. Work starts in earnest once the operating lists begin and continues until an hour or two after they finish. Emergency cases frequently occupy the evening hours, but at night only life-saving operations are performed. Recovery rooms may close at night[15], depend on help from theatre staff[21], or maintain a skeleton staff[14,22] during these hours. Fazio and Cottle[23] found a similar variety in the United States where only 16% of recovery rooms remained open at night and average opening hours were 12 daily, 6 days per week. Provision of a 24 hour service may weigh heavily on full-time staff if a large proportion of part-time nurses is employed.

(II) THE PATIENT'S PROGRESS

(1) The reception area

This is usually operated by the recovery nurses who may also visit the patients on the wards beforehand[14,20]. It enables the work of the theatres to proceed smoothly even when the porters or the lift services are busy, by bringing the patients to the theatre in good time. It should be kept as quiet as possible, to allay the patients' anxieties. However, a telephone for communicating with the wards, laboratory, etc., and an intercom for communicating with the theatres, will be needed. Its most important function is the performance of a series of essential safety checks[14,21]. These can conveniently be managed with the help of a printed check list.

The following are the most important questions: (1) Has the identity of the patient been verified? (2) Has consent for the procedure been given by the patient and signed by a doctor? (3) Have pre-operative drugs been given, and if so, when? (4) Has the patient been weighed and the weight recorded? (5) Has any blood been ordered, and if so, is it available? (6) Have the results of investigations been recorded (e.g. haemoglobin level, urine analysis, plasma electrolytes)? (7) Have such items as jewellery, false teeth, wigs and other prostheses been removed? Have other such items been noted and securely fastened to the patient (e.g. wedding ring, hearing aid)?

(2) Anaesthetic room and theatre

The patient proceeds from the reception area to the anaesthetic room. Anaesthesia is induced followed by other essential preparations for operation, such as setting up a drip, shaving the skin, or placing a tourniquet. In hospitals without anaesthetic rooms the patient proceeds directly to the theatre for induction of anaesthesia.

(3) Transfer to the recovery area

At the end of the operation the recovery nurses are notified. Meanwhile the anaesthetist allows the patient to wake up. Drugs may be given to reverse the effects of agents used during the anaesthetic. The pharynx is carefully aspirated of saliva, etc., before an endotracheal tube is removed. The patient is whenever possible turned on to his side (tonsil position) to allow secretions to run out of his mouth and to assist the passage of air by allowing the tongue to fall to one side. The recovery nurse takes charge of the patient at this stage. She first assures herself that the patient is breathing adequately, is safely placed on the bed (with the head of the bed removed) or trolley and is preferably placed on his side. The surgeon or senior nurse tells her what operation was done and what drains and dressings, etc., were used. The anaesthetist tells her of any special problems and shows her that analgesic drugs and intravenous fluids have been prescribed. She is informed of any special instructions or dangers. If the recovery area is not adjacent to the theatre, a portable oxygen cylinder, suction apparatus and self-inflating resuscitating bag must accompany the patient during the move. The patient should be taken feet first, with the nurse following behind, supporting the airway.

(4) The recovery area

Patients are kept under observation in the recovery area until they are either well enough to return to their wards or are sent to an intensive care unit. The average length of stay is about 1 hour[10] although major or complicated cases are kept for 2 hours or more. Eltringham[15] showed that 62% of the patients having operations in a general hospital spent less than half an hour in the recovery room, 35.6% spent from half to 2 hours, while only 1.5% stayed more than 2 hours. On the other hand, Schweizer[17] stated, 'Although most patients were discharged within 24 hours after the operation, approximately 5% remained in the unit (which was combined with the ICU) for 2 days to several weeks'. However, most recovery rooms find it essential to transfer all patients by the end of the working day. Hudson[8] has pointed out the effect of staffing level on length of patient stay.

(5) Records

It is important that adequate records are kept of observations and events occurring during recovery. Their complexity is less than that of the ICU records. In our recovery room the observations are recorded in red ink on the anaesthetic record sheet. This has the advantages of employing the same time scale and of avoiding an additional sheet of paper. Arterial pressure and heart rate are plotted routinely, while events such as arrival in the recovery room, recovery of consciousness or the giving of drugs are recorded. For patients who receive short-term intensive care in the recovery room, the ICU record chart may be used. Basic information about each patient passing should be entered in a book. This obviously applies only to a proper recovery room. It is useful to have a record of the patient's name, number, operation, times of arrival, awakening and discharge and of complications and treatment. This gives a good idea of the work done and the complications encountered. The figures may be the basis of an annual report[10].

(6) Discharge criteria

Discharge from the recovery room is considered when the patient has recovered consciousness, his general condition is satisfactory, with no circulatory or respiratory depression, and his observations have been stable for at least half an hour after arrival or receiving any drug. Return to the ward should be on the instruction of a doctor. Medical staff are seldom assigned to recovery areas and medical cover usually depends on the ready availability of the anaesthetists and surgeons concerned. In the absence of specific instructions, a nurse should take the record chart to the doctor and ask to send the patient back, or else ask him to come to see the patient.

(III) COMPLICATIONS AND TREATMENT IN THE RECOVERY PERIOD

The main object of the service is to care for patients recovering from anaesthesia and surgery, in the certain knowledge that some will suffer from serious and potentially fatal complications. Indeed, so predictable are many of these effects that they might be better regarded as inevitable consequences rather than complications. Much treatment during recovery is directed at the prevention of complications, which may only be noted when treatment fails. Although complications are common enough to cause alarm even with a well-run recovery nursing service, they are certain to be every bit as common, albeit less obvious, when no proper service is provided. In the latter case they may only become apparent when a patient has a cardiac arrest. Complications may be due to the anaesthetic or to the operation or to a combination of the two, while conditions unrelated to either of these factors may also give rise to problems during the recovery period. To understand all the complications which may be encountered it is necessary to have an extensive knowledge of anaesthesia, surgery and medicine. Clearly it is beyond the scope of this chapter to include all these, and the reader is referred to standard texts on these subjects. From the practical point of view the simplest and safest approach to the treatment of unexpected complications is to seek the help of the appropriate specialist. In this section a physiological classification is used to deal with complications and their prevention and treatment. However, a series of events may involve many physiological systems. Respiratory obstruction leads to hypoxia, which leads to cardiac arrest; cardiac arrest leads to metabolic acidosis, which will depress neuromuscular transmission, and so on.

An idea of the frequency of complications is given by Farman[10]. In a 5 year period 29 583 patients passed through the recovery room of a large general hospital. Of these 5349 had complications of some sort, an average of one patient in 5.5. Of these 2458 were circulatory and 987 were respiratory, while 740 vomited. There were other complications of various sorts in a further 1664 patients. Eltringham[24] in a survey of 10 000 similar patients, found an almost identical incidence. Incidentally, 8.5% of his patients were over 60 years old; the majority of surgical patients in the United Kingdom are elderly, with a greater tendency to suffer from complications than young subjects. Further evidence of the incidence of complications may be obtained from a study of the treatment given to patients during the recovery period[15]. While some of those procedures simply mark the end of treatment (e.g. tracheal extubation or removal of packs) and others represent routine care of drips, drains and dressings, the majority are aimed at preventing or treating complications. Table 18.1 lists 5643 procedures performed during the course of a year on the 7053 patients who passed through a typical recovery room[10]. In this instance 80% of patients received some special care, treatment or investigation during their stay, in

Table 18.1 Some therapeutic and investigative procedures noted on the 7053 patients passing through a general hospital recovery room in 1 year

Respiratory	
Oxygen given	2128
Oral suction	338
Artificial respiration	22
Reintubation of trachea	13
Physiotherapy	16
Monitoring and investigations	
E.c.g. monitoring	167
X-rays	59
Blood samples	33
Neurological observations	58
Drug therapy	
Analgesics	1627
Anti-emetics	161
Other drugs	200
Surgical procedures	
Bladder irrigation	252
Attention to dental packs	371
Redressing of wound	33
Bladder catheterization	21
Drips set up or taken down	33
Tepid sponging	8
Passage of nasogastric tube	5
Total	5547

addition to their routine care, observation and monitoring.

(1) Circulatory complications

These are the commonest of all, accounting for more than half of all complications. The commonest single complication is hypotension, occurring in 4.6% of our patients[10]. Other authors[24,25] reported a similar incidence, while Gordon[22] observed that more than 30% of cases showed a significant period of hypotension during recovery from anaesthesia. Altogether, circulatory complications of all types were seen in 8.3% of the 29 583 patients in Farman's series. These are listed in Table 18.2. Fortunately most circulatory disorders encountered in the recovery period respond to simple measures. There is little that can be done at this stage to prevent trouble, although the nurses are instructed to give oxygen on the least indication; Andrewes[3] indeed gave oxygen to 95% of patients. The foot of the bed may be raised to assist venous return, and the nurses are encouraged to do this if systolic arterial pressure falls below 100 mmHg.

Table 18.2 Cardiovascular complications recorded in 29 583 patients in the recovery rooms at Addenbrooke's Hospitals in a 5 year period

Hypotension	(< 100mmHg systolic)	1355	(1:22)
Hypertension	(> 150mmHg systolic)	485	(1:61)
Bradycardia	(< 60 beats/min)	288	(1:103)
Tachycardia	(> 150 beats/min)	209	(1:142)
Haemorrhage		74	(1:400)
Irregular pulse		33	(1:896)
Cardiac arrest (four deaths)		14	(1:2113)
Total		2458	(1:12)

Hypotension

The commonest cause of hypotension (systolic pressure below 100 mmHg) in the recovery period is the residual effect of general anaesthetic agents, particularly halothane. These agents depress myocardial contractility and reduce peripheral vascular tone. This effect wears off as the agent is excreted and seldom lasts more than half an hour. Patients who have received only light general anaesthesia with nitrous oxide and oxygen, combined with a relaxant and artificial respiration, show a rise in arterial pressure when the nitrous oxide is discontinued. Patients to whom supplementary agents are given show a gentler rise. By contrast, patients who breathe spontaneously during anaesthesia require higher concentrations of general anaesthetics, with a correspondingly longer period of recovery. No special treatment is required and the pressure recovers spontaneously if the patient is given oxygen and the foot of the bed is raised. Recovery usually follows return of consciousness.

Surgical bleeding, if more than 10% of the patient's calculated blood volume (approximately 80 ml/kg), will lead to pallor, vasoconstriction, tachycardia, and finally hypotension. Hypotension will develop earlier in patients receiving higher concentrations of general anaesthetics. Significant bleeding may continue after the operation and will appear in drainage containers, on the dressings, in the bed or as increasing girth. Operative blood loss is commonly estimated by weighing of swabs and by measurement of suction bottle contents (with allowance for other fluids present) or more rarely by diluting in a haemolysing fluid, combined with measurement of the optical density of the resulting mixture. All methods tend to underestimate the loss. Losses should be replaced with whole blood wherever possible. Concentrated cells require the addition of plasma or plasma substitute. Where blood transfusion is contra-indicated, plasma protein solutions or plasma substitute must be given to restore blood volume. The use of electrolyte solutions for this purpose is undesirable (see p. 423). Surgical bleeding may, of course, require operative treatment.

Spinal (subarachnoid) and epidural anaesthesia above the second lumbar segment are accompanied by sympathetic blockade, the level of which extends above that of the sensory block. Vessels in the blocked area relax, allowing pooling of blood with reduction of venous return, heart rate and cardiac output. Compensatory vasoconstriction in the unblocked area maintains arterial pressure, until the block reaches the region of the fifth thoracic segment[26], provided that the blood volume remains normal. The patient is very sensitive to position; raising the upper half of the body leads to gravitational pooling and the sudden outset of hypotension. The treatment is to give oxygen and raise the patient's legs until the block wears off. Hypotension may be accompanied by nausea. A vasopressor (e.g. ephedrine 0.5 mg/kg) may be given once posture and blood volume have been corrected. Movement, for example lifting or turning, may induce hypotension in any patient recovering from anaesthesia.

Adrenal cortical deficiency is a rare but important cause of hypotension in the postoperative period. Addisonian crisis may cause nausea and vomiting, which are in any case common at this time, and hypoglycaemia[27]. Patients who are or who have recently been receiving steroid treatment are given additional doses to cover the operative period. Twice the normal morning dose may conveniently be given by mouth as part of pre-operative medication and hydrocortisone is given intravenously during major operations, in which the stress response is likely to be great. Hypotension and bradycardia occurring in the absence of other obvious cause in a patient known to be at risk, should be treated with intravenous hydrocortisone, 100 mg.

Myocardial insufficiency, associated with ischaemic heart disease or severe metabolic disturbances, can develop during or after operation. Dysrhythmias may be caused by anaesthetic drugs, carbon dioxide retention or metabolic acid-base abnormality and will reduce cardiac output. Myocardial infarction is extremely rare during anaesthesia, in which metabolic demand is reduced and the patient well-oxygenated, but may occur in the recovery period. However, Gordon[22] found only one death from this cause in 77 143 patients. The problem of anaesthesia and cardiac disease has been reviewed by Clement[28].

Hypertension

This is a common observation in the recovery period. A systolic pressure above 150 mmHg was recorded in 1.6% of patients in Farman's series[10], while Eltringham[15] found a pressure above 170 mmHg in 5% of recovering patients. When hypertension occurs in a previously normotensive patient it will often be accompanied by other signs of sympathetic activity, such as tachycardia, sweating and pallor. The commonest cause is pain[29] while respiratory depression, bladder distension and overtransfusion may also be responsible. Patients in whom hypertension persists in the absence of these factors should be treated with great respect, particularly when the systolic pressure is over 250 mmHg. Eltringham[15] reported two such cases (out of 10 013), one of whom died in spite of active treatment and was found at postmortem to have had an unsuspected phaeochromocytoma.

Dysrhythmias and cardiac arrest

Only very rarely will rate changes require specific treatment, although Eltringham[24] found that atropine had been given to most of the 176 bradycardia patients in their series. Rhythm changes may be associated with changes in arterial pressure, as described above, and use of antidysrhythmics is more common. In any group of patients with severe cardiovascular disturbances, there will be some who proceed to cardiac arrest. In the recovery period there is the risk of cardiac arrest in fit patients with healthy hearts who develop respiratory obstruction, bleeding or occasionally drug effects. Eltringham[15] found five cases in 10 013 (1:2003) with two deaths, while Farman[10] reported 14 cases in 29 583 patients (1:2113) with four deaths, an almost identical incidence. Gordon[22] reported 39 deaths in the recovery room at the Toronto General Hospital, out of

77 143 patients. The death rates in these three series are 1:5006, 1:7396 and 1:1978 respectively. Careful attention must be paid to post-arrest management. Hypoxic brain damage must be assumed to have occurred unless the patient awakens immediately. The treatment follows that employed in any other type of brain injury. The patient is ventilated artificially so as to reduce $PaCO_2$ to 3.5 kPa (26.3 mmHg). Mannitol 10% (1 g per kg) is infused intravenously over 2 hours to avoid sudden expansion of vascular volume. This will reduce cerebral oedema and stimulate osmotic diuresis. A catheter is inserted into the bladder. Frusemide (20 mg) is given if urine output is less than 50 ml in the first hour and may be repeated later. Dextrose with 0.18% saline is infused in a volume equal to the urinary loss. This will maintain a negative fluid balance, particularly important in view of the normal postoperative salt and water retention. The role of steroids in the treatment of brain injury remains controversial, while barbiturates should be given only in severe cases. Treatment should continue until it is clear that the fullest possible recovery of cerebral function has occurred.

Conventional cardiopulmonary resuscitation has a very good chance of success if the precipitating cause of the arrest can be corrected. Deaths are most likely to occur in severely ill patients with multiple pathology. Gordon[22] emphasized that no patient in the Toronto group 'died as a result of postoperative or postanaesthetic accident which could be avoided or treated'.

(2) Respiratory complications

Respiratory obstruction is an obvious and justly feared complication of the recovery period. Respiratory depression and apnoea, although equally dangerous, are fortunately rarer. The commonest respiratory complication is hypoxia, which is present in most patients, even in the absence of obstruction or respiratory depression[30]. Complications recorded by the nursing staff in one recovery unit are shown in Table 18.3 and give some idea of their relative incidence. However, it must be remembered that preventative treatment, particularly airway care, will have a significant influence on this incidence, and that many patients suffer minor degrees of hypoxaemia, insufficient to cause cyanosis.

The recovery nurse is trained to look for signs of air passing in and out of the lungs. While supporting the jaw from the head end of the bed she can feel the patient's warm breath on her hand. She watches the movement of the chest and the colour of the skin, mucosae or nail beds. An oral airway is usually present but is removed as soon as the patient shows signs of rejecting it.

Hypoxaemia

Nunn and Payne[30] showed that the arterial oxygen tension is depressed for 12–24 hours after anaesthesia. Cyanosis is evident only when the tension falls below 8 kPa (60 mmHg). Nevertheless it was seen in 488 out of 29 583 patients (1:61); see Table 18.3. Lesser degrees of hypoxaemia are so common as to be considered inevitable. It can usually be corrected by the use of oxygen[31]. A flow of 4 l/min via a simple mask such as the OTU is sufficient. There is no single cause of postoperative hypoxaemia, but a number of factors have been identified.

Table 18.3 Respiratory complications recorded in a 5 year period in the recovery rooms at Addenbrooke's Hospitals

Cyanosis	488	(1:61)
Obstruction	288	(1:103)
Respiratory depression, apnoea	158	(1:187)
Coughing, bronchospasm	53	(1:558)
Total	987	(1:30)

Arterial oxygen tension declines with age: Nunn[32] found a mean postoperative tension of 11 kPa (83 mmHg) at the age of 20, falling to 8 kPa (60 mmHg) at 70. Patients who have received nitrous oxide, which is very much more soluble than nitrogen, may become hypoxic at the end of anaesthesia[33]. The explanation is that the volume of nitrous oxide passing out through the lungs is so great that there is a net outward flow of gas, which displaces the incoming air. The effect lasts only a few minutes and may be prevented by giving a high oxygen concentration at the end of the anaesthetic. Underventilation is an obvious possibility, although the majority of reports show normal carbon dioxide tensions, suggesting other causative factors[34]. However, carbon dioxide tension may be little altered in the presence of gross hypoxaemia due to underventilation[35] because the effect of CO_2 washout during some types of anaesthesia is that carbon dioxide is maintained at a normal tension by a low level of ventilation[36]. Causes of respiratory depression are discussed later. Spence and Alexander[37] drew attention to the reduction in functional residual capacity (FRC) which occurs during anaesthesia and persists into the postoperative period. They showed that FRC falls by 25% in patients having upper abdominal operations, by 15% in herniorrhaphy patients and least in those having limb operations. They suggested that patients who have had abdominal operations breathe at lower than normal lung volumes as the result of pain, which limits muscle movement. Small airway closure is likely to be widespread at low lung volumes and may be encouraged by high oxygen mixtures[38]. Closure occurs only when the lungs are nearly empty in normal subjects, but elderly patients and those with lung disease may exhibit this within the tidal range. The result of these changes is a deterioration in the ventilation/perfusion relationship with increasing venous admixture. Desaturated blood will pass through the lungs in greater quantity to dilute the normally oxygenated blood from better ventilated regions. Arterial oxygen tension will therefore be depressed. Any patient in whom lung expansion is hindered by external factors will be at risk. Possible causes are discussed in subsequent sections. A further complication is the effect of a deterioration in pulmonary blood flow in a patient who already has increased venous admixture. This causes an even greater fall in arterial oxygen tension. The hypotension which is so common at this stage is likely to be associated with a fall in cardiac output, suggesting that this vicious combination is not rare. An important contributory cause of venous admixture and hypoxaemia is airway obstruction due to pulmonary aspiration or secretions. Aspiration is discussed later.

Respiratory obstruction

Obstruction of the air passages occurs when consciousness is lost, particularly if the subject is supine. This is mainly due to the tongue falling back against the posterior pharyngeal wall, although the soft palate and lips may also contribute, especially in edentulous patients. Partial obstruction causes snoring but complete obstruction is silent. In an obstructed patient with good muscular tone the diaphragm contracts powerfully, drawing down the mediastinal structures, including the trachea (tracheal tug)[39] and sucking in the intercostal muscles. Airway obstruction should be regarded as inevitable in the unconscious patient, rather than as an occasional complication. Relief of airway obstruction is fundamental to the care of the patient, whether anaesthetized, recovering from anaesthesia or unconscious from any other cause. Anatomical obstruction can be relieved by a series of manoeuvres which every recovery nurse should know. The nurse should stand behind the patient's head. The head is extended and the jaw supported, either from the point or by lifting the angles. The effect of these movements is to lift the tongue off the posterior pharyngeal wall. In patients with normal dentition this is usually enough to clear the air passage[11]. If snoring continues an oral airway should be inserted, although in many cases the anaesthetist will already have done this. Occasionally a nasopharyngeal airway will prove more tolerable. Whenever possible the patient should be turned on to his side into the 'tonsil' position. This is essential in all patients in whom there is any bleeding into the mouth (e.g. after oral or nasal operations) and those in whom there is the slightest risk of regurgitation from the stomach. In some cases (e.g. those placed in orthopaedic traction frames) it may be impossible to turn the patient. Where there is any doubt it is wise to pass a nasogastric tube to aspirate the stomach while the patient is still anaesthetized. The other advantage of the tonsil position is that the tongue is less likely to fall back, although obstruction may still occur.

Occasionally obstruction is due to the presence of more solid objects, such as regurgitated food particles, chewing gum, teeth, etc. In such cases the patient's life may be saved by the prompt use of a laryngoscope and Magill's forceps, assisted by pharyngeal suction[40]. Obstruction at the glottic level will result from paralysis of the vocal cords due to damage to the recurrent pharyngeal nerves or from oedema following operations on the neck, such as thyroidectomy or parathyroid exploration. Deep haemorrhage in the neck may compress the trachea after thyroidectomy, while a soft or deviated trachea may collapse. Tumours of the larynx or base of the tongue may very rarely cause obstruction in the recovery period. The treatment is immediate reintubation, which has largely replaced the use of helium–oxygen mixture and of emergency tracheostomy. As the patient recovers consciousness, the tone of the pharyngeal muscles recovers and the cough and laryngeal reflexes return. Stridor at this stage is likely to result from the presence of mucus or other fluids, requiring pharyngeal suction. Oxygen will be needed in the obstructed patient. Airway obstruction was recorded in 288 cases in Farman's series[10], an incidence of 1:103, which occurred in spite of routine use of the manoeuvres described above.

Respiratory depression and apnoea

Although due to a variety of causes, these together are sufficiently common to justify the recovery service. One patient in 187 in Farman's series[10] was affected; of 158 cases, 81 were actually apnoeic and needed artificial respiration. The relative incidence of causative factors is for the most part unknown. The commonest factor is probably the use of opioids, given as premedication, as part of the anaesthetic or for relief of postoperative pain. The cause may be overdosage or individual hypersensitivity[41]. Anaesthetic techniques which employ very large doses of opioids have been advocated. Lowenstein *et al.*[42] used up to 200 mg of morphine for open heart surgery; in such patients artificial respiration will continue into the postoperative period. Fentanyl has been employed to supplement nitrous oxide anaesthesia in doses of approximately 1 μg/kg per hour. Very much larger doses 10–15 μg/kg have also been advocated to depress sympathetic activity (stress-free anaesthesia). Although originally presented as short-acting, fentanyl has been shown to act for more than 4 hours, at least as long as morphine[43]. Adams and Pybus[44] have described cases of respiratory depression occurring some hours after fentanyl was given, in patients who made a good initial recovery. No obvious explanation is forthcoming, although Cormack[45] has suggested that the stimulus of pain may lessen within a short time, leaving the depressant effect of the opioid unopposed. Although gross respiratory depression is revealed by a slow frequency of breathing[46], minor degrees of depression may remain unnoticed, although the patient is unable to overcome a minor degree of obstruction. Fentanyl has minimal sedative effect and the patient appears awake and alert. By contrast, buprenorphine, morphine and pethidine have an obvious sedative effect which alerts the nursing staff to the state of the patient. Prevention is better than cure, and it behoves the anaesthetist to moderate the use of opioids in premedication and anaesthesia. Most opioids are reversible by naloxone, but this acts for only 45 minutes[47]. Continuous injection via a syringe pump of 0.005–0.01 (mg/kg)/hour is preferable. Doxapram or amphetamine may be effective in stimulating respiration[48,49], particularly in the case of buprenorphine which is not antagonized by naloxone. Eltringham et al.[15] found that naloxone was used in 92 patients, anticholinesterases in 34, nalorphine in seven and doxapram in six, out of 10013 cases. Anaesthetic drugs can depress respiration. Barbiturates used in premedication or for induction of anaesthesia may be responsible, particularly in repeated doses. Respiration may be depressed by inhalation agents, particularly halothane and enflurane[50], which thereby delay their own excretion via the lungs. Marshall and Millar[36] showed that patients anaesthetized with the aid of muscle relaxants who are hyperventilated, will suffer from carbon dioxide depletion. When the relaxant is reversed, spontaneous respiration is depressed by the effect of the low $PaCO_2$. Anaesthetized patients have metabolic rates around 80% of basal or less if body temperature falls, so carbon dioxide production is likely to recover only slowly[51]. Although washout of carbon dioxide is rapid, its replacement by underventilation is in any case slow[52]. Cormack[45] has pointed out that under such circumstances a normal $PaCO_2$ indicates underventilation, and that hypoxaemia may be present.

Neuromuscular blocking effects are familiar to anaesthetists. If a relaxant is not adequately reversed the patient will show signs of muscle weakness. He will be unable to lift his head and in extreme cases will show tracheal tug with indrawing of the intercostal spaces during inspiration. All muscle movements are jerky and the patient appears distressed, a picture aptly described by Robertson as 'fighting for breath'. The diagnosis may be confirmed with the aim of a simple nerve stimulator[53]. Non-depolarizing relaxants such as curare, gallamine, pancuronium and alcuronium are partially reversible by neostigmine. Atropine is given at the same time to prevent the muscarinic effects of the acetyl choline which is released. Depolarizing relaxants are not reversible by neostigmine, which may actually increase the block. A number of other factors may affect the degree or duration of neuromuscular block. At temperatures below 32°C non-depolarizing drugs are potentiated. This may affect neonates in whom body temperature falls readily[11]. All non-depolarizing relaxants are excreted in the urine, while tubocurarine and pancuronium are also excreted in bile. Renal or hepatic failure may therefore prolong their duration of effect. Aminoglycoside antibiotics also have a neuromuscular blocking action and will potentiate relaxants. Acidosis, whether of respiratory or metabolic origin, will potentiate tubocurarine. This gives rise to the picture of neo-stigmine-resistant curarization, in which the patient shows the signs of inadequate reversal, often getting progressively worse when breathing spontaneously; a period of hyperventilation may lead to temporary improvement. Blood gas analysis reveals metabolic acidosis and recovery usually follows correction with sodium bicarbonate. Some volatile anaesthetics, particularly diethyl ether, potentiate non-depolarizing relaxants. Suxamethonium is widely used a short-acting relaxant to assist endotracheal intubation, to modify e.c.t and for other short procedures which require profound relaxation. Its short action is due to breakdown by plasma or pseudocholinesterase, which is made in the liver. Patients with hepato-cellular failure, those who have been receiving anticholinesterase drugs in the treatment of glaucoma or have been poisoned with organophosphorus insectides and those with congenitally abnormal enzymes, will all show a prolonged response to suxamethonium. Although a human cholinesterase extract is available[54] to reverse this effect, the duration of apnoea is seldom above an hour and it is usually simplest to ventilate the patient artificially until muscle tone recovers. Any patient showing a prolonged response should have his plasma cholinesterase level measured and genotype determined. In the case of a genetic variant other members of the patient's family should also be investigated and any carriers of the abnormal gene given written warning of the danger of receiving suxamethonium. The reader is referred to the excellent description by Feldman[53] for details of the mode of action of and complications of muscle relaxants.

Respiratory depression may be the result of physical factors. Pneumo-thorax, rib fractures, pleural fluid and deficiences of the diaphragm permitting bowel to pass into the thorax, may all cause collapse of the lungs. Tension pneumothorax may develop rapidly and unexpectedly; if the patient is severely dyspnoeic an axillary chest drain should be inserted immediately. Obesity, ascites, bowel gas, abdominal tumours, pneumoperi-toneum[55], the use of relaxants in upper abdominal surgery and external bandaging may all prevent movement of the diaphragm and expansion of the chest, with basal atelectasis. Besides specific treatment it is usually a help to sit the patient up. Respiratory excursions may be limited by pain, particularly after upper abdominal and thoracic operations. Paradoxically, the use of opioids will often improve respiratory depression in these cases, while Spence and Smith[56] have demonstrated the value of extradural analgesia.

The effects of severe respiratory depression are so grave that rather than spend time on diagnosis it is often best to institute immediate treatment. The patient may need to be ventilated, at first with a mask and self-inflating bag, later with an endotracheal tube and ventilator, using an oxygen-rich mixture. Further investigation of possible causes can then be undertaken at leisure. In many cases underventilation is due to a combination of factors rather than to a single cause. It is a common observation that a patient will breathe without difficulty after a night on a ventilator in the ICU and in cases of doubt it is usually wise to arrange this.

Other respiratory complications

Coughing and bronchospasm were rarely noted as complications in Farman's[10] and Eltringham's[24] series. The recovery of the cough reflex is regarded more as a sign of recovery than as a complication, and only persistent coughing will be remarked. The use of an endotracheal tube or bronchoscope will often leave the patient with discomfort in the trachea, with perhaps a hoarse voice and a cough. This usually disappears in a few hours. Wheezing and true bronchospasm have a number of causes and almost invariably cause hypoxaemia. Asthmatic patients who are under treatment seldom develop bronchospasm during anaesthesia, while inhalational anaesthetics tend to relax bronchioles. Untreated asthmatics may be treated with intravenous salbutamol or with an aerosol of the drug, via an endotracheal tube. The commonest cause of wheezing in an anaesthetized or recovery patient is compression of the lungs by an attenuated attempt to cough. This will contribute to the reduced FRC and small airway closure that has long been appreciated[57]. It may be diminished by the use of a local anaesthetic spray to the trachea before intubation, but this is contraindicated in many cases. A small dose of intravenous opioid may be needed to prevent this straining. 5% carbon dioxide inhalation was at one time recommended to prevent atelectasis.

The most serious cause of persistent cough and wheeze is the presence in the lungs of foreign material such as mucus, blood, or stomach contents. The patient should be kept on the side, head down, and given oxygen. The pharynx should be aspirated. It may be necessary to pass an endotracheal tube to permit repeated suction, while occasionally artificial respiration is needed to maintain oxygenation. If the lungs are not cleared and there is reason to believe that solid or semi-solid matter has entered them, a bronchoscope should be passed. A ventilating bronchoscope is preferred so that an assistant can assist or control ventilation with the oxygen jet during the procedure. A chest X-ray is taken once the patient's condition is stable. Physiotherapy will be helpful at this stage. Mendelson[58] described the effects of the aspiration of acid gastric contents, in which pulmonary

419

oedema develops in addition to wheezing and hypoxaemia. This condition is a much feared complication of obstetric operations. Doughty[59] recommends the use of steroids, with artificial respiration and correction of any acid–base abnormality. Bronchial lavage with 1.4% sodium bicarbonate was at one time recommended although large volumes of fluid may lead to further hypoxia and the method is seldom used now. Antibiotics may be required to treat secondary infection.

(3) Neurological aspects

The pattern of recovery

Recovery of consciousness after general anaesthesia is assessed at regular intervals by the nursing staff. The usual criteria are spontaneous activity on the part of the patient and the ability to open the eyes on command. Patients who have had light general anaesthesia combined with relaxants will usually be awake on arrival in the recovery room, while those who breathed spontaneously (which paradoxically requires a greater concentration of anaesthetic) will take rather longer. The average waking time in our recovery room was $8\frac{1}{2}$ minutes after arrival, while in Eltringham's[24] it was 9 minutes. However, a proportion of patients take longer than this, as many as one patient in 89 taking more than 30 minutes[14]. Recovery of consciousness at most involves a progression from a deep plane of anaesthesia characterized by absent reflexes, reduced muscle tone and perhaps depressed cardiorespiratory function. The tracheal cough reflex and later the laryngeal response return, followed by pharyngeal reflexes (swallowing). Muscle tone recovers and the jaw may no longer need support, while limb rigidity may be prominent. The patient may vomit at this stage. The speed of recovery will depend on the duration and depth of anaesthesia and on the agents used. Respiratory depression will delay excretion of inhaled drugs. Their rate of excretion also depends on their aqueous solubility; the body has a very large capacity for highly soluble agents such as diethyl ether and trichloroethylene and recovery is correspondingly slow. The anaesthetist tries to anticipate the end of the operation, turning the agent off well beforehand, but this is difficult to judge correctly. Drugs of intermediate water solubility, typically halothane and enflurane, are characterized by average recovery times, while recovery from nitrous oxide and cyclopropane, both insoluble agents, is rapid. The role of metabolism is probably unimportant to recovery except in the case of the most soluble agents. These are in part degraded in the liver. Ether is converted to CO_2 and water via ethanol, and is a powerful hepatic microsomal enzyme inducer[60]. Trichloroethylene is broken down to both trichloroethanol and trichloracetic acid. Variations in hepatic enzyme pathways will perhaps account for the occasional patient in whom recovery is very prolonged. Patients receiving local anaesthesia will return to the recovery room conscious though possibly drowsy from sedation. Whatever the site of the block, recovery of motor function precedes recovery of sensation. Indeed, use of low concentrations of local anaesthetics will produce only a sensory block. Very low concentrations will merely block the unmyelinated autonomic fibres. During the recovery period the patient will therefore pass through a stage of full motor recovery with incomplete sensory recovery. Pain will be absent even when touch sensation is present. Last of all to recover is sympathetic function. The significance of this is that after spinal (subarachnoid) or epidural block, the patient will be functionally sympathectomized even when other modalities have returned to normal. This will render him incapable of vasoconstricting in response to blood loss or resumption of the upright posture and so liable to become hypotensive.

Pain

Pain is the dominating aspect of the postoperative return of sensation. Although ether, trichloroethylene or opioids given during anaesthesia will still be effective during recovery, many patients experience pain within a short time. Pain is worse after upper abdominal and intrathoracic than lower abdominal operations, least after superficial operations. Men experience greater pain than women. In most cases pain is at its worst initially and recedes over 12–24 hours, longer after abdominal or thoracic operations. There is considerable individual variation. Conventional pain relief is based on the use of morphine, 0.1 mg per kg, every 4 hours or so. Pethidine 1 mg per kg is also satisfactory and may be given at similar intervals. Buprenorphine (0.0075 mg per kg) is a promising new analgesic which has the advantage of very long duration of action, up to 12 hours or more[61]. It is a partial agonist and so is not addictive, which simplifies dispensing. The average patient requires a repeat dose after 6–8 hours. These doses all refer to intramuscular injections. Masson[62] obtained superior pain relief by titrating the dose to suit the individual patient; an initial dose is given slowly intravenously until analgesia is achieved. Subsequent intramuscular doses are related to the patient's initial requirement. A similar approach was adopted by Rutter[63]. All opioids are capable of causing nausea, vomiting, drowsiness and respiratory depression. Continuous infusion of opioid has considerable advantages in major cases in which analgesia is needed for long periods and in which good supervision is available. Fentanyl 0.5–1 (μg/kg) hour is effective without causing nausea or undue sedation. Rutter[63] and Bryan-Brown[64] have observed similar advantages when using morphine. Lower total doses are required and

421

tolerance does not appear to be a problem.

Entonox 50:50 nitrous oxide–oxygen mixture is a useful 'bridging' analgesic in the recovery period while an injection of opioid is taking effect. The demand flow apparatus is not suitable, most recovering patients being unable to co-operate in its use. It can be given via a simple oxygen mask at 5 l/min. This is quite safe when used under the supervision of a trained recovery nurse. Local anaesthetics may be used in the production of analgesia. Bupivicaine is the agent of choice, having a duration of action of up to 6 hours. Injections may be made by the anaesthetist or surgeon either before the operation, as a component of the anaesthetic, or afterwards. Caudal epidural block is suitable for perineal operations, while intercostal block is effective after abdominal or thoracic operations[64]. A catheter may be placed in the epidural space for repeated doses or continuous infusion of local anaesthetic. This produces excellent analgesia at the expense of sympathetic blockade (see above), causing hypotension, which may have fatal consequences. Simpson et al.[65]. showed that smaller volumes of solution are needed for analgesia if the catheter is placed in the thoracic region, but even so the technique is not without danger. More recently the injection of opioids into the subarachnoid space[66] or epidural space[67] has been reported. This produces effective analgesia without loss of other modalities and in particular without sympathetic blockade; this technique is still under trial. No local injection of drug will control the discomfort associated with nasogastric tubes, drips, oxygen masks and pain in areas remote from the operation site.

Shakes

The term 'shakes' describes a common combination of shivering and rigidity of skeletal muscles seen during recovery from general anaesthesia. It is most often seen after halothane but may occur after any inhalational agent. 41 patients in Farman's series[10] were noted to have shivering and rigidity, an incidence of 1:55 patients. In the case of halothane, such shivering is associated with a fall in core temperature[68]. Bay et al.[69] pointed out the danger of hypoxaemia in patients with respiratory depression or a fixed low cardiac output. The duration of shakes is usually short, a few minutes and oxygen should be given although no specific treatment is indicated.

Restlessness and agitation

There are several possible causes of these, which were noted in 197 of our cases (1:150)[10]. The most common is discomfort from pain, hypoxia, full bladder, nasogastric tube, backache or headache. This is confirmed by the success of appropriate treatment. Young patients may be distressed on awakening, women and children crying, men tending to thrash about and shout. In resistant cases this can be treated with droperidol (0.1 mg/kg) or halperidol (0.1 mg/kg) intravenously.

Vomiting

This is considered here because it is almost always unrelated to surgical factors. It relates to the drugs used, to the operation site and to the patient's sex and personality. The incidence in the Addenbrooke's series was 1:40 cases[10]. There was a difference between the old hospital which handled mainly gynaecological patients (1:33) and the new hospital which took general, orthopaedic and dental cases, in which only one patient in 50 was noted to vomit. The overall incidence is similar to that observed by Lee and Atkinson[70] but less than the 5% reported by Gold and Ruy[71]. Drugs which increase the tendency to vomit are opioids, whether used for premedication or injected later, and cyclopropane, trichloroethylene and ether in larger doses. Low concentrations of trichloroethylene and ether used in combination with relaxant do not increase the tendency to vomit[72]. However, no drug or combination of drugs is immune in this respect. Females are more likely to vomit than males[27], particularly those inclined to vomit in other circumstances or who have a previous history of post-operative vomiting. Patients having abdominal operations are more likely to vomit than those having most superficial operations. Middle ear surgery is a notorious exception in which nausea may persist for days. Treatment is based on the use of anti-emetic drugs, which were used in 1 in 44 of Farman's[10] patients and 1 in 24 of those reported by Eltringham et al[15]. Perphenazine 0.1 mg/kg intramuscularly is usually effective. Metoclopramide 0.2 mg/kg was preferred by Breivik and Lind[73]. Some anaesthetists give patients injections during the anaesthetic with the aim of preventing this complication. If vomiting is persistent a search for a more serious underlying cause should be made.

(4) Fluid and metabolic balance

There are some important aspects of early postoperative care which are not incuded in the earlier sections because they seldom cause immediate complications. All the same, anyone dealing with patients recovering from operation should be aware of the effects of anaesthesia and surgery on fluid and electrolyte balance and on metabolism. These effects may well be super-imposed on disturbance due to pre-existing disease. The reader is referred to recent reviews by Horsey[74] and Bevan[75] for more complete descriptions. This section will serve mainly to draw attention to the importance of careful early postoperative management in the prevention of later complications. Surgery and trauma give rise to intense responses from the pituitary and adrenals, unless prevented by regional conduction anaesthesia or by the use of large doses of opioids. Antidiuretic hormone is secreted by the posterior pituitary[76] and levels remain high in the early postoperative period[77]. It is almost certainly the main cause of the normal postoperative oliguria. Growth hormone release is greatly increased and will lead to hyperglycaemia by antagonizing insulin[78]. ACTH is also released in large amounts in response to surgical stimulation[79]. As a result plasma levels of cortisol rise and remain elevated for days[80]; it is customary to mimic this response in patients who are on therapeutic or replacement steroid therapy, by giving additional dosage during this period. Aldosterone secretion may increase tenfold during surgery[81] and is an important contributory cause of postoperative sodium retention[82]. Plasma levels of catecholamines increase during surgery, particularly if ether or cyclopropane are used, and will contribute to gluconeogenesis and hyperglycaemia.

Patients who are about to undergo surgery are starved and given no drink for some hours, to allow their stomachs to empty and so to reduce the risk of vomiting, particularly during induction of anaesthesia. Although 4–6 hours is generally considered adequate, patients on a morning operating list are commonly given nothing to drink from the previous evening[11]. It may well happen that a patient may only reach the theatre late in the morning. After an operation of only moderate severity, the patient may receive an opioid which will suppress his thirst for some hours. He may be able to take a little to drink that evening and it will then be the next day before he can once again drink freely. Such a patient may therefore have a fluid deficit of 0.5–1.0 litre, depending on body and environmental temperature, in addition to measurable losses in urine, etc. Patients who have been vomiting will already have lost fluid, although postoperative vomiting usually entails little actual fluid loss. Abdominal operations are associated with fluid loss from the bowel surface, while absorption of fluid from the intestine is depressed for many hours afterwards[83]. Wound drains may account for further appreciable losses. The trauma of the operation itself has been blamed for a futher functional loss of extracellular fluid in the form of localized oedema[84]. These losses are commonly underestimated. Common humanity prompts the use of a measure which will prevent the patient suffering the discomfort of a dry mouth and intense thirst, so it is reasonable to put up a drip in any patient having anything more than a minor operation.

The question of exactly what the patient needs in the drip in addition to water has been the subject of considerable argument. The uncomplicated patient will exhibit a phase of oliguria and reduced sodium excretion, with increased potassium loss, in the recovery period. It would seem sensible to aim to maintain a normal volume of water in the body, with normal concentrations of solutes. Regimens which contain considerable amounts of sodium will induce a markedly positive balance; water is retained and ECF osmolarity remains near normal. Eventually such a patient will exhibit signs of oedema, either peripheral or pulmonary. By contrast patients who are given only 5% dextrose will become hyponatraemic; because water is retained this introduces the risk of water intoxication. Fortunately in the majority of patients, having operations of intermediate severity, these dangers are minimal. In the more severely ill patient or one who is having a major operation, the correct choice of fluid may determine survival. Ideally, precise fluid and electrolyte balances should be kept, but this ideal is seldom achieved. The reasons are that in the pressure of day to day work there is no time for it and that in any case much fluid loss is not measurable. In major cases such formal studies should nevertheless be undertaken. Estimation of immeasurable losses must in any case be made. The volume of fluid given should be that needed to restore or maintain normality, usually of the order of 50 (ml/kg)/day. Additional volume is given during operation for the indications mentioned above. After the initial recovery period further evidence is sought from clinical signs such as mouth dryness, vein filling and skin perfusion. During operation isotonic saline or Hartmann's solution may be used, but afterwards dextrose with 0.18% saline (30 mmol/l) and 0.15% (20 mmol/l) potassium chloride is preferable. This approach is likely to lead to a normal serum sodium level throughout the postoperative period[77]. In a major operation in which the patient may require plasma, albumin or sodium containing drugs, particularly if more than one drip is running, care must be taken not to overload the circulation. Use of a loop diuretic or mannitol will ensure a satisfactory urine output. This is particularly important in patients with obstructive jaundice[85]. In veiw of the wide range of sodium intakes in normal life (from less than 1 mmol per day to over 200 mmol per day) and of the ability of the renal tubules to reabsorb the sodium in the glomerular filtrate, it would seem wise to err on the side of undersalting rather than oversalting.

(5) Surgical complications

It is beyond the scope of this chapter to deal even with the early complications of the vast range of operations that are performed. It is the responsibility of the surgeon to warn the recovery nurses of particular problems. The only complication in the recovery period common to all operations is bleeding (discussed above). Occasionally wound haematoma, wound disruption and surgical emphysema will be encountered.

Nevertheless the recovery staff have a valuable part to play in the surgical care of the patient. In many cases, for example, bladder irrigation after transurethral resection of the prostate, their attention is vital to the success of the procedure.

(6) Miscellaneous complications

Statistically it is likely that almost any sudden cause of deterioration in a patient's condition will occur occasionally in the recovery period. Many patients have pre-existing disease which is not related to their surgical condition and which may require special care in the recovery period. A high index of suspicion should be maintained in any patient who fails to respond to routine treatment of what may appear to be a common complication. Expert help should be summoned at an early stage. Examples of such occurrences are convulsions (five patients out of 30 000 in our series) and

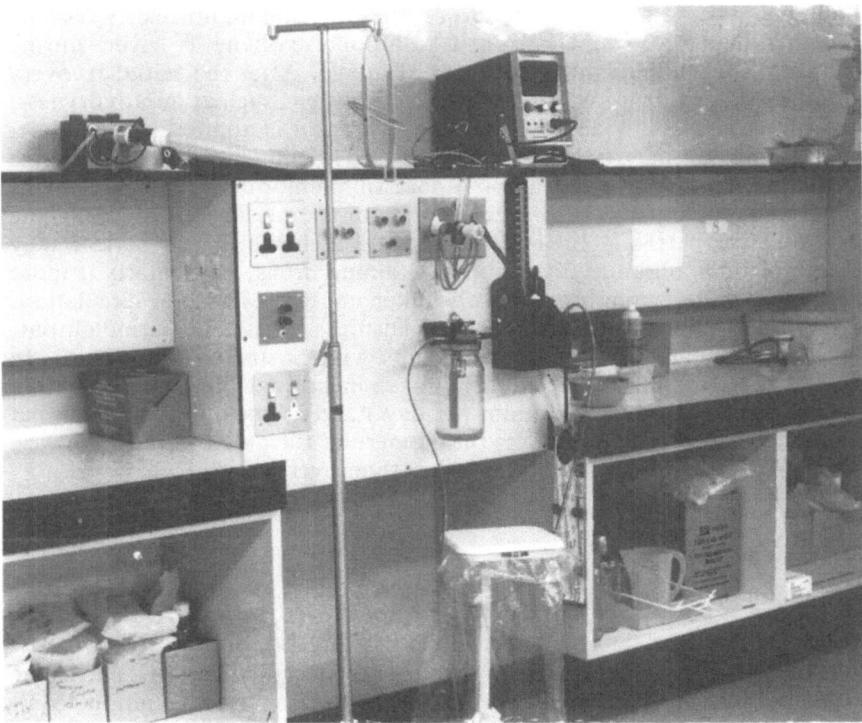

Figure 18.1 Bedhead services: all outlets are grouped on panels, leaving the shelves free for equipment and notes

426

unexplained fever. Drug and transfusion reactions should be suspected. Regrettably a number of patients suffer from traumatic episodes, some of which occur in the theatre but may also become apparent on recovery. These include corneal abrasions, damage to teeth and lips, nerve palsies from pressure applied during operation and injury from falls.

ACKNOWLEDGEMENT

I should like to express my thanks to Michael Lindop and Patricia Holister for their kindness in scrutinizing the text and for their helpful suggestions.

References

1. Nightingale, F. (1863). *Notes on Hospitals*. 3rd Ed. (London: Longman)
2. Stephens, D. S. B. and Boaler, J. (1977). The nurse's role in immediate post-operative care. *Br. Med. J.*, **1**, 1199
3. Andrewes, S. J. (1979). The recovery room as a nursing service. *J. R. Soc. Med.*, **72**, 275
4. Wylie, W. D. (1975). There but for the grace of God ... *Ann. R. Coll. Surg. Engl.*, **56**, 171
5. Lim Poh Vs Camden and Islington Area Health Authority (1979). *1 All ER 332*
6. Fisher, T. L. (1970). Responsibility for care in recovery rooms. *Can. Med. Assoc. J.*, **102**, 78
7. Fisher, T. L. (1972). Responsibility for care in recovery rooms – again. *Can. Med. Assoc. J.*, **107**, 348
8. Hudson, R. B. S. (1979). The pattern of work in the recovery room. *J. R. Soc. Med.*, **72**, 273
9. Department of Health and Social Security. (1967). *Hospital Building Note 26: Operating Departments*. (London: HMSO)
10. Farman, J. V. (1978). The work of the recovery room. *Br. J. Hosp. Med.*, **19**, 606
11. Farman, J. V. (1962). Heat losses in infants undergoing surgery in air-conditioned theatres. *Br. J. Anaesth.*, **34**, 543
12. Shepherd, L. C. and Kirklin, J. W. (1974). Cardiac surgical intensive care computer system. *Fed. Proc.*, **33**, 2326
13. Mason, J., Price, D. J. and Trimnell, S. (1980). Closed-loop control of intracranial pressure. In Becker, D. P. and Miller, J. D. (eds.). *Intracranial Pressure* IV. (Berlin: Springer-Verlag)
14. Farman, J. V. (1979). Do we need recovery rooms? *J. R. Soc. Med.*, **72**, 270
15. Eltringham, R. J., Coates, M. B. and Hudson, R. B. S. (1978). Observations in 10000 patients in the immediate post-operative period. *Resuscitation*, **6**, 45
16. Hedstrand, U. and Holmdahl, M. H. (1976). Organisation of postoperative care. Presented at a *Symposium of the Faculty of Anaesthetists, Royal College of Surgeons*, London

17. Schweizer, O. (1970). The recovery and intensive care unit, a clinical laboratory. *Anaesthesiology*, **32,** 247
18. Stead, B. R. (1977). Personal communication
19. Aw, A. C. (1977). The recovery room. *NAT News*, **14,** 15
20. Wallis, D. (1979). The recovery room. *NAT News*, **16,** 10
21. Renfrew, M. J. and McManus, R. (1975). Recovery and reception area. *NAT News*, **12,** 13
22. Gordon, R. A. (1963). The postanaesthetic recovery room. *Can. Anaesth. Soc. J.*, **10,** 140
23. Fazio, A. N. and Cottle, B. (1968). Survey of recovery rooms shows staffing, utilisation patterns. *Hosp. Top.*, **46,** 90
24. Eltringham, R. J. (1979). Complications in the recovery room. *J. R. Soc. Med.*, **72,** 278
25. Barbour, C. M. and Little, D. M. J. (1957). Postoperative hypotension. *J. Am. Med. Assoc.*, **165,** 1529
26. Shimosato, S. and Etsten, B. E. (1969). The role of the venous system in cardiocirculatory dynamics during spinal and epidural anaesthesia in man. *Anaesthesiology*, **30,** 619
27. Gregory, I. C. (1978). Anaesthesia and the endocrine glands. In Churchill-Davidson, H. C. (ed.). *A Practice of Anaesthesia.* (4th Ed). pp. 1529–1584. (London: Lloyd-Luke)
28. Clement, A. J. (1978). Anaesthesia and Cardiac disease. In Churchill-Davidson, H. C. (ed.). *A Practice of Anaesthesia.* (4th Ed). pp. 530–593. (London: Lloyd-Luke)
29. Gal, T. J. and Cooperman, L. H. (1975). Hypertension in the immediate post-operative period. *Br. J. Anaesth.*, **47,** 70
30. Nunn, J. F. and Payne, J. P. (1962). Hypoxaemia after general anaesthesia. *Lancet*, **2,** 631
31. Conway, C. M. and Payne, J. P. (1963). Postoperative hypoxaemia and oxygen therapy. *Br. Med. J.*, **1,** 844
32. Nunn, J. F. (1965). Influence of age and other factors in hypoxaemia in the postoperative period. *Lancet*, **2,** 466
33. Fink, B. R. (1955). Diffusion anoxia. *Anaesthesiology*, **16,** 511
34. Mathias, J. A. (1978). Oxygen and associated gases. In Churchill-Davidson, H. C. (ed.). *A Practice of Anaesthesia.* (4th Ed.) pp. 180–210. (London: Lloyd-Luke)
35. Cooper, E. A. (1972). Postoperative lung dysfunction: predisposing factors. *Proc. R. Soc. Med.*, **65,** 10
36. Marshall, B. E. and Millar, R. A. (1965). Some factors influencing post-operative hypoxaemia. *Anaesthesia*, **20,** 408
37. Spence, A. A. and Alexander, J. (1972). Mechanisms of postoperative hypoxaemia. *Proc. R. Soc. Med.*, **65,** 12
38. Prys-Roberts, C., Nunn, J. F., Dobson, R. H., Robinson, R. H., Greenbaum, R. and Harris, R. S. (1967). Radiologically detectable pulmonary collapse in the supine position. *Lancet*, **2,** 399
39. Rees, J. G. (1960). Quoted in *Anaesthesia and Respiration*. Gray, T. C. *Triangle*, **4,** 259
40. Silverstone, N. A. (1978). Personal communication

41. Stoetling, R. K. (1977). Ventilatory arrest after meperidine. *Anesth. Analg.*, **56**, 727
42. Lowenstein, E., Hallowell, P., Levine, F. H., Daggett, W. M., Austen, W. G. and Laver, M. B. (1969). Cardiovascular response to large doses of intravenous morphine in man. *N. Engl. J. Med.*, **281**, 1389
43. Rigg, J. R. A. and Goldsmith, C. H. (1976). Recovery of ventilatory response to carbon dioxide after thiopentone, morphine and fentanyl in man. *Can. Anaesth. Soc. J.*, **23**, 370
44. Adams, A. P. and Pybus, D. A. (1978). Delayed respiratory depression after use of fentanyl during anaesthesia. *Br. Med. J.*, **1**, 278
45. Cormack, R. S. (1980). Postoperative recovery. In Gray, T. C., Nunn, J. F. and Utting, J. E. (eds.). *General Anaesthesia*. (4th Ed.) Vol. II, pp. 1061–1078. (London: Butterworths)
46. Lindop, M. J. (1980). Personal Communication
47. Evans, J. M., Hogg, M. L. J., Lunn, J. N. and Rosen, M. (1974). Degree and duration of reversal by naloxone of effects of morphine in conscious subjects. *Br. Med. J.*, **2**, 589
48. Gupta, P. K. and Dundee, J. W. (1974). The effect of an infusion of doxapram on morphine analgesics. *Anaesthesia*, **29**, 40
49. Forrest, W. H., Brown, B. W., Brown, C. R., De Falque, R., Gold, M., Gordon, H. E., James, J. E., Katz, J., Mahler, D. L., Schroff, P. and Tentsch, G. (1977). Dextroamphetamine with morphine for treatment of postoperative pain. *N. Engl. J. Med.*, **296**, 712
50. Coleman, A. J. (1978). Inhalational anaesthetic agents. In Churchill-Davidson, H. C. (ed.). *A Practice of Anaesthesia*. (4th Ed.) pp. 238–303. (London: Lloyd-Luke)
51. Nunn, J. F. and Matthews, R. L. (1959). Gaseous exchange during halothane anaesthesia: the steady respiratory state. *Br. J. Anaesth.*, **31**, 330
52. Ivanov, S. D. and Nunn, J. F. (1968). Influence of duration of hyperventilation on rise time of PCO_2 after step-radiation of ventilation. *Respir. Physiol.*, **5**, 243
53. Feldman, S. A. (1978). Neuromuscular blocking drugs. In Churchill-Davidson, H. C. (ed.). *A Practice of Anaesthesia*. (4th Ed.), p. 865 (London: Lloyd-Luke)
54. Doenicke, A. M., Schmidinger, St. and Krumey, L. (1968). Suxamethonium and serum cholinesterase. *Br. J. Anaesth.*, **40**, 834
55. Bevan, P. G. (1961). Postoperative pneumoperitoneum and pulmonary collapse. *Br. Med. J.*,**2**, 609
56. Spence, A. A. and Smith, G. (1971). Postoperative analgesia and lung function: a comparison of morphine with extradural block. *Br. J. Anaesth.*, **43**, 144
57. Beecher, H. K. (1933). Effect of laparotomy on lung volume: demonstration of a new type of pulmonary collapse. *J. Clin. Invest.*, **12**, 651
58. Mendelson, C. L. (1946). Aspiration of stomach contents into the lungs during obstetric anaesthesia. *Am. J. Obstet. Gynecol.*, **52**, 191
59. Doughty, A. (1978). Anaesthesia for operative obstetrics and gynaecology. In Churchill-Davidson, H. C. (ed.). *A Practice of Anaesthesia*. (4th Ed.) pp. 1355–1395. (London: Lloyd-Luke)

60. Brown, B. R. and Sagalyn, A. M. (1974). Hepatic microsomal enzyme induction by inhalation anaesthetics: mechanism in the rat. *Anaesthesiology*, **40**, 152

61. Harcus, A. H., Ward, A. E. and Smith, D. W. (1980). Buprenorphine in postoperative pain: results in 7500 patients. *Anaesthesia*, **33**, 383

62. Masson, A. H. B. (1971). Postoperative pain relief. *Int. Anesthesiol. Clin.*, **9**, 247

63. Rutter, P. C., Murphy, F. and Dudley, H. A. F. (1960). Morphine: controlled trial of different methods of administration for postoperative pain relief. *Br. Med. J.*, **280**, 12

64. Moore, D. C. (1975). Intercostal nerve block for postoperative somatic pain following surgery of thorax and upper abdomen *Br. J. Anaesth.*, **47**, 284

65. Simpson, B. R. J., Parkhouse, J., Marshall, R. and Lambrechts, W. (1961). Extradural analgesia and the prevention of postoperative respiratory complications. *Br. J. Anaesth.*, **33**, 628

66. Wang, J. K., Nauss, L. A. and Thomas, J. E. (1979). Pain relief by intrathecally applied morphine in man. *Anaesthesiology*, **30**, 149

67. Behar, M., Magora, F., Olshwang, D. and Davidson, J. T. (1979). Epidural morphine in treatment of pain. *Lancet*, **1**, 527

68. Jones, H. D. and McLaren, A. M. (1965). Postoperative shivering and hypoxaemia after halothane, nitrous oxide, oxygen anaesthesia. *Br. J. Anaesth.*, **37**, 35

69. Bay, J., Nunn, J. F. and Prys-Roberts, C. (1968). Factors influencing arterial PO_2 during recovery from anaesthesia. *Br. J. Anaesth.*, **40**, 398

70. Lee, J. A. and Atkinson, R. S. (1973). *Synopsis of Anaesthesia*. (7th Ed.), p. 805 (Bristol: John Wright)

71. Gold, M. I. and Ruy, B. P. (1966). Efficacy of thiethylperazane as a recovery from anti-emetic. *Br. J. Anaesth.*, **38**, 380

72. Holmes, C. McK. (1965). Postoperative vomiting after ether-air anaesthesia. *Anaesthesia*, **20**, 199

73. Breivik, H. and Lind, B. (1971). Anti-emetic and propulsive peristaltic properties of metoclopramide. *Br. J. Anaesth.*, **43**, 400

74. Horsey, P. J. (1978). Parenteral fluid therapy. In Churchill-Davidson, H. C. (ed.). *A Practice of Anaesthesia*. (4th Ed.) pp. 678–704 (London: Lloyd-Luke)

75. Bevan, D. R. (1980). Metabolic response to anaesthesia, surgery and trauma. In Gray, T. C., Nunn, J. F. and Utting, J. H. (eds.). *General Anaesthesia*. (4th Ed) Vol. II, pp. 1017–1036. (London: Butterworths)

76. Oyama, T. and Sato, K. (1970). Plasma levels of antidiuretic hormone in man during methoxyflurane anaesthesia and surgery. *Anaesthesia*, **25**, 500

77. Thomas, T. H. and Morgan, D. B. (1979). Post-surgical hyponatraemia; the role of intravenous fluids and arginine vasopressin. *Br. J. Surg.*, **66**, 540

78. Davies, A. G. (1972). Antidiuretic and growth hormones. *Br. Med. J.*, **2**, 282

79. Ganong, W. F., Alper, L. C. and Lee, T. D. (1970). ACTH and the regulation of adreno-cortical secretion. *N. Engl. J. Med.*, **290**, 1006

80. Vandam, L. D. and Moore, F. D. (1960). Adrenocortical mechanisms related to anaesthesia. *Anaesthesiology*, **21**, 531

81. Casey, J. H., Bickel, E. Y. and Zimmerman, B. (1957). The pattern and

significance of aldosterone secretion in the postoperative patient. *Surg. Gynecol. Obstet.*, **105**, 179

82. Bevan, D. R., Dudley, H. A. F. and Horsey, P. J. (1973). Renal function during and after anaesthesia and surgery. *Br. J. Anaesth.*, **45**, 263
83. Bunch, G. A. (1971). The intestinal response to surgery. *Br. J. Surg.*, **58**, 755
84. Shires, T. and Jackson, D. E. (1961). Postoperative salt tolerance. *Arch. Surg.*, **84**, 703
85. Davison, J. L. (1965). Postoperative renal function in obstructive jaundice: effect of a mannitol diuresis. *Br. Med. J.*, **1**, 82

19
Training the nurse – UK style

PAT ASHWORTH

(I) ROLE OF THE TRAINED NURSE

It has become widely recognized that good, well-prepared nursing staff are essential for good intensive care. Although doctors and others should be readily available, and may even provide continuous service on the unit, yet nurses are usually the only staff providing direct supervision and care of individual patients throughout the 24 hours[1]. Their functions in direct patient care include:

(1) Supporting vital functions such as ventilation, sometimes by mechanical means, and maintaining therapeutic regimes.

(2) Monitoring physiological functions both by use of their senses and the effective use of electronic and other equipment.

(3) Maintaining records of their observations which readily show any changes in the patient's condition, whether improvement or deterioration.

(4) Taking appropriate action in response to changes, whether this is giving nursing care, treatment according to standard protocols, or seeking help from medical staff.

(5) Giving basic nursing care, which includes both prevention of the complications which may occur due to the pathological condition

432

present or the treatment regimes, and substituting for the patient in those activities of daily living contributing to his health 'which he would perform for himself if he had the necessary will, knowledge and strength'. And doing this in such a way that he regains independence as soon as possible[2].

(6) Promoting and/or maintaining the patient's integrity as a whole human being, rather than just a set of biological systems. Even if survival were to be seen as the only objective of intensive care this function is essential, since physiological and social systems are interdependent[3]. Since most patients have family, spouse, and/or friends who are an important part of their support system in normal life, help must also be provided for them, so that they can continue their support to the patient.

(7) Co-ordinating treatment and care activities to achieve maximum benefit to the patient.

In addition to these direct patient care activities the nursing staff usually play a large part in: (a) management of the unit in terms of staffing, supplies and maintenance, and co-ordination of activities. Even in hospitals where there are independent systems for supply and maintenance, it usually falls to the nurses to ensure that these are adequate and effective and to take action when they are not; (b) training and education of personnel. There is mutual benefit when experienced members of various disciplines each contribute to the education of others as well as their own students. Nowhere is good teamwork more essential than in an intensive care unit (ICU), and for this to happen members of each discipline must have knowledge of and respect for the roles and functions of others.

How then should nurses be prepared for their work in an intensive care unit? Experience, personal communication and available literature suggest that in other countries problems similar to those in Britain have to be faced and overcome before appropriate and effective educational courses are achieved[4-6]; this chapter describes British practice. The chapter is based on 13 years as an intensive care nurse together with experience as a teacher and university lecturer in nursing.

(II) EVOLUTION OF TRAINING

As intensive care units began to develop in the 1950–1960s it became obvious that the basic training of a state registered nurse was inadequate preparation for nursing patients needing specialized care aided by modern technology. Some in-service training was done by doctors and nurses but this tended to be rather unsystematic, and was often geared to the provision of immediate manual skills, rather than including the basic sciences necessary for intelligent patient care.

By the mid-1960s a number of units in Britain ran courses, but these were unsatisfactory in several ways: (1) The education content was very variable and often unbalanced. The content was mainly physiology, technical skills, and information on various pathological conditions likely to be seen in the unit. The wider nursing content was often not well-defined and taught. (2) The value of the certificate given at the end of the course was only as great as the degree to which other hospitals, where the nurse might wish to work, knew and respected the unit issuing it. (3) Courses were often a device to attract 'pairs of hands' to work in the unit rather than being designed as an educational experience, and there was little involvement of nurse education departments. While it is true that many of the nurse tutors knew little about intensive care, equally many of the intensive care staff knew little about educational principles and strategies.

(III) NATIONAL COURSE

In March 1970 the Joint Board of Clinical Nursing Studies (JBCNS) was set up by the Secretary of State for Social Services and the Secretary of State for Wales: 'To consider and advise on the needs of nurses and midwives for post-certificate clinical training in specialized departments of the hospital service in England and Wales and to co-ordinate and supervise the courses provided as a result of such advice, and to discharge such other functions as the Secretaries of State may assign to them'[7]. Scotland has a separate but similar body. A survey conducted by the JBCNS revealed that there were 350 courses offered in 47 specialties, distributed very unevenly over the country. Once a standard list of names for courses had been compiled and some order of priority determined, the first advisory panels were set up.

Each specialist panel was composed of doctors and nurses experienced and working in the specialty, plus a member of the Joint Board staff. The General Intensive Care Panel was one of the first to start work, and met regularly over a period of some months to draw up an Outline Curriculum, first for a course for registered nurses[8] (Figures 19.1 and 19.2) and then for enrolled nurses. This includes the course content and objectives, length (24–27 weeks), criteria for entry, clinical experience required, and time required for the theoretical programme (at least 28 days). Any centre, deciding to start a course, designs a course (Figure 19.3) based on the outline curriculum, submits this to the JBCNS with assurances that there are adequate funds and clinical experience, and is visited by a JBCNS officer and a doctor and nurse from a specialist list. If the centre is approved it must apply for reapproval after a limited number of courses, often after about 3 years. The first courses were approved in 1972, and so, through reapproval visits and informal visits by a JBCNS officer, progress can be monitored, and the quality maintained or improved.

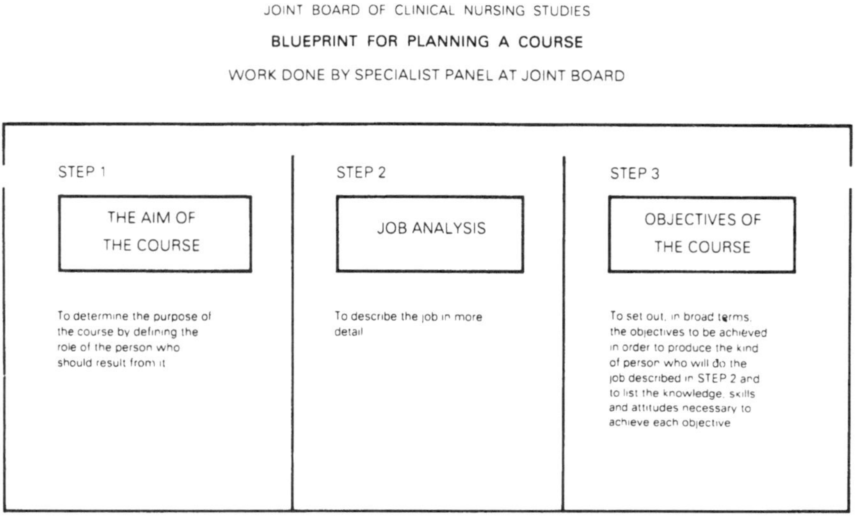

TRAINING THE NURSE - UK STYLE

JOINT BOARD OF CLINICAL NURSING STUDIES

BLUEPRINT FOR PLANNING A COURSE

WORK DONE BY SPECIALIST PANEL AT JOINT BOARD

STEP 1

| THE AIM OF |
| THE COURSE |

To determine the purpose of the course by defining the role of the person who should result from it

STEP 2

| JOB ANALYSIS |

To describe the job in more detail

STEP 3

| OBJECTIVES OF |
| THE COURSE |

To set out, in broad terms, the objectives to be achieved in order to produce the kind of person who will do the job described in STEP 2 and to list the knowledge, skills and attitudes necessary to achieve each objective

Figure 19.1

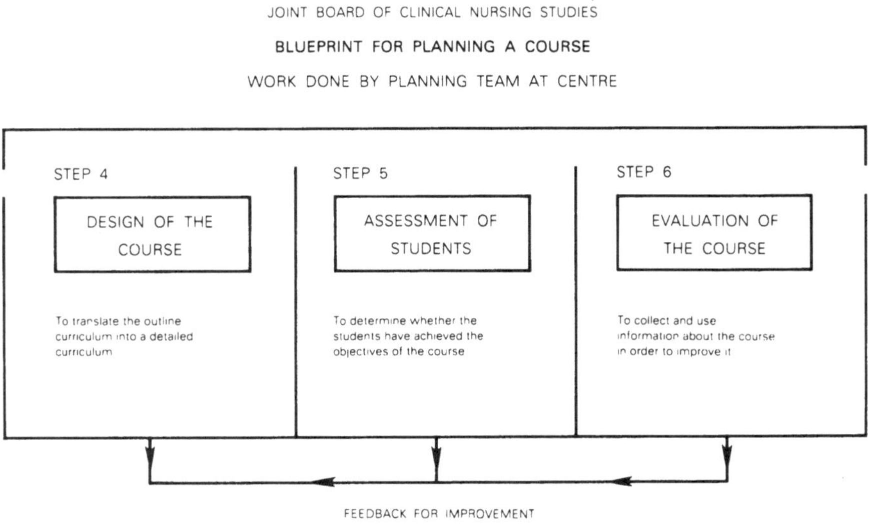

JOINT BOARD OF CLINICAL NURSING STUDIES

BLUEPRINT FOR PLANNING A COURSE

WORK DONE BY PLANNING TEAM AT CENTRE

STEP 4

| DESIGN OF THE |
| COURSE |

To translate the outline curriculum into a detailed curriculum

STEP 5

| ASSESSMENT OF |
| STUDENTS |

To determine whether the students have achieved the objectives of the course

STEP 6

| EVALUATION OF |
| THE COURSE |

To collect and use information about the course in order to improve it

FEEDBACK FOR IMPROVEMENT

Figure 19.2

435

JOINT BOARD OF CLINICAL NURSING STUDIES

STEP 4 – DESIGN OF THE COURSE

ORDER IN WHICH THE OUTLINE CURRICULUM CAN BE TRANSLATED INTO A
DETAILED CURRICULUM

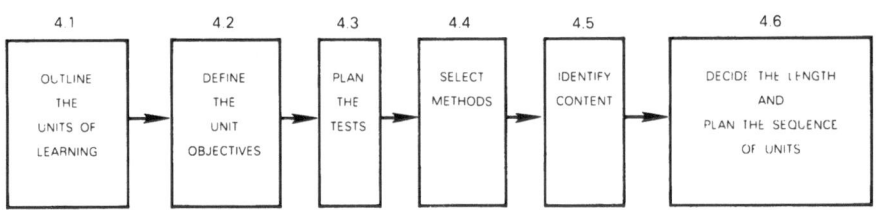

Figure 19.3

(1) Objectives

The outline for the course is set out in skills, knowledge and attitudes required to meet the five major objectives. Because it is only an outline, individual centres can add new material according to developing knowledge and changing technology. In the past, content designed to meet the first two objectives was much better taught and assessed than that required for the others. As in other countries the emphasis was almost entirely cure oriented. Yet achievement of the other three objectives is just as important to the development of good nurses who can function well as team members in a specialized unit. Each of the objectives will be considered in relation to current progress.

First objective

'At the end of the course the nurse will be skilled in giving total nursing care to patients undergoing intensive therapy.'

The content required to meet this objective includes all the various technical procedures such as cardiopulmonary resuscitation, use of

436

ventilators and defibrillators, tracheal aspiration and many more, together with care and treatment related to specific diseases such as acute poisoning or major trauma. To use such skills effectively and intelligently the nurse needs a variety of knowledge of physiology, pathology, body mechanics, and electrical and microbiological hazards. She also needs to learn to adapt basic nursing skills to the intensive care situation. For example, patients still develop pressure sores while in intensive care units and suffer unnecessarily, and may have further sepsis and tissue damage, and delayed rehabilitation. While it is recognized that poor circulation and other factors contribute to decubitus ulcers, yet these could be prevented by nurses with sufficient skill, ingenuity and motivation. To change the position of a critically ill patient without disrupting vital equipment or causing harm and still leave him comfortable is not easy. It requires manual skill, knowledge and intelligence to learn how best to do this for each patient, since not all will react in the same way.

Although attitudes such as 'respect for the human dignity of every patient and relative' are probably 'caught rather than taught', yet knowledge may contribute to changes in attitude. For example, there is now considerable literature relating to physical and psychological stress in the intensive care unit and the possible effect on both staff and patients[9]. An understanding of this may result in changes in behaviour and perhaps attitude.

Second objective

'At the end of the course the nurse will be skilled in making clinical observations, taking measurements, interpreting these and taking appropriate action.'

Methods of measuring and recording physiological functions are constantly developing. As the nurse develops skills in the use of this equipment, so she becomes involved in using the information obtained. The use of the Swan–Ganz catheter and measurement of cardiac output are now commonplace in many units. According to such measurements, the nurse is expected to regulate the treatment by following a prescribed regime. But however sophisticated the methods become, the principles to be learned remain the same. The nurse must be able to use the equipment safely and effectively, interpret observations accurately and intelligently and then respond appropriately. There are electrical hazards with monitoring equipment, and dangers of infection or haemorrhage from intravascular lines. Good oscilloscope displays are of little value unless the nurse can interpret what she sees, understand its significance, the reasons for the actions she is expected to undertake, and her responsibility. Good records are essential to obtain trends which indicate the patient's response to treatment or to factors in his environment. If the recordings are merely an automatic routine they are likely to become inaccurate or incomplete, or show deterioration without appropriate action. Perhaps one of the most important principles to be learned is never to look at one recording or parameter in isolation. It is the composite picture of all the observations and the trends which indicates progress.

It is equally important to recognize that 'we see what we look for and we look for what we know'[10] but this must not be allowed to prevent early observation of the unexpected.

Third objective

'At the end of the course the nurse will be skilled in communication and in establishing good relationships with the patient and his family and with colleagues.'

In the small area of an ICU there are many people each with their own absorbing and sometimes anxiety-provoking preoccupations, and each with expectations of each other. For example, the doctor may have been operating for some hours and be anxious about the success of the operation; the nurse may be trying to do numerous measurements and recordings, plus keeping an eye on another patient whose condition is worrying; the patient, anxious and uncomfortable, may be making demands which the staff feel unable to fulfil; the relatives are worried, bewildered by what is going on and want someone to spend time listening and explaining. In this situation good communication and an understanding of the interactions between people are essential to the good relationships so necessary for good care. In the past, teaching of communication has usually been almost entirely anecdotal. This has its uses, but if students are to learn and apply the principles of good verbal and non-verbal communication, then some theoretical background and practical exercises are necessary. Communication is impaired in many ICU patients. They often cannot speak, cannot see because of eyelid swelling or paralysis, cannot hear well and may be disorientated due to deprivation or overload[11]. Verbal and non-verbal communication skills should be refined in intensive care so that communication is precise and perceptive, because it is often limited by short visiting periods, mechanical interference, disruption of consciousness, or sensory distortion[12]. The nurse needs to be able to assess the patient, define communication input and output problems and find ways to overcome or compensate for them. The basic principles apply between staff and patient, staff and patient's visitors or staff-to-staff communication. The work initiated by the JBCNS on the best ways of teaching communication skills aims to improve patient care, but should also improve relationships with others. Only when communication is taught and assessed, as are other skills and knowledge, will its importance be fully recognized by both course members and experienced staff.

Fourth objective

'At the end of the course the nurse will have an understanding of: the management and organization of the unit, the principles of design of an intensive therapy unit and an appreciation of research.'

While many of the principles of managing an ICU are the same as for any other unit, yet there are certain aspects which are particularly important. The consequences of management failure can be more devastating because most of the patients are critically ill. Some of the important aspects are: supplies – the patient's treatment may be urgently needed and delay may be dangerous; domestic cleanliness, awareness of infection hazards and well-defined policies for avoiding infection or cross-infection; good personnel policies and management – intensive care nurses are scarce and often work under pressure, and patients' survival may depend on retaining them and maintaining a high standard of welfare and performance; staff development and education – an environment which promotes continued learning and personal development is likely to promote good patient care and job satisfaction.

The way in which the area is managed will affect not only the environment and resources but also the way in which care is performed. While it is recognized that there may not always be a one-to-one nurse–patient ratio, it seems inconceivable that care and treatment in such a specialized unit could be organized on a task assignment basis, e.g. one nurse going round doing all the medications, or doing all the observations. Yet this has been observed in some ICUs, particularly at night. If the patient is to receive optimum care then this must be planned by one nurse, at least on a shift basis and preferably for longer. Then medical requirements are fulfilled and the patient is seen as a whole so that nursing needs and problems are defined and care planned to meet them.

Knowledge of the principles of design of the unit and equipment are not only necessary for those who will plan new units, but also for the constant review of the design and use of the services and equipment. Steps can then be taken to improve them where necessary or at least to use them in the most effective way.

The expectation that nurses should appreciate and be actively involved in research is a recent innovation; it still does not occur in some countries. Relatively few nurses will initiate and undertake full research projects. Far more will be involved when medical research is being carried out on their patients and they may be expected to obtain data. All professional nurses should be looking at relevant research, whether performed by nurses or

439

others, to see whether it should modify their current practice in any way.

For example, one of the most obvious actual or potential problems is deprivation of sleep and rest[13], which can have serious consequences. Care must be planned so that there are periods when the patient will be undisturbed and where possible the patient should know when these occur. The hyper-vigilant patient who cannot sleep is sometimes an iatrogenic phenomenon, though nurses are often as guilty in this respect. They should also be aware of ethical issues[14], and learn to criticize nursing practices. The ICN Code[15] says that nurses have a responsibility to play ' . . . the major role in determining and implementing desirable standards of nursing practice and nursing education. The nurse is active in developing a core of professional knowledge.' If nurses are to do this, then they need help to read research reports critically, understand the basic terminology and pick out what is valid and useful to them. They also need information on sources of relevant literature and the use of a library. This is best taught by the following methods: teachers to the course quoting relevant findings and references; expecting course members to search out information in a library or other source; applying the problem-solving process to small projects; discussing the ethics of research as well as practice. These are the tools for continued learning after the end of the course.

Fifth objective

'At the end of the course the nurse will have an understanding of the basic methods of learning and teaching and will be able to pass on skills and knowledge effectively to staff.'

An understanding of the teaching and learning process is an asset to any nurse. The ICU nurse should not only help patients and their visitors to learn how best to help themselves and each other, but also share her expertise and experience with others less experienced in the care of critically ill patients, both within and outside specialized units. Patients transferred from ICUs still suffer from unskilled nursing. For example, patients with tracheostomies have commented how unsafe they felt when transferred to a general ward. Intensive care nurses can raise the standard of nursing within their hospital by helping others to use modern techniques and technical equipment, while at the same time recognizing and seeking to meet the needs of the individual. Attention to the patient should never be obscured by concentration on the equipment, but an inexperienced or harassed nurse may be so anxious about the machinery that she has no time or energy left to attend to the patient as a person. These are skills and concepts which can be transferred from intensive care nursing to other settings.

(2) Assessment

Assessment is required to ensure that the students have achieved the objectives. Now this is done within each centre where continuous assessment is supplemented by three well-spaced examinations. There is also a course evaluation with each group so that the course can be improved as necessary. A very active research unit of the JBCNS has produced an evaluation 'package', in addition to studies on assessment, a booklet on the research objective within courses, and the follow-up of course members.

(3) The teachers

Since the course content is very varied it is best taught in the classroom and the clinical area by a variety of experts – doctors, nurses, physiotherapists, and possibly technicians. It is essential to have a course tutor who co-ordinates the training, takes part in clinical teaching, and is available for consultation by permanent staff and course members. Both the tutor and the clinical nursing staff provide role models (good ones, it is to be hoped) for the course members. The teachers can relate theory to practice, so that whatever the student needs to learn can be emphasized.

(4) Planning the tuition

It is essential to remember that in post-registration courses the students arrive with differing educational experience, both in time and content. They have differing educational backgrounds and may find it anxiety provoking to be students again. The state registered nurse may have qualified after 3 years of very didactic and sometimes limited teaching, from a 4 year Bachelor of Nursing programme, or from various other programmes. A pre-test is therefore a useful guide to the course member's knowledge. Teaching is then planned and performed in such a way that the nurse's confidence as a trained nurse is maintained, but gaps in necessary knowledge or experience are filled. If there is a conflict between theory and practice, the apprentice is more likely to practise that seen in the unit, rather than that taught in the classroom; a sobering thought, since bad practice is just as easily learned as good. Some of the essentials for post-basic education and training of the intensive care nurse have been described. The final and perhaps most important point is that this should take place in a unit with a high standard of practice and an 'atmosphere of learning' as well as the necessary available experience, for the best education prepares a practitioner to continue to learn and seek to improve patient care.

Since many of the unit nurses who will be teaching course members in the unit have had no training as teachers, it is useful to hold workshops such as those organized by the JBCNS. These are 2 day workshops designed to help the clinical staff to realize the importance of their contribution as teachers, and to develop their knowledge and skills in planning and conducting clinical teaching sessions, so that they can make the best use of available opportunities. They also have the opportunity to learn more about assessment of course members.

Apart from the basic course of 6 months for state registered nurses (SRNs) and state enrolled nurses (SENs) which leads to a certificate of competence in the specialty, and separate courses for specialties such as coronary care or neonatal intensive care, there are also short courses for experienced nurses leading to a certificate of attendance.

(IV) FUTURE TRENDS

There is yet far to go in Britain. Perhaps partly because of the much smaller numbers involved there is as yet nothing like the variety of continuing education programmes offered in the USA to critical care nurses. Because of the different education system in nursing in this country, it will be some time before there is a Master's Degree such as the Critical Care Clinical Specialist Program at California State University[5].

But within British courses described there are some of the same elements such as pathophysiology, physical assessment, behavioural science, communication, management, teaching and learning and research appreciation. Also the nursing process is evolving. So there is promise for the future that we will have programmes which produce nurses who 'bring the expertise of advanced educational preparation to the clinical area . . . deliver expert direct bedside care to critically ill patients . . . serve the overall patient population of the units where they are employed . . . in their roles as patient and staff educators and as clinical resources for care planning and implementation'; programmes which will also lead 'to critical analysis of nursing practice in critical care areas . . . ' and 'facilitate implementation of solutions to problems'[5]. Nursing in Britain is mature enough to recognize that increased theoretical knowledge can, combined with clinical experience, enhance rather than detract from practical expertise. There are many nurses with such practical expertise who give good intensive nursing care, but as we learn more it becomes more obvious that there is yet more to be learned. There is an exciting future ahead as we seek to develop educational programmes which will help nurses to give ever-improving patient care.

References

1. Bredenberg, P. (1979). Critical care nurse practitioner: Education expectation and implementation. *Heart Lung*, **8** (5), 939
2. Henderson, V. (1966). *The Nature of Nursing*, pp. 15–17. (London: The Macmillan Company: Collier-Macmillan Ltd.)
3. Maron, L., Bryan-Brown, C. and Shoemaker, W. (1973). Towards a unified approach to psychological factors in the I.C.U. *Crit. Care Med.*, **1** (2), 81
4. McLees, J. P. (1979). Critical care nursing: evolution towards unity. Introduction. *Heart Lung,* **8** (5), 873
5. Brault, G. L. and Pflaum, S. S. (1979). Planning and development of a masters degree in critical care. *Heart Lung,* **8** (5), 933
6. Kahn, J. M. (1975). Trends in the educational process for the critical care nurse. *Crit. Care Med.,* **3** (3), 123
7. Joint Board of Clinical Nursing Studies (1972). First Report
8. Joint Board of Clinical Nursing Studies. Outline Curriculum in General Intensive Care Nursing for State Registered Nurses Course No. 100. 178–202, Great Portland Street, London W1N 5TB
9. Ashworth, P. M. (1980). *Care to Communicate.* An investigation into problems in communication between Patients and Nurses in Intensive Therapy/Care Units. (London: Royal College of Nursing Research Series)
10. Harken, D. E. (1974). Post-operative care following open-heart surgery. *Heart Lung,* **3** (6), 109
11. Ashworth, P. M. (1979). Sensory deprivation: the acutely ill. *Nurs. Times*, **75** (7), 290
12. Reuther, M. A. (1979). Student experience in intensive care units: a faculty–staff collaborative venture. *Heart Lung*, **8** (5), 944
13. Barney, M. *et al.* (1971). The problems of sleep and rest in the intensive care unit. *Psychosomatics*, **12** (3), 155
14. Royal College of Nursing (1977). *Ethics Related to Research in Nursing.* (The Royal College of Nursing of the United Kingdom, Henrietta Place, London W1M 0AB)
15. International Council of Nurses (1973). *Code for Nurses. Ethical Concepts Applied to Nursing*

Other relevant reading

Darling, V. H. (1979). Through the eyes of continuing education – Post-basic education in clinical nursing specialties in England and Wales, the work of the Joint Board of Clinical Nursing Studies. *J. Contin. Educ. Nurs.*, **10** (5), 49

Finn, B. (1974). Special training for intensive care. *Nurs. Times,* **70** (48), 1868

Gardner, M. (1977). The history, philosophy and evaluation of the Joint Board of Clinical Nursing Studies. *J. Advan. Nurs.*, **2**, 621

20
Teaching the medical undergraduate

MAURICE RAPIN AND JEAN–ROGER LE GALL

During the past two decades there has been a large increase in the number of general or specialized intensive care units in university, community and district general hospitals. Therefore, specific training programmes in intensive care medicine have been organized in different countries in order to enable physicians to work in intensive care units at director or consultant level[1,2].

Nevertheless, in addition to this specialized training, it may be useful to teach intensive medicine to physicians working in other fields. Furthermore, the increasing number of patients with multiple organ failure has encouraged more and more medical students to search for complementary training. To fulfil such requirements, optional training in intensive care medicine at undergraduate level has been established by an increasing number of medical schools. This training does not need to reach the same standard as the postgraduate one. In 1974 we organized, at the School of Medicine of Creteil, an optional undergraduate training in intensive care medicine. It is not designed to train specialists, but, on the other hand, to study problems not usually known by the standard student.

(I) AIMS AND OBJECTIVES OF THE COURSE

Several preliminary aims have to be decided before setting up a training programme: to identify the trainee; to define the skills, knowledge and capacities that the trainee has to attain at the end of training (intermediate objectives); to define the knowledge required before starting the training; to test the candidate's prerequisite knowledge; to define the learning objectives of the training; to give to the students the means to reach the learning objectives; to verify that the learning objectives have been reached.

At the end of training the student must be able to:

(1) Diagnose acute life-threatening failures.
(2) Analyse pathophysiological mechanisms.
(3) Prevent acute system failures.
(4) Evaluate the advantages and disadvantages of numerous investigations and multiple treatments.
(5) Provide efficient management.

A list of 129 learning objectives is given to the students. This includes 21 practical and 108 theoretical objectives (Table 20.1). Examples of such learning objectives are shown in Tables 20.2 and 20.3. The students are arranged in groups of 12 to 15. Active learning and active participation are stimulated in several ways. Directed discussions on each subject are organized to explain theoretical objectives; active discussion of case records and direction participation in clinical activity in the intensive care unit are necessary.

Table 20.1 Training programme: learning objectives

	Practical objectives	Theoretical objectives	Total
Electrolyte disturbance	1	18	19
Acid–base disturbance	1	9	10
Acute renal failure	2	15	17
Acute respiratory failure	8	19	27
Shock	2	14	16
Circulatory failure	1	8	9
Nutrition		5	5
Haemostasis	1	4	5
Infections	4	9	13
Neurological problems		5	5
Acute poisoning	1	2	3
Total	21	108	129

Table 20.2 Problems related to infection: practical objectives

(i) Wash the hands correctly in order to avoid transfer of bacteria from a septic to a clean wound
(ii) Dress a septic wound avoiding self-contamination
(iii) Dress a clean wound avoiding patient contamination
(iv) Perform aerobic and anaerobic blood cultures

Table 20.3 Theoretical objectives

Acute respiratory failure: Enumerate the principal drugs that must be avoided in chronic respiratory failure and explain why.
Shock: Knowing the history, clinical features and haemodynamic data (MAP, CVP, PAWP, CI and SAR) of a patient in a state of shock, describe the pathophysiology of:

(a) Hypovolaemic shock
(b) Hyperkinetic (septic) shock
(c) Cardiogenic shock
(d) Vagal shock
(e) Shock due to pulmonary embolism

(II) PREREQUISITE KNOWLEDGE

The prerequisite knowledge has been acquired in the faculty of medicine during the preclinic stage of training in physiology, biochemistry, biophysics, pharmacology and microbiology. For example, the prerequisite knowledge required before studying shock states is listed in Table 20.4.

Table 20.4 Prerequisite knowledge: shock

(i) Haemodynamics: dynamics of the cardiac valves, filling pressures, the Frank–Starling law
(ii) Regulation of blood pressure (arterial pressure, cardiac output, systemic arterial resistance)
(iii) Regulation of cardiac output (cardiac output, cardiac frequency, stroke volume)
(iv) Action of catecholamines on cardiac and vascular receptors
(v) Normal values of central venous pressure, pulmonary artery pressure, pulmonary wedge pressure, mean arterial pressure, cardiac output, cardiac index, systemic vascular resistance, pulmonary vascular resistance

Before the start of training, a pretest is made to check the prerequisite knowledge, in order to inform teachers and students of the gaps to fill preliminarily. Multiple choice questions are used. In Table 20.5 are listed the mean percentages of correct answers obtained by this method during three consecutive years. It is worthwhile noting that the students only remember half the basic knowledge which clinicians judge necessary.

Table 20.5 Results of pretests (1975, 1976 and 1977)

Knowledge	Results: percentage mark awarded
Electrolyte equilibrium	51
Acid–base balance	62
Respiratory function	38
Cardiorespiratory function	55
Renal function	47

(III) CONTENTS

The training programme consists of ten topics as follows:

(1) Disturbance of the milieu intérieur; electrolyte and acid–base disturbances
(2) Acute renal failure.
(3) Acute respiratory failure.
(4) Shock.
(5) Circulatory failure.
(6) Nutrition in intensive care medicine.
(7) Disturbances of haemostasis.
(8) Infection in intensive care medicine.
(9) Neurological problems in intensive care medicine.
(10) Acute poisoning.

(IV) EVALUATION OF THE TRAINING

At the end of training, the objectives are evaluated by a set of questions requiring open and short answers. These questions are designed to verify that each objective has been reached. Two examples of such questions are shown in Table 20.6. Another kind of question consists of a short case record observed in the unit, capable of evaluating both theoretical knowledge and the ability of the student to analyse, synthesize and criticize the data from various clinical situations.

447

Table 20.6   Short essay questions

(i) *Neurological problem:* Enumerate the clinical and e.e.g. criteria for brain death.

(ii) *Shock:* On a ventricular function curve (work/filling pressure) insert the following points: (a) hypovolaemic shock before and after plasma volume expansion; (b) cardiogenic shock before and after inotropic drug therapy.

In emergency and intensive care medicine the objectives need to be exactly defined according to the learner. It must be designed in different ways; either it is designed for the physician, the internist, the anaesthesiologist or the future head of an ICU. We should define for each learner a desirable level of qualification.

Our training scheme leads the student to qualify in intensive care at a level superior to that reached by the family doctor but below that of the specialist. The outgoing students are capable of working in the emergency department of a general hospital. They can discriminate between patients treatable by ordinary methods or by themselves, from patients who have to be rapidly transferred to a general intensive care unit with sophisticated equipment. Thus, they can be left in charge of emergency patients without making serious professional mistakes.

References

1. Committee on training guidelines of the Society of Critical Care Medicine (1971). Guidelines for training of physicians in critical care medicine. *Crit. Care Med.*, **1**, 39
2. Safar, P. and Grenvik, A. (1977). Organization and physician education in critical care medicine. *Anaesthesiology*, **47**, 82

Index